Male **Fertility**
& **Infertility**

This contemporary account of male fertility provides a much needed bridge between those seeking to understand the subject from an evolutionary and biological perspective, and those with clinical responsibility for the investigation and treatment of infertility. Accordingly, the first half of the book deals with the evolutionary aspects of male reproduction and sperm competition, sperm production and delivery in man and other animals, spermatogenesis and epididymal function, sperm transport in the female tract, and the apparent decline in human sperm count. The second part of the book puts greater emphasis on clinical problems and opens with a discussion of intracytoplasmic sperm injection (ICSI), its value and limitations. This is followed by a review of modern developments in the genetics of male infertility and proceeds to a further chapter on the role of surgical procedures used in the treatment. Semen analysis is critically reviewed and the molecular techniques now being used in preimplantation diagnosis and in the study of mitochondrial inheritance are fully described.

Taken together, these chapters, written by an international team of authors, illustrate the breadth of vision needed to tackle the problem of male infertility.

Male **Fertility** & **Infertility**

Edited by TIMOTHY D. GLOVER
University of Leeds

and CHRISTOPHER L. R. BARRATT
University of Birmingham

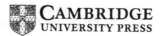

CAMBRIDGE
UNIVERSITY PRESS

CAMBRIDGE UNIVERSITY PRESS
Cambridge, New York, Melbourne, Madrid, Cape Town, Singapore, São Paulo, Delhi

Cambridge University Press
The Edinburgh Building, Cambridge CB2 8RU, UK

Published in the United States of America by Cambridge University Press, New York

www.cambridge.org
Information on this title: www.cambridge.org/9780521104005

First published 1999
This digitally printed version 2009

A catalogue record for this publication is available from the British Library

Library of Congress Cataloguing in Publication data
Male fertility and infertility/edited by Timothy D. Glover and
    Christopher L. R. Barratt.
        p.   cm.
    Includes index.
    ISBN 0 521 62375 8 (hardback)
    1. Infertility, Male.   2. Fertility, Human.   3. Generative organs,
Male – Evolution.   I. Glover, Timothy D.   II. Barratt, C. L. R.
    [DNLM: 1. Infertility, Male.   2. Fertility.   3. Fertilization in
Vitro – methods.   4. Microinjections.   5. Spermatozoa – physiology.
WJ 709 M2449   1999]
RC889.M335   1999
616.6′92 – dc21
DNLM/DLC for Library of Congress   98-55696   CIP

ISBN 978-0-521-62375-9 hardback
ISBN 978-0-521-10400-5 paperback

Contents

Contributors

C. L. R. BARRATT
Reproductive Biology and Genetics Group
Department of Obstetrics and
    Gynaecology
Birmingham Women's Hospital
Edgbaston
Birmingham B15 2TG, UK

T. R. BIRKHEAD
Department of Animal and Plant Sciences
The University
Sheffield S10 2TN, UK

D. BROOMFIELD
Department of Obstetrics and
    Gynaecology
Division of Human Reproduction
University of Pennsylvania Medical
    Center
Philadelphia
PA 19106–4283, USA

J. BROWN
School of Biological Sciences
University of Birmingham
Birmingham B15 2TT, UK

J. COHEN
Institute of Mathematics
University of Warwick
Coventry CV4 7AL, UK

J. M. CUMMINS
Division of Veterinary and Biomedical
    Sciences
Murdoch University
Perth, Western Australia
Australia

D. M. DE KRETSER
Institute of Reproduction and
    Development
Monash Medical Centre
Block E, Level 3
Clayton Road, Clayton
Victoria 3168, Australia

H. M. DOTT
Mammal Research Institute
Department of Zoology
University of Pretoria
Pretoria, South Africa

I. FINDLAY
Centre for Reproduction, Growth and
    Development, and Institute of
    Pathology
Algernon Firth Building
University of Leeds
Leeds LS2 9LS, UK

W. C. L. FORD
University Division of Obstetrics and
    Gynaecology
St Michael's Hospital
Southwell Street
Bristol BS2 8EG, UK

T. D. GLOVER
Department of Obstetrics and
    Gynaecology
University of Leeds
D Floor, Clarendon Wing
Leeds General Infirmary
Leeds LS2 9NS, UK

D. S. IRVINE
MRC Reproductive Biology Unit
Centre for Reproductive Biology
37 Chalmers Street
Edinburgh EH3 9EW, UK

A. M. JEQUIER
Department of Obstetrics and
    Gynaecology
King Edward Memorial Hospital
University of Western Australia
Perth, Western Australia
Australia

R. JONES
Laboratory of Sperm Function and
    Fertilization
The Babrahm Institute
Cambridge CB2 4AT, UK

K. L. LOVELAND
Institute of Reproduction and
    Development
Monash Medical Centre
Block E, Level 3
Clayton Road, Clayton
Victoria 3168, Australia

P. PATRIZIO
Department of Obstetrics and
    Gynaecology
Division of Human Reproduction
University of Pennsylvania Medical
    Center
Philadelphia
PA 19104-4283, USA

S. J. PUBLICOVER
School of Biological Sciences
University of Birmingham
Birmingham B15 2TT, UK

S. J. SILBER
Infertility Center of St Louis
St Luke's Hospital Medical Building
224 South Woods Mill Road
St Louis
MO 63017, USA

J. C. ST JOHN
Reproductive Biology and Genetics Group
Department of Medicine
University of Birmingham and Assisted
    Conception Unit
Birmingham Women's Hospital
Edgbaston
Birmingham B15 2TG, UK

H. TOURNAYE
Centre for Reproductive Medicine
University Hospital
Brussels Free University
Laarbeeklaan 101
B-1090 Brussels
Belgium

Foreword

The first part of this book is concerned with an account – comprehensive but sufficiently idiosyncratic to grip the reader's attention – of the evolution, anatomy and physiology underlying male fertility. The complexities of spermatogenesis are clearly explained. Few could fail to be intrigued by the discussion of penis length and its controversial evolutionary significance, or the information that rams can ejaculate thirty or forty times in one day, compared with a maximum of six for the human male.

Yet from the point of view of the book's editors, all this is mere background to their primary concern. As the second part of the book reveals, it is ICSI, the intracytoplasmic sperm injection procedure, in which they are really interested. Many of us were astonished when it became apparent that a single spermatozoon, selected by the practitioner and possibly malformed and immotile, could through ICSI achieve fertilisation and finally the birth of a healthy baby as readily as conventional IVF. This remains true; but there is now abundant evidence that the genetic defects which may be responsible for the infertility of the ICSI patients may also be transmitted to their sons – hence the need for careful genetic counselling (and perhaps testing) of ICSI patients. Other problems with ICSI, and other challenges and opportunities for andrology in general, are discussed in the later chapters.

There may be a danger that biologists interested in understanding more about sex and male sexual function will wish that the first part of this book had been published as a separate volume, while clinicians concerned with their patients and geneticists specializing in the Y chromosome may harbour similar thoughts about the second part. But biologists today, however pure their field, must surely spare a thought for possible implications for human welfare; while clinicians ignore basic biology at their peril. So I urge evolutionists, reproductive biologists, geneticists, molecular biologists, andrologists, clinicians, and indeed anyone interested in male fertility, to read this book themselves and recommend it to their students.

Anne McLaren

Preface

Intracytoplasmic sperm injection, or ICSI, represents the greatest single technological advance in human-assisted reproduction since the advent of *in vitro* fertilization (IVF). So many problems associated with female infertility were solved with IVF, yet male infertility remained an intractable problem. Today, however, because of the use of ICSI, pregnancies are achievable when even the most severe forms of male infertility are encountered. Moreover, as both Herman Tournaye and Sherman Silber have pointed out in this book, ICSI has provided us with new knowledge of, or potential areas of investigation into, several aspects of molecular genetics that were hitherto unavailable to us.

Yet, as with many new developments in science and technology, there is often a tendency for the interested scientific or clinical community to find these results so exciting that they fail to be sufficiently critical or sufficiently aware of drawbacks and limitations. Frequently, the latter may be obscured from our view in the first instance, but we are dealing with human lives here and so it is surely prudent for us to be extra vigilant. Furthermore, it should be recognized that most couples would prefer to reproduce by conventional means, so disorders of male fertility still need to be diagnosed correctly, treated and rectified if at all possible. This demands further research into testicular function and semen production. It is impossible that any one technique will be a panacea.

The technical finesse that is required for ICSI is to be greatly admired and a new offer of hope for couples with a male problem on their hands is most gratifying. But what are the hidden long-term hazards of these latest developments or is there none? These are questions worth asking and it is our belief that a broad biological perspective is a good starting point. This is why the first half of this book is so titled.

Part 1 opens with a discussion by Jack Cohen on the evolution of male sex. This author has a wide knowledge of his subject and manages to turn some conventional ideas about it on their head. He provides new and interesting angles, which are really worth digesting. Tim Birkhead continues this biological saga by discussing the role of sperm competition in the evolution of male reproductive activity. Then Hector Dott and Tim Glover follow with some of the fundamentals of mammalian male reproduction. They encourage us to jettison some of our shibboleths and question a number of our modern assumptions. They also indicate some of the lessons about human reproduction that can be learned from work on animals.

In Chapter 4, Kate Loveland and David de Kretser explain the local control of spermatogenesis and discuss aspects of its molecular basis. The intricate character of intratesticular events involved in the production of spermatozoa is revealed. Roy Jones contributes the next chapter, in which he presents a very persuasive case for including the epididymis in our deliberations on male fertility. He gives a clear account of the importance of sperm maturation in the epididymis, including that of man.

Jackson Brown, Steve Publicover and Chris Barratt continue by reminding us how little is known about sperm transport in the human female tract compared with that in many other mammals. They bring us up to date on the problems of oocyte penetration by spermatozoa and focus especially on the part played by calcium ions in the acrosome reaction. They end with brief but useful suggestions about future research in this area.

The problem of a possible decline in sperm numbers in human ejaculates and other changes in human male reproductive health is next debated by Stewart Irvine as a conclusion to this first part of the book.

Part 2 deals with recent technological advances in the field of assisted conception in humans. Herman Tournaye opens the section by giving us the pros and cons of ICSI. He does so with remarkable clarity and his chapter is followed by a most valuable and informative account by Pascuale Patrizio of some of the latest work on the genetics of male infertility. Sherman Silber takes the issue of human male infertility further in Chapter 9, by looking at it from a surgeon's point of view and Chris Ford presents a critical survey of semen analysis as it stands in the light of so much new and emerging knowledge and understanding of the reproductive process.

Ian Findlay and Justin St John bring us fully into the contemporary scientific world by explaining how molecular techniques, especially those involving the polymerase chain reaction (PCR), have contributed to the study of human fertility. They have interesting things to say about mitochondrial inheritance and preimplantation diagnosis. Thus, they provide a good perspective on some of the new developments in reproductive medicine.

Finally, Jim Cummins and Anne Jequier bring it all together and try gazing into the crystal ball. They help us to look into the future and give us clues as to possible developments in the coming century.

Some overlap of subjects may be detected in different chapters, but this has been permitted only in order to allow different viewpoints to be put on some subjects. However, we have made every effort to avoid repetition.

Some conflict of opinion between different authors may also be evident and what each has to say does not necessarily reflect the views of the editors. After all, we are only editors and we must allow our authors a free rein! We trust, though, that this book will be seen as a broad narrative rather than as a series of unconnected chapters simply strung together.

We hope too that, as a start to the next millennium, the book will offer some new ideas, some food for thought and a few pointers to the future. If it succeeds in this, it should provide new horizons for the study of male fertility and for the treatment of infertile male patients.

TIM GLOVER

CHRIS BARRATT

Acknowledgements

The editors wish to thank Dame Anne McLaren of the Wellcome Trust, Cambridge, for kindly consenting to write a Foreword for this book and Professor Roger Gosden of the Department of Obstetrics and Gynaecology, University of Leeds, for his interest and encouragement.

Part 1 **Biological perspectives**

1   The evolution of the sexual arena

JACK COHEN

Introduction: the *Scala Naturae* of reproduction

In the early 1950s, a *Scala Naturae* view of the evolution of sex was fashionable and alas it still survives in some quarters 40 years on. The *Scala Naturae* embodied a ladder of 'improvements' in our evolution, exemplified by a succession of modern species. Its peak of reproductive sophistication was seen as being a man and a woman. Primitive asexual creatures such as bacteria, plants and coelenterates, which simply bud or divide into two, provided the first steps of the ladder. An excess of cell division leads to their multiplication, thereby providing safety in numbers.

The next steps on the *Scala* constituted protection of the reproductive products, spores and seeds. Dormancy is the reproductive tactic, especially among primitive bacteria, fungi and even plants such as angiosperms. Viviparity was seen as showing the 'highest' form of care and protection and its peak was achieved in mammals, although a few other species also show this form of reproduction.

However, diversity was seen to be a 'Good Thing', partly because it dealt with variable or patchy environmental conditions, partly because nature was varied in time and space and needed to be kept track of. So mutations suddenly became useful on the evolutionary scene. Before this point they could simply be considered as 'useless' mistakes in genome replication, which primitive creatures could not avoid. However, they landed simple asexual creatures into Muller's ratchet trouble if you were a clone (Morell, 1997). We find meiosis and fertilization on the next step of the ladder, their purpose being to recombine 'good' mutations (and also to maintain ploidy).

Eventually, it was claimed, anisogamy was followed by isogamy and, in turn, the next step up showed the beauties of oogamy and the evolutionary advent of spermatozoa and eggs, which was considered to be the ultimate in reproductive sophistication. Some individuals at the next level specialized in very small gametes and became males, whilst others went in for yolky eggs and became females. Dalcq (1957) described this level in a fashion typical of his time: 'The puzzle for embryology is to determine how the fussy mobility of the sperm and the deep and perilous inertia of the egg contrive between them to animate a new individual.'

Some of these creatures, which were basically sexual, nevertheless reverted to parthenogenesis. Perhaps they did better without sex and, for example, produced well-camouflaged stick insects. Some either lost part of their sexuality by having haploid males (hymenopterans) or alternated sex with parthenogenesis, e.g. *Daphnia* and aphids) (Cohen, 1977).

The top steps were occupied by mammals, which acquired internal fertilization and viviparity and this was the 'best' way to reproduce. But large numbers of spermatozoa and oocytes (even though many oocytes became atretic) were difficult to understand in this context. 'There seems no reason for this prodigality under the conditions of mammalian reproduction', wrote Asdell in 1966.

It is now recognized that, as a result of the oddities of modern organisms being chosen to represent steps on the evolutionary ladder, practically all of these assumptions were wrong.

A better history of reproduction

Graham Bell's scholarly book *Masterpiece of nature* (not to mention my own textbook *Reproduction*) took these older ideas apart. Some criticisms of the old ideas are set out below.

'Primitive' organisms

In 1911, Dobell pointed out that to refer to the 'man-like ancestor of apes' is as correct as the more usual 'ape-like ancestor of man' and he even suggested a re-evaluation of the status of the 'primitive' protista in the evolutionary argument (protista being the group containing the amoeba, with some human-like aspects of its biochemistry). Also, Margulis (1981) emphasized the 'sexual' nature of *all* bacteria and reminded us that even the archaea swap DNA strands. The first two-thirds of organisms in the evolutionary story (all prokaryotes) apparently had rampant sex and recombination, including variants which looked, and still look like some of today's prokaryotes, very similar to male/female differentiation and spore production (Catcheside, 1977). Thus, today, there are no modern representatives of the lowest steps of the reproductive *Scala* and those for the higher levels are, at least, misleading.

Spermatozoa may well have evolved from early infective prokaryote symbionts that had acquired a genome-carrying role. Today's protozoans, especially ciliophorans such as suctoria, have a most advanced reproductive system, which includes viviparity and meiotic processes that are much more complex than our own (Roeder, 1997). So we cannot use contemporary protista (which were among the earliest eukaryotes) to illumine or exemplify steps in our own evolution. They have their own ways of doing things.

Provision for propagules

Bacterial organization increases simply so that the cells can multiply; that is, the bacterium continues its vegetative, trophic physiology and this results in two individuals arising from one. Cell wall, cell contents and genome are added continually until splitting or budding occurs. This is true vegetative (trophic) reproduction, as in the grasses. We should note that such bacterial daughters (and, indeed, viral particles) are the products of two genomic generations. The daughter bacterium has its own genome, of course, but most of its cell contents and wall are inherited directly from the mother and are thus not specified by its own genome; viral particles also have their infective mechanism and protein coat specified by earlier DNA and not by their own integral genome. This is true of most propagules (Cohen, 1977). They have at least two generations of genomes contributing to their fitness. Parents not only donate genome (usually recombined), but, of greatest importance to the early life of the offspring, they also provide mitochondria, a complete working cellular machinery, a DNA readout and replication kit, yolk or starch. According to Mendel, peas had 'factors' carried on the chromosomes and a 'packed lunch' from mother in their cotyledons. This is the 'privilege' story emphasized elsewhere in connection with the maternal contribution to reproduction (Cohen, 1979). It represents the *other* secret of successful reproduction.

Sex is not simply a recombination of mutations

The best criticism of naïve *Scala* thinking is Bell's (1982) the *Masterpiece of nature*, which is what Erasmus Darwin called sexuality. To put it briefly, it had been thought that sexual creatures went out and conquered the variable and unpredictable world by their own versatility, providing a few progeny with matching adaptations. But Bell cited a host of examples in the literature, demonstrating that it is the *asexual* forms (parthenogenetic, amazonogenetic, and many other forms that had lost the ability to reproduce sexually) which actually go out and conquer. Sexual creatures related to these forms are found only in glacial relicts and equally stable ecologies. Bell found about a hundred cases of sexual forms going out to conquer diverse habitats (and he deals adequately with the probability of asymmetry in the reporting), compared with thousands of asexual forms. So the real world told us that the story of stick insects giving up sex in favour of better camouflage had to be re-evaluated; at this point the whole concept of sex being maintained in order to give versatility in a hostile world had to be rethought. A good overview of the classical position is provided by Smith (1972), but it is well worth reading Bell (1982) to put sex and spermatozoa into a more modern context.

Spermatozoa and eggs are not the 'ultimate development'

Many reproductively successful creatures, however, have avoided simple sexual reproduction. Non-cellular protistans had different sexual problems, which have been explored elsewhere by Bell (1989). Further, the persistence of sexual dimorphism cannot be attributed merely to history ('we've got it right, so we might as well get on with it'), because the diversity of spermatozoa and egg-like forms among animals and plants suggests that loss or gain of sexual function has occurred many times during their evolution. Red algae and some ascomycete fungi, for example, have complex sexual systems with no motile stages, and ciliate protozoa have developed a vegetative macronucleus for multiplication between episodes of sexual reproduction. Eggs have different systems also, with those of nematodes, spiralia and frogs differing as much as angiosperm embryo sacs from fern archegonia. There seemed to be no alternative to the view that sex was useful, but was often lost and sometimes reacquired as a new adaptation. We could not, however, explain why. Certainly, the idea that our sperm/egg system was the goal to be achieved explains nothing.

Mammals have not got the best method of reproduction

The suggestion derived from nineteenth century natural history books that mammals have the best and most sophisticated mode of reproduction does not hold up in the face of knowledge of the variety of reproductive strategies and tactics elsewhere in the animal kingdom (Cohen, 1977). Giraffes and gnus, for instance, are impressive in that they produce big, well-programmed young that are able to recognize their mothers and are afraid of wild dogs and hyaenas (frequently the subject of television natural history programmes). But the parasitic flatworm *Gyrodactylus* is much *more* viviparous. Its uterus has two generations of progeny at the same time and sometimes even three. In this respect, even the tsetse fly *Glossina* may be regarded as being more viviparous than a mammal, because its larva is fully developed when it is laid and it burrows, pupates and emerges as a full-sized fly without feeding after it leaves the oviduct.

Revolutions in reproductive theory

There have been further revolutions in our thinking that are even less easy to relate to naïve nineteenth century views, because there are a number of questions that had not occurred to us until DNA-based genetics developed in the 1950s. At least three of these questions are relevant in the context of this book and need to be considered alongside the evolution of sex and spermatozoa. The prevalence of heterozygosity (that is, too many mutant alleles occurring at too many loci) is one. Canalization (the standardization of phenotypes in spite of heterozygosity) and 'gene conversion' (the non-reciprocal nature of genetic recombination) are others. These new ways of thinking, based in part on molecular biology, are very relevant to sperm function. Thus, we find, that many earlier views are no longer valid in today's world.

In the late 1950s (see Haldane, 1957; Fisher, 1958) and even as recently as the mid 1990s (Korol *et al.*, 1994), it was assumed that all members of each species had much the same genome, except for those with mutations (either 'good' ones coming into the population or 'bad' ones being lost by death or reduced breeding of the organisms carrying them). Whether alleles were 'good' or 'bad' was measured by one-dimensional 'fitness'. However Lewontin & Hubby (1966) turned this view over. They showed, and it has been amply confirmed since then, that about a third of protein-specifying loci (genes) have variants somewhere in the population, even in parthenogenetic species, and that about 10% of loci are heterozygous in individual wild animals. This means that organisms in that population, represented by parents of the 10% heterozygotes, have different alleles at approximately 10% of their loci (Lewontin, 1974). Unlike Mendel's pea plants, laboratory mice or *Drosophila*, nearly all wild animals and angiosperms produce gametes which differ across many axes, with multiple alleles occurring at many of them. Some lengths of chromosome are inhibited from crossing over and have sets of alleles that are haplotypes (as in the histocompatibility loci of mammals). In addition, some animals, such as the cheetah, are surprisingly homozygous even in the wild. But the reproductive message is that, contrary to the Haldane, Fisher and laboratory models, genotypes within a species are amazingly varied (Rollo, 1995).

What needs to be explained, therefore, is the *phenotypic* similarity of organisms in a population, despite their different genetic blueprints (Rollo, 1995). Waddington (1956) had laid the foundations of this in his concept of 'canalization'. Wild species had 'balanced genomes', so that a frog developing at 8 °C ended up looking like the same animal that it would have been had it developed at 28 °C, by using a different developmental route and by using different variants of temperature-sensitive enzymes. Equally, the same frog would be produced even if there were several 'less useful' alleles present and, indeed, there usually are (Rollo, 1995).

In Birmingham, we had three populations of zebra fishes. First, there were wild (pet shop!) *Danio (Brachydanio) rerio*, whose developmental stability resistant was 500 rad of X-rays. Fifty per cent of these failed to develop, but few of the rest had overt abnormalities. In a long-finned domestic variant, whose canalization was compromised by inbreeding, 50–100 rad resulted in 50% abnormal developments, including enlargement of the pericardium, as well as eye and blood vessel abnormalities. The third population comprised 'zebra crossings', whose five-generation-back ancestors had been crossed with *Danio nigropunctatus*, then consistently back to *Danio rerio*. These crossings destroyed the balance of their genomes, so that without irradiation, they produced about 50% abnormal developments. What had happened is that they had lost their canalization of development and showed noticeable asymmetry of fin ray number and other abnormalities.

The general lessons to be learned from these observations are that genetics in natural populations is much more variable than we had thought and that phenotypic stability is hard won. So, for gamete biologists, minds should be kept open to the possibility that, at least in K-strategist species (those producing relatively few zygotes), gametes are selected to construct or maintain balanced genomes.

The third revolution is still proceeding. The Mendelian recombination model for meiotic processes has been an accepted textbook diagram for almost 80 years. It claims that homologous chromosomes associate into bivalents, each forming two chromatids. Non-sister chromatids then break and rejoin, without any interpolations or deletions, forming a new chromosomal array for assortment into spermatids, ootids or polar bodies. These meiotic products can easily be examined in mycelial ascomycetes. In these organisms there is a postmeiotic mitosis, which allows any mispairing in postmeiotic products to be discriminated, so that each makes two ascopores. It can be observed that non-reciprocal exchange, called 'gene conversion', appears in up to a third of asci (each containing 8 ascospores). This is best explained by the resolution of heteroduplex DNA segments (whose bases do not pair properly) into neighbouring ascospores by postmeiotic mitosis. This non-reciprocal exchange can be seen in ascomycete fungi, but there is good evidence that such non-Mendelian repairs or reconstructions occur *wherever* there are meiotic processes (Smith *et al.*, 1995; Roeder, 1997). The relevance here is that if ascomycetes do indeed show us the general meiotic picture in detail, then most spermatozoa and ootids have unresolved heteroduplexes, because unlike ascomycetes they do not have postmeiotic mitosis, which could resolve them into two different DNA duplexes in the daughter cells. Hanneman *et al.* (1997) have recently published an analysis of this in mouse spermatids. Cohen (1967) showed that this could explain sperm numbers if those spermatozoa with heteroduplexes were not used for fertilization. Cross-species comparisons showed that, as the number of recombination events rises linearly, the number of spermatozoa offered for each fertilization rises logarithmically. If a large proportion of spermatozoa are not to fertilize, the reciprocal of this, at least, would have to be offered at copulation. For example, if only 6 per 1000 spermatozoa were permitted to reach the site of fertilization, at least a thousand would have to be offered for six fertilizations to be accomplished. (It would be expected that *all* spermatozoa *could* fertilize, if they reached the right place at the right time; a 'confession mechanism' for heteroduplexes – if that is what caused the problems – would prevent most spermatozoa from getting the chance.)

Reproduction and redundancy

Charles Darwin, Wallace and the early twentieth century embryologists were all impressed by the 'profligacy of Nature'. They were impressed, also, by the beauty of biological adaptation: Nature, it was believed, was profligate with well-adapted organisms, rather than most organisms being mistakes of the evolutionary process. The number of spermatozoa, for example, was seen as another indication of Nature's overprovision, not as a profligacy error. Only in the period of material shortage after the Second World War were biologists to begin to question this philosophy. Typical of the reversal of thought is Saunders' (1970) statement that 'The egg has solved its problem'. Almost without fail, each egg produced in the right environment forms a new individual, which in turn makes sperm or eggs that begin another generation. In this new paradigm, the overwhelming numbers of spermatozoa were seen as a puzzle to be explained, because biological efficiency, not profligacy, was the expectation. Two classes of explanation were offered, paralleling the ecological explanations of prodigality of, for example, fish eggs (the female cod fish lays about 40 million eggs in her life, of which only two, on average, survive to breed). It was considered that gametes were either being offered up to a dangerous world (Antonie van Leeuwenhoek in 1658 had said that 'There must be many adventurers, when the task is so difficult...') or the process of their production (like that of some early computer chips) was such that a vast excess of failure was an inevitable outcome (Cohen, 1967, 1971, 1973, 1975a). Bishop (1964), for example, suggested that most spermatozoa had defects inherited from the male that produced them, but in the female tract were winnowed down to useful ones. This could be explained, however, as being due to heteroduplexes in DNA.

[An interesting error was that large numbers of spermatozoa were necessary to expose the range of Mendelian possibilities. But if, for instance, only 10 spermatozoa are used, it makes no difference to the assortment of genes in each spermatozoon, whether 10, 20 or 30 million spermatozoa are offered in the first place. In other words, you do not have to deal all the cards to guarantee that each hand is random.]

Nature's overproduction is now seen in a new light by ecologists, and we should perhaps take this new way of thinking on board for spermatozoa too. The energetic 'costs' of reproduction, which in the 1960s and 1970s were seen as the major currency of ecology (Philippson, 1964) are now, with the demise of 'balance' ecological models, regarded as impossible to calculate. Here is an example other than that of spermatozoa. Nauplius larvae of barnacles contribute greatly to the spring zooplankton of the North Sea and they include those of *Sacculina* (aberrant barnacles, which are parasitic on crabs), as well as the larvae of the acorn barnacle *Chthamalus*. Who pays energetically for these larvae? Is it perhaps the crabs, because parental barnacles provide yolk more in the parasite than in the free-living organisms? Alternatively, could it be the bounty of the sun via phytoplankton? How do we calculate the energetic cost of a human ejaculate with 200 million spermatozoa in it, relative to that individual's physiological arithmetic? It is about 5% of skin cell loss, 3% of gut cell loss, or less than 1% of erythrocyte turnover (but these are anuclear and cost less). In such an economic biological model, spermatozoa have been supposed to contribute to female nutrition. But, except for a few cases such as leaf-eating monkeys (which are deficient in nucleic acids), and some queen termites (which receive only sugar solutions from the workers and need spermatozoa from the kings to make eggs), arithmetic of this kind is clearly inappropriate. Surely the cost of ejaculates to a man, or to a bull, is incalculable (but see Dewsbury, 1983, for a good comparative attempt). So how can profligacy or efficiency be measured against loss, sperm heterogeneity or sperm effectiveness as a reproductive strategy?

In recent years, the community at large has been encouraged to avoid thinking about the real, that is the actual, arithmetic of ecology. Some wildlife films may have encouraged the belief that animals in the wild live long, happy and fulfilling lives compared to those in, for example, agriculture or laboratories (Cohen, 1996). However, the real arithmetic resembles that of spermatozoa, rather than of well-balanced accounts of a corner store. Even K-strategists, such as starlings, lay about 16 eggs in their lives, of which about 2 survive to breed. For some frogs, the figure is 10 000 eggs, of which 2 survive to breed, and for cod 39 999 998 eggs contribute to food chains in order to produce 1 pair of parents. Darwin told us this, but the lesson has been greatly diluted by the great amount of attention devoted to geneticists' experiments with fruit flies or mice. Breeders are selected and are on average different from the rest. This was not what laboratory *Drosophila* tell us, but it is true in Nature. Equally, the possibility that there is sorting among gametes, not merely profligacy, cannot be ignored.

For many years it was believed that Mendelian ratios were proof that the genetic constitution of an egg or a spermatozoon did not affect its chances of fertilization. The 3:1 ratio or 9:3:3:1 proportions showed that, for those particular alleles, there was no discrimination, no bias. They demonstrated further that this was true for many alleles. However, many loci (such as the t-locus in the mouse, SD in *Drosophila* and HLA in humans) did not behave in a Mendelian fashion. Perhaps there could be genetic situations, produced as a result of meiosis, that need not be represented by zygotes. Cohen (1967) came up with the suggestion that the meiotic non-reciprocity in ascomycetes gene conversion could account for sperm redundancy in a new way, if it occurred in all other meioses and prohibited access to fertilization for spermatozoa with problems of this type. C (chiasma number at meiosis) and R (sperm redundancy) data were collected for a wide variety of organisms. Oocyte redundancy in some females was also included. The conclusion drawn from these data (Cohen, 1973) was that spermatozoa were mostly badly made. They needed a test-and-select process to allow some (the few effective ones) to reach the site of fertilization. This initiated a successful research programme, which, unfortunately, has remained a bywater of reproductive theory (Cohen & Adeghe, 1987; Cohen, 1992).

Sperm competition

The concept of sperm competition, which is discussed in more depth in Chapter 2, arose partly because a clever set of observations had led Parker

(1970, 1984) to propose that the major reason for large numbers of spermatozoa being produced by one male was so that they could compete successfully in the female with those from other males. Males who won this battle, like those who won courtship competitions and had successful female-guarding strategies, became ancestors. The others were lost to posterity. The obvious way to compete was to produce more of the cheap-to-produce spermatozoa. More and more evidence in support of this accumulated (see Smith, 1984); for example, in 1979, Short demonstrated that testis size and sperm output in the gorilla, the chimpanzee and man were each related to mating strategies, with the chimpanzee's ten times larger ejaculate having predominated evolutionarily because of the multimale copulations that occur when a female is in oestrus. Gorillas rarely have sperm competition and, accordingly, they have very small testes. Man is intermediate between these two apes with regard to testis size. It has been discovered that there is extra-partner mating in several monogamous species of birds (Birkhead, Chapter 2). Furthermore, DNA paternity assignments in other wild species have shown diversity of paternity and this has indicated that sperm competition (that is, the presence of spermatozoa from two or more males inside a female at the time of ovulation) is much more common than had been thought, perhaps even among mammals (Møller & Birkhead, 1989).

There has been a great deal of recent work documenting sperm competition in insects and birds. Here, the geometry of the female tract determines whether spermatozoa are stacked in a cul-de-sac spermatheca, so that last-male precedence occurs, or whether spermatozoa queue in a tube, so that there is first-male precedence. In their ejaculates some males mimic substances normally used by the female to cause ovulation, and so presumably achieve more ovulations at the expense of subsequent males. A variety of these postcopulatory tactics is seen in animals, ranging from female guarding to copulatory locks and plugs, offensive substances exuded from the mated female to deter further matings, and substances in ejaculates which subvert rejection in the female tract. These have been comprehensively reviewed by Andersson (1994). Darwin (1871) believed that male–male competition for females was a major factor in the evolution of male display, especially in human evolution. But the tactics have turned out to be more detailed and devious than even he would have guessed. Whether they are as devious as Baker & Bellis (1995) supposed is a matter of debate, but, if their data are to be believed, there is a case for sperm competition in man. It is unlikely, however, that it has the baroque theoretical basis which they propose, with 'kamikaze' spermatozoa and other fanciful ideas.

There is one further twist to the story, which pushes Andersson's review into the same historical context as that of Darwin. It is perhaps because we are now beginning to bring context into scientific explanations (Cohen & Stewart, 1994). This has happened later in molecular biology than in some other areas of science (Cohen & Rice, 1996), but the authors of some of the earlier papers on sperm competition realised that the female tract was a necessary and important variable (see Austad, 1984; Eberhard, 1985). Eberhard (1996) has now produced a very convincing monograph that firmly sets sperm competition in the context of so-called 'cryptic female choice'. In many species (especially insects, arachnids and some birds), the female makes the choices and sets the scale of the stakes. Moreover, she often decides who will win, in advance of the game being played. As in human sports, the arena managers (in this case the females) control the male competition games in many important ways.

Female management of males and sperm competition

Female management makes good evolutionary sense. The female progeny of a female will impose more or less the same obstacle courses as their mother and male progeny will be derived from males that were successful earlier against these obstacles. That set of progeny will, on average, do well in the mating games of the next generation, promoting females with discriminating obstacle courses and males who beat other males in traversing them. This is multidimensional, multigenerational analogue selection. It is much more complicated than the Darwinian principle of female peacocks choosing males with long tails and being selected to choose them. This was a one-dimensional concept, with only winners and losers in a race. Here, we are talking rather in terms of sports stadia, with managers competing to have the highest diving boards, the longest athletic tracks and the most exciting courses, all of which will discriminate between, and select, the best players. So males who succeed will have sons who are 'better' in the next generation's female tracts. In addition, the female's daughters will up the stakes in future generations.

Sex organs differ in all kinds of ways and males have found many special ways of 'cheating'. These cheats either become the regular courtship pattern (they determine ejaculate composition or sperm head shape in all males of a given species), or they are rejected within a very few generations. All these dimensions are refined, as males are required to produce gametes further out along all the axes, as the female tracts require more spermatozoa and as more is required of spermatozoa. This could explain the rather strange morphologies of spermatozoa in general, especially those of species that have internal fertilization (Cohen, 1977; Jamieson, 1987), and also sperm competition (if indeed it is present in mammals). It could similarly explain the peculiar shapes of rodent sperm heads if their female ancestors had the choice of competing sperm from different males.

Because such a discriminating female appears to exert physiological control on the reproductive process, once spermatozoa (or spermatophores) are deposited her utilization of those spermatozoa can be modified only by the male who is copulating with her, if he is able to modify her behaviour or her physiology to his advantage. This selection of male behaviour to control the female is a good candidate for the origin of copulation (Cohen, 1971, 1977). As a theory of copulation it has the advantage that it can be tested and lends itself to comparative studies. Eberhard's comparison of tube lengths to and from the spermatheca of spiders is one such test. If the tube leading from the spermatheca to the site of fertilization is extra long and tortuous, then spermatozoa from several different males will probably have to compete. On the other hand, if the proximal tube leading to the spermatheca (along which males must pass their sperm packages) is long as well as tortuous, it is likely to be the males themselves rather than their spermatozoa which are being discriminated. From 314 species of spider with such ducts, the proximal ducts were equal in length in 6 species, slightly shorter in 40 and longer in all the rest. The conclusion is that most spiders exhibit 'cryptic female choice' and discriminate against those males that cannot get their sperm packets to reach the spermatheca. An alternative is that spermatozoa compete by differences in function in the second (higher) part of the tract. When all the physiological ways in which a female can bias the outcome are taken into account, however, it is clear that there are other parts of the story. Among insects and arachnids many cases have been documented in which females use the spermatozoa of some males but not of others, by rejecting spermatophores, failing to move spermatozoa along the tract or not ovulating. Even in mammals, a female in early pregnancy may resorb her embryos if she encounters and smells a male that she considers to be more attractive than her first mate (the Bruce effect). This is a form of female choice that occurs later in the reproductive process, but there are many mammals with multimale copulations where female choice might occur in the same way as in arthropods.

We should not go overboard on this new step towards an evolutionary explanation of sexual behaviour and sperm morphology and physiology. But the generality which it embraces is that females of many animal species make their tracts as difficult to traverse as is required to discriminate between their males. Such a suggestion is welcome because it gives another explanation of the large number of spermatozoa that are offered by males and includes an explanation of oddities like the lepidopterans producing apyrrhene spermatozoa (spermatozoa without nuclei). It does not explain why sperm redundancy correlates with chiasma number, however, so it is still possible that most spermatozoa are excluded from fertilizing and that most female tracts have some form of sperm-selecting mechanism, as well as a male-discriminating function.

Conclusions: simplexities and complicities in the evolution of sexuality

We should beware of single-cause explanations, especially in evolutionary biology. While science should seek simple explanations, it is rarely the case that simple variables such as sperm number can be tied to a single parameter of difference between species (Cohen, 1973), or between copulations, as suggested by Baker & Bellis (1995). More usually, the pattern of biological variability is evident in several directions, which in the present discussion might be chiasma-associated redundancy, male competition and/or female control (see Cohen, 1975*b*).

Any pattern of evolutionary differences among organisms results from an interaction between at least two phase spaces. First, the possibilities available to DNA sequences (only a tiny proportion of which can be functional) overlap with those developmental possibilities in the environment, as this changes through evolutionary time. This means that if the organism is to be successful, its DNA prescription and its environment must interact. This kind of interaction, with all its recursions and strange loops, has been called a 'complicity' by Cohen & Stewart (1991, 1994). It is the most fruitful of the ways in which complex patterns can be produced from simple causes. The other type of interaction is 'simplexity' which is the development of simple systems into more complex ones through the operation of internal rules. These rules, in their turn, take the systems into a new set of rules. Male–male competition within a species (which results in more and more spermatozoa being produced) is an example of a simplectic process. But discrimination by successive female tracts, which produces a lineage of males that are best able to negotiate ever more elaborate obstacles, is a complicity.

Unless we see and learn to understand the constraints on sperm function and the new possibilities arising from these interactions, our attempts to describe and understand the ways in which spermatozoa perform *in vivo* must be futile. For instance, models of spermatozoa that owe more to salmon swimming upstream to breed than to female choice are not helpful, even for today's molecular biology. Questions *can* be produced which derive a reductionist picture of sperm function ('How can Ca^{2+} be involved in the acrosome reaction?', for example). We all know that spermatozoa do not just 'swim upstream' and that it is only the continually changing context of sperm physiology in female tracts (or some other arcane factor) that is likely to yield better explanations and thus enlighten us. We need a sperm's eye view of the female tract and the tract's view of the spermatozoa. Personally, I look forward to spermatozoa being investigated in more biologically natural circumstances than hitherto, such as in coagulated human semen or in reacted cervical mucus, rather than in physiological salines. Only by this sort of approach, it seems to me, can the theories we generate have relevance to real life (Pandya & Cohen, 1985; Cohen, 1990).

References
Andersson, M. (1994). *Sexual selection.* Princeton: Princeton University Press.
Asdell, A. A. (1966). Evolutionary trends in physiology of reproduction.
Symposium of the Zoological Society London, **15**, 1–14.

Austad. S. N. (1984). Evolution of sperm priority patterns in spiders. In *Sperm competition and the evolution of animal mating systems*, ed. R. C. Smith, pp. 223–50. London: Academic Press.

Baker, R. R. & Bellis, M. A. (1995). *Human sperm competition: copulation, masturbation and infidelity.* London: Chapman & Hall.

Bell, G. (1982). *The masterpiece of nature.* London: Croom Helm.

   (1989). *Sex and death in protozoa.* Cambridge: Cambridge University Press.

Bishop, M.W. H. (1964). Paternal contribution to embryonic death. *Journal of Reproduction and Fertility,* **7**, 383–96.

Catcheside, D. G. (1977). *The genetics of recombination.* London: Edward Arnold.

Cohen, J. (1967). Correlation between chiasma frequency and sperm redundancy. *Nature,* **215**, 862–3.

   (1971). The comparative physiology of gamete populations. *Advances in Comparative Biochemistry and Physiology,* **4**, 267–380.

   (1973). Cross-overs, sperm redundancy and their close association. *Heredity,* **31**, 408–13.

   (1975*a*). Gamete redundancy: wastage or selection? In *Gamete competition in animals and plants*, ed. D. Mulcahy, pp. 99–112. Amsterdam: Elsevier.

   (1975*b*). Gametic diversity within an ejaculate. In *Functional morphology of the spermatozoon*, ed. B. Afzelius, pp. 329–39. Oxford: Pergamon Press.

   (1977). *Reproduction. Textbook of animal and human reproduction.* London: Butterworths.

   (1979). Introduction: maternal constraints on development. In *Maternal effects on development*, ed. D. R. Newth & M. Balls. *British Society for Developmental Biology Symposium,* **4**, pp. 1–28. Cambridge: Cambridge University Press.

   (1990). The function of human semen coagulation and liquefaction *in vivo*. In *Advances in in vitro fertilization and assisted reproduction technologies*, ed. S. Mashiach, Z. Ben-Rafael, N. Laufer & J. G. Schenker, pp. 443–52. New York: Plenum Press.

   (1992). The case for and against sperm selection. In *Comparative spermatology – twenty years after*, ed. B. Baccetti, *Ares-Serono Symposia,* **75**, pp. 759–64. New York: Raven Press.

   (1996). Reproductive fallacies. *Proceedings of the Royal Institution,* **67**, 171–92.

Cohen J. & Adeghe, J.-H. A. (1987). The other spermatozoa; fate and functions. In *New horizons in spermatozoal research*, ed. H. Mohri, pp. 125–34. Tokyo: Japanese Science Societies Press.

Cohen, J. & Rice, S. H. (1996). Where do biochemical pathways lead? In *Molecular biology*, ed. J. Collado-Vides, B. Mayasnik & T. F. Smith, pp. 239–51. Cambridge, MA: MIT Press.

Cohen, J. & Stewart, I. (1991). Chaos, contingency and convergence. *Non-linear Science Today,* **1**(2), 9–13.

   (1994). *The collapse of chaos; simple laws in a complex world.* New York: Penguin, Viking.

Dalcq, A. M. (1957). *Introduction to general embryology.* London: Oxford University Press.

Darwin, C. (1871). *The descent of man and selection in relation to sex.* New York: Modern Library (Reprinted).

Dewsbury, D. A. (1983). Ejaculate cost and male choice. *American Nature*, **119**, 601–3.

Dobell, C. (1911). The principles of protistology. *Archiv für Protistenkunde*, **21**, 269–310.

Eberhard, W. G. (1985). *Sexual selection and animal genitalia*. Cambridge, MA: Harvard University Press.

(1996). *Female control: sexual selection by cryptic female choice*. Princeton, NJ: Princeton University Press.

Fisher, R. A. (1958). Polymorphism and natural selection. *Journal of Ecology*, **46**, 289–93.

Haldane, J. B. S. (1957). The cost of natural selection. *Journal of Genetics*, **55**, 511–24.

Hanneman, W. H., Schimenti, K. J. & Schimenti, J. C. (1997). Molecular analysis of gene conversion in spermatids from transgenic mice. *Gene*, **200**, 185–92.

Jamieson, B. G. M. (1987). A biological classification of sperm types, with special reference to annelids and molluscs, and an example of spermiocladistics. In *New horizons in sperm cell research*, ed. H. Mohri, pp. 31–54. Tokyo: Japanese Science Societies Press.

Korol, A. B., Preygel, I. A. & Preygel, S. I. (1994). *Recombination, variability and evolution: algorithms of estimation and population-genetic models*. London: Chapman & Hall (adapted from the 1990 Russian version).

Lewontin, R. C. (1974). *The genetic basis of evolutionary change*. New York: Columbia University Press.

Lewontin, R. C. & Hubby, J. L. (1966). A molecular approach to the study of genic heterozygosity in natural populations. II. Amount of variation and degree of heterozygosity in natural populations of *Drosophila pseudoobscura*. *Genetics*, **54**, 595–609.

Margulis, L. (1981). *Symbiosis in cell evolution*. San Francisco: Freeman.

Møller, A. P. & Birkhead, T. R. (1989). Copulation behaviour in mammals: evidence that sperm competition is widespread. *Biological Journal of the Linnean Society*, **38**, 119–31.

Morell, V. (1997). Sex frees viruses from genetic ratchet. *Science*, **278**, 1562–3.

Pandya, I. J. & Cohen, J. (1985). The leucocytic reaction of the human cervix to spermatozoa. *Fertility and Sterility*. **43**, 417–21.

Parker, G. A. (1970). Sperm competition and its evolutionary consequences in the insects. *Biological Review*, **45**, 525–67.

(1984). Sperm competition and the evolution of animal mating strategies. In *Sperm competition and the evolution of animal mating systems*, ed. R. C. Smith, pp. 2–61. London, Academic Press.

Philippson, R. D. (1964). *Ecological energetics*. London: Edward Arnold.

Roeder, G. S. (1997). Meiotic chromosomes: it takes two to tango. *Genes and Development*, **11**, 2600–21.

Rollo, C. D. (1995). *Phenotypes*. London: Chapman & Hall.

Saunders, J. W. Jr. (1970). *Patterns and principles of animal development*. London: Macmillan.

Short, R. V. (1979). Sexual selection and its component parts, somatic and genital selection, as illustrated by man and the great apes. *Advances in the Study of Behaviour*, **9**, 131–58.

Smith, G. R., Amundsen, S. K., Dabert, P. & Taylor, A. F. (1995). The initiation and control of homologous recombination in *Escherischia coli*. *Philosophical Transactions of the Royal Society of London*, B, **347**, 13–20.

Smith, J. M. (1972). The origin and maintenance of sex. In *John Maynard Smith on evolution*, pp. 115–25. Edinburgh: Edinburgh University Press.

Smith, R. C. (ed.) (1984). *Sperm competition and the evolution of animal mating systems*. London: Academic Press.

Waddington, C. H. (1956). *Principles of embryology*. New York: Macmillan.

2 The role of sperm competition in reproduction

TIM BIRKHEAD

Introduction

Why is it that a male chimpanzee (*Pan troglodytes*) ejaculates an average of 600×10^6 spermatozoa, whilst humans ejaculate fewer than 200×10^6 and the gorilla (*Gorilla gorilla*) 65×10^6? This question can be answered in a number of different ways, depending on one's perspective. A reproductive physiologist or clinician might answer by describing the mechanisms of sperm production, storage in the epididymal cauda and vas deferens and ejaculation. An evolutionary biologist, on the other hand, might answer by discussing the selection pressures that have been responsible for shaping chimpanzee reproductive anatomy and physiology and how individuals producing ejaculates containing this number of spermatozoa left the most descendants. Both answers are correct, but they are concerned with different levels of analysis: mechanisms and function (or adaptive significance), respectively (Alcock & Sherman, 1994). The type of question we ask and how we go about answering it depend very much on our background training. Recently, though, behavioural ecologists have started to integrate evolutionary ideas and physiological mechanisms in a highly productive way (see Krebs & Davies, 1997) and this approach has been particularly successful in elucidating many of the factors which determine fertilization success.

Animal characteristics such as morphology, physiology and many types of behaviour, have evolved in response to both natural selection and sexual selection. Sexual selection is defined as the selection of any trait that enhances an individual's reproductive success relative to others in a population (Darwin, 1871; Andersson, 1994). It comprises intrasexual selection, usually competition between males, and intersexual selection, usually female choice of male. Male–male competition is often obvious and sometimes brutal; female choice is more subtle and hence more difficult to observe, but there is now abundant evidence for its occurrence (Andersson, 1994). The early view of sexual selection was that it ended once an individual had acquired a partner. However, in a ground-breaking paper, Parker (1970) showed that sexual selection, specifically male–male competition, could continue after insemination, through the competition between spermatozoa to fertilize a female's ovum. Subsequently it was proposed that female choice may also occur following insemination, through the differential utilization of spermatozoa by females (Eberhard, 1996). Sexual selection may even continue beyond fertilization, through the differential abortion of embryos or the differential investment in offspring (Møller, 1994).

The traditional view of reproduction was that it was a cooperative venture between male and female. A moment's reflection, however, suggests that it may not be cooperative and that the processes of courtship, copulation and fertilization can be sources of potential conflict between male and female. Austin & Bishop (1957) and Bedford (1970) hinted at this many years ago when they referred to the journey of spermatozoon to ovum as a saga, thereby raising the question of why females make it so difficult for spermatozoa to fertilize their ova (Roldan *et al.*, 1992; Birkhead *et al.*, 1993). The answer lies in an evolutionary perspective: individuals of each sex have evolved to maximize their own reproductive success (Williams, 1966; Dawkins, 1976). In other words, it is in the evolutionary interests of each individual, male or female, to retain control over reproductive events that affect their genetic contribution to subsequent generations. Selection will favour those males that fertilize many females, and should favour those females who discriminate between males and produce successful offspring. This conflict of interest between the sexes has undoubtedly been responsible for shaping many aspects of sexual reproduction. Many reproductive traits are likely to be the result of a coevolutionary arms race between males and females as they grapple for control (Bedford, 1991; Rice, 1996). However, identifying the traits that have evolved in response to these selection pressures is not easy (see e.g. Rice, 1996).

The second factor that is thought to have affected the evolution of reproductive traits is seasonality of reproduction. Some species are sexually active throughout the year, others only for a relatively short period. Ecological factors dictate when successful breeding can occur. Species constrained to breed over a relatively short period of time must be under selective pressure to produce ejaculates of sufficient size and quality to ensure fertilization (Gibson & Jewell, 1982; Bedford *et al.*, 1984; Harcourt *et al.*, 1995; A. P. Møller, unpublished results).

The third factor to influence reproduction is competition between males. Contrary to what is commonly assumed, the females of many species are not sexually monogamous and typically copulate with more than one male during a single reproductive cycle. When this occurs, and it is extremely widespread across the entire animal kingdom, the result is sperm competition (Smith, 1984*a*; Birkhead & Møller, 1998). Sperm competition has been defined as the competition between the ejaculates of different males for the fertilization of a given set of ova (Parker, 1970; Birkhead & Parker, 1997): this implies a male-driven phenomenon, but there is increasing awareness that differential utilization of spermatozoa by females may also be important (e.g. Eberhard, 1996). Here I use the term sperm competition in its broadest sense (see Birkhead, 1996) to encompass both intra- and intersexual processes.

How do we know that sperm competition occurs and how can we measure its intensity, and hence its likely power in shaping reproductive features? There are two main lines of evidence for the existence of sperm competition: (1) observations of females copulating with more than one male during a reproductive cycle, and (2) the occurrence of offspring in the same litter fathered by different males. In this respect the recent advent of molecular techniques such as DNA-fingerprinting have revolutionized this area of study (Schierwater *et al.*, 1994). The intensity of sperm competition can be estimated from observations of the proportion of females copulating with multiple males, or by the proportion of litters with multiple paternity, or the overall proportion of offspring fathered by a male other than the female's main suitor. However, these two measures tell us different things. Observations of copulation tell us about the behaviour of individuals; for example, whether males or females are more active in initiating multiple mating. Because many mammals are nocturnal and/or secretive, witnessing copulations can be difficult and this is therefore an unreliable way of assessing sperm competition. Molecular techniques, on the other hand, although expensive and time consuming, are more reliable in telling us about the outcome of multiple mating. For example, a female may copulate with several males, but her ova may be fertilized by only one of them. Both measures therefore provide only an index of the intensity of sperm competition. However, in terms of evolutionary significance, paternity determines a male's genetic fitness and is of fundamental importance. The extent of multiple paternity varies markedly between species. For example, among rodents, in the Oldfield mouse (*Peromyscus polionotus*), no multiple paternity was detected in 220 litters (Foltz, 1981). At the other extreme, in Gunnison's prairie dog (*Cynomys gunnisoni*), one-third of all litters were sired by two or more males and 61% of all offspring were fathered by males from other territories (Travis *et al.*, 1996).

The power of male–female conflict and of sperm competition in shaping reproduction has been elegantly demonstrated in the fruit fly *Drosophila*. At first sight it might seem that what happens in the fruit fly has little bearing on reproduction in our own species or other mammals. However, this example provides compelling evidence that some male and female reproductive traits coevolve in response to sperm competition. As in a number of organisms, male fruit flies father more offspring the more females they inseminate. In contrast, female reproductive success is not increased by the female fly copulating with more than one male, although multiple mating by females is relatively common (Bateman, 1948). This means that males frequently inseminate females that are already carrying spermatozoa inseminated by other males. However, the last male to inseminate a female typically fertilizes the majority (>90%) of her eggs. The mechanism responsible for this appears to be the inclusion of substances in the seminal fluid, inserted ahead of the sperm, which disable previously stored spermatozoa (Harshman & Prout, 1994; Chapman *et al.*, 1995). The ability of males to disable the spermatozoa of competitors is an adaptation to sperm competition. However, the substances that damage stored spermatozoa are also toxic to females and reduce their survival: the more frequently a female mates, the shorter is her lifespan (Fowler & Partridge, 1989). There is thus a clear conflict of interest between the sexes which arises from sperm competition: males benefit from frequent copulations, females do not.

The coevolutionary nature of the relationship between male and female *Drosophila* was demonstrated by an elegant experiment. Rice (1996) allowed male fruit flies to evolve over successive generations independently of females. By keeping females evolutionarily 'static', males and females were prevented from coevolving. When individuals of the two lines were subsequently allowed to copulate, the selected males were disproportionately successful in sperm competition compared with those from control lines, an effect due to toxins in their seminal fluid. As a consequence, however, the females inseminated by these males suffered higher mortality. This indicates that male and female traits coevolve: males are under strong selection to be effective in disabling the sperm of competitors, and females are under strong selection to minimize the damage caused by toxic substances in seminal fluids. This is an extreme example, but the principles may be identical, albeit more subtle, in other animal groups. It is not appropriate therefore to discuss the evolutionary factors that have influenced the reproductive system of one sex, without reference to the other. The aim of this chapter is to examine the evolutionary forces, including female interests, that have shaped the male reproductive system in different mammalian species.

The male reproductive system in mammals

The male reproductive system comprises the testes, epididymides, vasa deferentia, accessory sex glands and penis, which together produce and transfer the ejaculate which comprises spermatozoa and seminal fluid. Within any particular taxon, all of these features show considerable variation in size, although there is less variation than between taxa. Much of this variation has evolved in response to sexual selection and the best way to appreciate it is through interspecific comparisons (Harvey & Pagel, 1991). Although the patterns discussed below occur in a wide range of species, including fish, reptiles and birds, attention is focused on mammals, and on primates in particular.

The testis

The testes are responsible mainly for the production of spermatozoa and hormones. As with many other organs, testes size in mammals scales allometrically with body mass, with an exponent close to three-quarters (Calder, 1984; Møller, 1989). This is not surprising since a large number of spermatozoa is required in larger animals because of dilution effects (Short, 1981). Residuals from the relationship between log body mass and log testes mass provide an index of relative testes mass. In several animal taxa, relative mass of the testes appears to be related to the mating system and the intensity of sperm competition (see e.g. Parker, 1970; Short, 1979; Harcourt *et al.*, 1995; Møller & Briskie, 1995). This is hardly surprising, given that sperm numbers play an important role in determining the outcome of sperm competition (Martin & Dziuk, 1977; Huck *et al.*, 1989).

Two factors are likely to have been particularly important in the evolution of relative testes size: sperm competition and sperm depletion. Sperm competition is likely in mammals with multimale social systems, in which females typically copulate with more than one male. Sperm depletion is likely when males are polygynous (e.g. species where males hold large harems of females, as in some ungulates and seals), and copulate with several females over a short period of time (e.g. during a short breeding season).

A comparative study of primates (Fig. 2.1) showed that species with multimale mating systems, in which females typically copulate with more than one male, had relatively larger testes than those in single-male and monogamous mating systems (Harcourt *et al.*, 1995). Similarly Møller (1989) showed that some species in which females copulated with several males had

Fig. 2.1. Relationship between log body weight and log testes weight in mammals. Different symbols represent different families: filled symbols are multimate groups, open symbols are one-male primate families and are less likely to experience sperm competition. The value for *Homo sapiens* falls very close to the fitted regression line. (Redrawn with permission from Harcourt *et al.* (1995) *Functional Ecology*, 9, 472.)

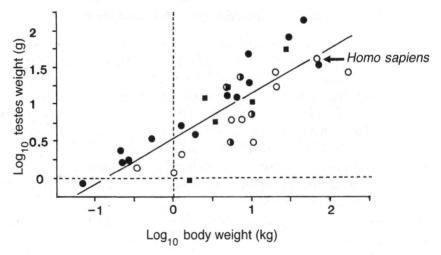

significantly higher ejaculation rates (which implies relatively larger testes) than polygynous species. While sperm competition has clearly been important in determining the evolution of testes size, sperm depletion mediated through polygyny and/or a short breeding season has therefore been much less important (Harcourt *et al.*, 1995).

Epididymis

The epididymis is the site in which spermatozoa mature and are stored (see Chapters 3 and 5). Interspecific differences in the relative size of the epididymis, and hence sperm reserves, are considerable (Møller, 1989) and means that different species have different capacities to make successive ejaculates (Bedford, 1994). The relative size of the male's epididymal sperm store can be expressed two ways.

1 Relative to testes mass (Møller, 1989). Species with large testes have correspondingly large sperm stores, and hence a greater capacity to produce successive ejaculates. Moreover, overall, species with large testes also produce ejaculates with large numbers of spermatozoa (Møller, 1989).

2 The ratio of sperm numbers in the caudal region of the epididymis to the rate of daily sperm production (DSP) (Bedford, 1994). The ratio varies by a factor of 3 or 4 across domestic mammals, from about 13 in the sheep to about 5 in the rat and 4 in humans (Bedford, 1994). For example, in rams the epididymis contains $165\,000 \times 10^6$ spermatozoa, and a ram can ejaculate 30–40 times in one day (Lindsay, 1991). In contrast, the human epididymis contains just 440×10^6 spermatozoa and (some) males can make a maximum of just six ejaculations per day (Bedford, 1994). Obviously, this difference is determined by the fact that sheep are polygynous and, in the wild, experience intense sperm competition (Salamon, 1962; K. Wilson, personal communication). This subject is further examined in Chapter 3.

A factor that enhances a male's ability to produce a succession of high-quality ejaculates is the temperature at which epididymal spermatozoa are stored. The location of the epididymis in the scrotum maintains sperm at temperatures 2–6 deg.C lower than that in the abdominal cavity (Carrick & Setchell, 1977). Initially, biologists had asked why some mammals, including ourselves, have scrotal testes while others (i.e. the Testiconidae, e.g. elephants, hyraxes, cetaceans) have abdominal testes. Glover (1973) and Bedford (1977) recast the question however, and shifted the focus from the testes to the epididymis. Both these workers have shown that the location, and hence temperature, of the testes has little bearing on their ability to produce spermatozoa, but has a profound effect on the viable lifespan of spermatozoa in the tail of the epididymis. For example, in the rabbit, spermatozoa in the scrotal cauda epididymidis remain viable for more than 3 weeks, but in experimental artificial cryptorchidism they show distinct signs of degeneration after only 8 to 9 days (Glover, 1960). Similarly, in the rat, the viability of the spermatozoa under the same conditions is 21 days and 3–4 days, respectively (Bedford, 1977). The question of the location of mammalian testes still remains: there have been a number of hypotheses, but no consensus (Bedford, 1977; Freeman, 1990; Chance, 1996). The various ways in which cauda epididymal sperm are kept at lower than body temperature are remarkable (Bedford, 1977). For example, the arrangement in hyraxes is unique among mammals: the testes are abdominal, but the epididymis lies in the pelvic cavity, close to the body surface (Glover & Sale, 1968), an arrangement virtually identical with that in passerine birds (Wolfson, 1954; Birkhead & Møller, 1992). In some rodents, the testes are scrotal, but the cauda epididymidis resides in an additional and hairless projection of the scrotum (Fig. 2.2), presumably an additional cooling device. The most likely explanation for the evolution of a cool epididymis is the ability to produce a succession of high-quality ejaculates (see Chapter 3). The two factors that favour this ability are polygyny and sperm competition: males that need to inseminate a number of females over a short period of time, and males inseminating females that are likely to have mated (or to mate) with other males (i.e. sperm competition).

Penis

The main roles of the penis are the transfer of semen from male to female and the excretion of urine. As with other male reproductive morphol-

Fig. 2.2. The scrotum (left-hand side) and testis and cauda epididymidis (right-hand side) of a wood mouse (*Apodemus sylvaticus*), showing the hairless extension of the scrotum in which the cauda lies (see the text). (Photograph by H. D. M. Moore.)

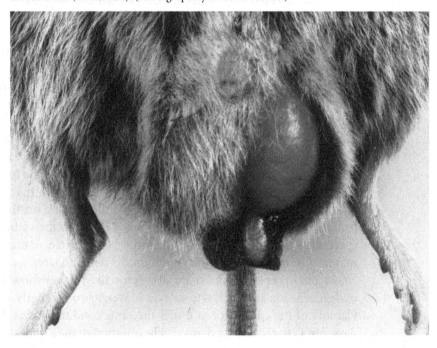

ogy, relative penis size and form show considerable variation in mammals. Indeed, the variation is so striking that several authors have speculated that the penis must have additional functions (Gomendio *et al.*, 1998). Two additional functions have been suggested,

  1 That the penis has evolved in an intrasexual context; that is, in male–male display (Wickler, 1967).
  2 That the penis has evolved in an intersexual context through internal 'courtship' of the female; that is, as a device for persuading the female to accept a male's ejaculate (Eberhard, 1985; Dewsbury, 1988; see also Chapter 3).

Since a longer penis may allow a male to place his ejaculate in a relatively more favourable position within the female reproductive tract, sperm competition may have favoured increased penis length. As predicted, primates in which sperm competition is likely have a longer (and more structurally complex) penis than monandrous species (Dixson, 1987; Verrell, 1992; see also Harcourt & Gardiner, 1994). However, it also seems likely that the dimensions of the penis and the female reproductive tract have coevolved. For example, whether a male can place semen in an optimal position may depend to some degree on the dimensions of the vagina (Brown *et al.*, 1995) and it is possible that the sexual swellings that occur in some primates (Sillén-Tullberg & Møller, 1993), and which functionally extend the length of the female tract, represent an evolutionary attempt by females to counter male control (Brown *et al.*, 1995).

The size and form of the penis may also be associated with the placement of the ejaculate. In mammals semen is deposited either in the vagina (e.g. in cattle, sheep, goats) or in the uterus (e.g. in horses, pigs, dogs and rodents). In the domestic pig, for example, the terminal spiral morphology of the penis enters the cervix, and ejaculation occurs only once this interlocking has been achieved (Hunter, 1995). Sperm competition may have been responsible for the evolution of penis design, the location of semen placement and ejaculate features.

Ejaculate

Ejaculates comprise spermatozoa and seminal fluids and both these features show considerable interspecific variation. The numbers of spermatozoa per ejaculate, the frequency of ejaculation and the quality of ejaculates are all likely to have been influenced by a species' mating system and by the intensity of sperm competition.

A. P. Møller (unpublished results) examined five ejaculate features (volume, sperm concentration, proportion of morphologically normal spermatozoa, proportion of motile spermatozoa and total number of spermatozoa per ejaculate) in a comparative study of mammals. He found that several features scaled allometrically with body size (presumably, in part, because of dilution effects in the female tract) and more closely with testes

mass. Two features in particular, ejaculate volume and total number of spermatozoa per ejaculate, were significantly related to the likelihood of sperm
competition. Seasonality of reproduction had no effect on any ejaculate
feature.

The mean volume of mammalian ejaculates varies considerably, from as
much as 400 ml (containing 10×10^6 to 100×10^6 spermatozoa) in the domestic pig (Dziuk, 1991) to 2.5 ml (containing approx. 175×10^6 spermatozoa) in
humans, to 0.4 ml (approx. 65×10^6 spermatozoa) in the gorilla (Smith,
1984b). Much of this variation is attributable to variation in the relative
amount of seminal fluid. In mammals, the composition of seminal fluid is
incompatible with prolonged sperm survival in the female tract or elsewhere, but the adaptive significance of interspecific variation in seminal
fluid volume remains to be explored (Møller, 1988). In some taxa (e.g. bats,
rodents), the seminal fluid forms a 'copulatory plug'. The adaptive
significance of these plugs is unclear: they may, as claimed in Chapter 3,
prevent sperm leakage, or they may have evolved through sperm competition to prevent or hamper inseminations by other males (Hartung &
Dewsbury, 1978). They could serve both functions.

In *Drosophila* and a number of other invertebrates, seminal fluids have
been shown to contain a cocktail of substances that affect or 'manipulate'
female reproductive physiology in different ways. These include the disabling of previously inseminated spermatozoa (Harshman & Prout, 1994;
Chapman *et al.*, 1995), increasing the rate of egg production (Loher *et al.*,
1981) and a reduction in female libido (Reiman *et al.*, 1967). All of these features are thought to have evolved through sexual selection (e.g. Eberhard,
1996). Such effects are not confined to invertebrates; it is well known that
prostaglandins in mammalian semen stimulate smooth muscle in the female
tract and may influence sperm transport and this has been clearly demonstrated in primates (Kelly *et al.*, 1976). Moreover, a recent study of domestic
pigs demonstrated that substances in the seminal plasma advanced the
timing of ovulation by 8 to 10 h following the onset of oestrus (Waberski *et
al.*, 1997).

The quality of an ejaculate, in terms of the motility and velocity of spermatozoa, the proportion of live spermatozoa, and the ability of spermatozoa
to penetrate the vestments of ova are all likely to be subject to strong selection, especially when females typically copulate with more than one male
(Møller, 1988; Gomendio *et al.*, 1998).

Spermatozoa

The main function of the spermatozoon is to activate the egg to complete meiosis and form a zygote. The diversity of sperm size and morphology
across the animal kingdom is remarkable. Even within the primates, mean
sperm length varies from 50.0 to 93.6 μm (Cummins & Woodall, 1985) and
some of this variation may be explicable in terms of sperm competition.

Polyandrous primates (and rodents) have longer spermatozoa than monandrous species (Gomendio & Roldan, 1991), and because, in these taxa at least, longer spermatozoa swim faster than shorter ones they are likely to be at a competitive advantage (Gomendio *et al.*, 1998). However, more information is needed to verify this.

Sperm competition in humans

In the preceding sections of this chapter it is has been argued that two components of sexual selection, intersexual conflict and sperm competition have been powerful, if rather subtle selective forces shaping reproductive features. An obvious question is the extent to which these factors have shaped human reproductive biology. There is rather little information regarding intersexual selection in humans and what there is is embodied in studies of sperm competition. In the sense that females sometimes copulate with a male other than their regular partner, or sometimes produce extra-pair offspring, sperm competition undoubtedly occurs in humans. However, there is controversy over its intensity and hence its likely influence on reproductive function and morphology. The incidence of extra-pair paternity in humans has been reported in a number of studies (for reviews, see Smith, 1984*b*; Baker & Bellis, 1995), none of which has been published in detail, making it difficult to assess their accuracy or reliability (MacIntyre & Sooman, 1991). The most commonly cited estimates are around 10%. This value is relatively low compared with many other mammals (Birkhead & Appleton, 1998) and many birds (Birkhead & Møller, 1992), but still sufficient to increase the variance in male reproductive success and hence constitute a non-trivial component of sexual selection.

However, a relatively low intensity of sperm competition is consistent with the results from comparative analyses (see above). First, as Fig. 2.1 shows, human testes size is close to that expected from body mass, compared with other primate species, indicating neither particularly intense nor weak sperm competition. It is also worth noting that testes size in humans shows considerable variation between different races (Diamond, 1986), for which there has been no satisfactory functional explanation. A comparative study of ejaculate size and testes mass (both log-transformed) in primates showed that in humans the number of spermatozoa per ejaculate is also very close (residual: -0.17) to that expected from their body mass (A. P. Møller, personal communication). Secondly, the rate at which the human testes produce sperm (expressed as daily sperm production (DSP)) per gram of testis tissue (4.4×10^6 is lower than that of any other mammal investigated so far (range: 13×10^6 to 25×10^6; Knobil & Neil, 1994, p. 1373). Thirdly, the storage capacity, the ability to store spermatozoa in a viable state and produce successive ejaculates, is also extremely limited in humans compared with most other mammals (Bedford, 1990, 1994). Fourthly, sperm quality in humans is also

relatively poor compared with other primates, with as many as 50% of spermatozoa in normally fertile men showing gross morophological abnormality (see e.g. Mortimer, 1994, p. 25). The poor sperm quality in humans is also
reflected by the fact that sperm dimensions are extremely variable between
ejaculates (Harcourt, 1991). Fifthly, the total length of the human spermatozoon (mean 58.4 μm) is shorter, albeit not by much, than that of most other
hominids (Smith, 1984b). Finally, perhaps surprisingly, erect penis size in
humans is absolutely longer than in any other ape (Short, 1979). In summary,
with the exception of penis size, virtually all this evidence (see also
Gomendio et al., 1998) suggests that, for humans, sperm competition has
been a relatively weak force in the evolution of morphological reproductive
traits.

Contrary to the view presented above, there have been a number of
claims that sperm competition in humans is intense (Smith, 1984b; Baker &
Bellis, 1995). The issue of sperm competition in humans is highly charged,
partly because we are all interested in how we operate, and partly because of
novel but controversial work conducted by Baker and colleagues, which has
been given considerable positive and often uncritical media attention. These
authors have made a number of assertions regarding the importance of
sperm competition in human reproductive biology. Baker & Bellis (1995)
proposed that: (1) females actively seek extra-pair copulations at the time
that maximizes their likelihood of fertilization; (2) females influence paternity by the differential retention of spermatozoa, often via female orgasm;
(3) male and female reproductive processes have coevolved, and that males
attempt to counter female strategies by adjusting ejaculate size and quality,
in part by masturbation, to maximize their likelihood of achieving fertilization in a sperm competition situation; (4) different sperm morphs are not
production errors, as was once thought (Cohen, 1969), but are adaptive and
have evolved to assume different roles in 'sperm warfare'.

All of these novel assertions are consistent with predictions from sperm
competition theory. However, data which are merely consistent with predictions constitute rather weak evidence (Birkhead et al., 1997). So far none of
Baker & Bellis' ideas has been substantiated by rigorous experimentation,
and indeed some have been refuted (Harcourt, 1989, 1991; Birkhead et al.,
1997; Gomendio et al., 1998; A. P. Møller, unpublished results). The issue is
not whether sperm competition occurs in humans (it undoubtedly does),
but its intensity and hence its importance in shaping our reproductive
morphology and behaviour.

Conclusions

Studying a single species can provide a distorted, or at best a myopic
view of the world. Comparing ourselves, or indeed, any other species with a
range of others allows us to view biological features in a broad, evolutionary

context and in so doing we are less likely to jump to erroneous conclusions. Three selection pressures that might have shaped reproductive morphology (and behaviour) were identified in the Introduction: male–female conflict, seasonality and sperm competition. While sexual conflict undoubtly occurs, its role in influencing reproductive features is largely unknown, especially in mammals. As far as seasonality is concerned, it is perhaps surprising that this has had so little evident effect on reproductive traits. On the other hand, the evidence that sperm competition has been a powerful selective force is very strong.

It is relatively easy to see how the risk of sperm competition has favoured relatively large testes, sperm stores and ejaculates: a male inseminating more spermatozoa is more likely to father offspring. However, it is less obvious why, even when the risk of cuckoldry is absent or relatively low, reproductive traits should be reduced in size. The answer to this is that there are also costs to producing and maintaining these structures. These costs include: (1) the metabolic costs of developing and maintaining morphological features; (2) the costs of sperm production and storage (generally regarded as trivial, but never accurately measured); and (3) immunological costs. Sperm production is controlled by testosterone, and high levels are required to maintain high levels of sperm production. However, because testosterone suppresses the immune system, high levels are potentially costly, particularly for individuals in poor condition (Folstad & Skarstein, 1997; Hillgarth *et al.*, 1997).

The traits that evolve are those that represent the optimum evolutionary compromise between different selection pressures and the optimal balance between the costs and benefits. In the absence of sperm competition, we predict that the relative size of reproductive organs will be reduced to that which is adequate to achieve efficient fertilization. At the other extreme, when sperm competition is intense, sexual selection will have favoured those individuals with a suite of traits that enables them to compete effectively for fertilizations. This is exactly what the comparative studies described in this chapter demonstrate.

Acknowledgements

I thank J. M. Bedford, A. P. Møller and A. Pacey for helpful comments on the manuscript, and A. Harcourt, A. Purvis and L. Liles for permission to reproduce Fig. 2.1, which was redrawn by E. J. Pellatt.

References

Alcock, J. & Sherman, P. W. (1994). The utility of the proximate–ultimate dichotomy in ethology. *Ethology*, **96**, 58–62.

Andersson, M. (1994). *Sexual selection*. Princeton, NJ: Princeton University Press.

Austin, C. R. & Bishop, M. W. H. (1957). Fertilization in mammals. *Biological Reviews*, **32**, 296–349.

Baker, R. R. & Bellis, M. (1995). *Human sperm competition*. London: Chapman & Hall.

Bateman, A. J. (1948). Intra-sexual selection in *Drosophila*. *Heredity*, **2**, 349–68.

Bedford, M. J. (1970). The saga of mammalian sperm from ejaculation to syngamy. In *Mammalian reproduction*, ed. H. Gibian & E. J. Plotz, pp. 124–82. Berlin: Springer-Verlag.

   (1977). Evolution of the scrotum: the epididymis as the prime mover. In *Reproduction and evolution*, ed. J. H. Calaby & C. H. Tyndale-Biscoe, pp. 171–82. Canberra: Australian Academy of Sciences.

   (1990). Sperm dynamics in the epididymis. In *Gamete physiology*, ed. R. H. Asch, J. P. Balmaceda & I. Johnson, pp. 53–67. Norwell, MA: Serono Symposia.

   (1991). The coevolution of mammalian gametes. In *A comparative overview of mammalian fertilization*, ed. B. S. Dunbar & M. G. O'Rand, pp. 3–35. New York: Plenum Press.

   (1994). The status and state of the human epididymis. *Human Reproduction Update*, **9**, 2187–99.

Bedford, J. M., Rodger, J. C. & Breed, W. G. (1984). Why so many mammalian spermatozoa – a clue from marsupials? *Proceedings of the Royal Society of London*, B, **221**, 221–33.

Birkhead, T. R. (1996). Sperm competition: evolution and mechanisms. *Current Topics in Developmental Biology*, **33**, 103–58.

Birkhead, T. R. Appleton, A. (1998). Multiple paternity in mammals. In *Sperm competition and sexual selection*, ed. T. R. Birkhead & A. P. Møller, pp. 752–6. London: Academic Press.

Birkhead, T. R. & Møller, A. P. (1992). *Sperm competition in birds: evolutionary causes and consequences*. London: Academic Press.

Birkhead, T. R. & Møller, A. P. (eds.). (1998). *Sperm competition and sexual selection*. London: Academic Press.

Birkhead, T. R. & Parker, G. A. (1997). Sperm competition and mating systems. In *Behavioural ecology: an evolutionary approach*, ed. J. R. Krebs & N. B. Davies, pp. 121–45. Oxford: Blackwell.

Birkhead, T. R. & Møller, A. P. & Sutherland, W. J. (1993). Why do females make it so difficult for males to fertilize their eggs? *Journal of Theoretical Biology*, **161**, 51–60.

Birkhead, T. R. Moore, H. D. M. & Bedford, J. M. (1997). Sex, science and sensationalism. *Trends in Ecology and Evolution*, **12**, 121–2.

Brown, L., Shumaker, R. W. & Downhower, J. F. (1995). Do primates experience sperm competition? *American Naturalist*, **146**, 302–6.

Calder, W. A. I. (1984). *Size, function and life history*. Cambridge, MA: Harvard University Press.

Carrick, F. N. & Setchell, B. P. (1977). The evolution of the scrotum. In *Reproduction and evolution*, ed. J. H. Calaby & C. H. Tyndale-Biscoe, pp. 165–70. Canberra: Australian Academy of Sciences.

Chance, M. R. A. (1996). Reason for externalisation of the testis in mammals. *Journal of Zoology, London*, **239**, 691–5.

Chapman, T., Liddle, L. F., Kalb, J. M., Wolfner, M. F. & Partridge, L. (1995). Cost of mating in *Drosophila melanogaster* females is mediated by male accessory gland products. *Nature*, **373**, 241–4.

Cohen, J. (1969). Why so many sperms? An essay on the arithmetic of reproduction. *Science Progress, London*, **57**, 23–41.

Cummins, J. M. & Glover, T. D., (1970). Artificial cryptorchidism and fertility in the rabbit. *Journal of Reproduction and Fertility*, **23**, 423–33.

Cummins, J. M. & Woodall, P. F. (1985). On mammalian sperm dimensions. *Journal of Reproduction and Fertility*, **75**, 153–75.

Darwin, C. (1871). *The descent of man, and selection in relation to sex*. London: John Murray.

Dawkins, R. (1976). *The selfish gene*. Oxford: Oxford University Press.

Diamond, J. M. (1986). Variation in human testis size. *Nature*, **320**, 488–9.

Dewsbury, D. A. (1988). Copulatory behaviour as courtship communication. *Ethology*, **79**, 218–34.

Dixson, A. F. (1987). Observations on the evolution of the genitalia and copulatory behaviour in male primates. *Journal of Zoology, London*, **213**, 423–43.

Dziuk, P. J. (1991). Reproduction in the pig. In *Reproduction in domestic animals*, ed. P. T. Cupps, pp. 471–89. San Diego, CA: Academic Press.

Eberhard, W. G. (1985). *Sexual selection and animal genitalia*. Cambridge, MA: Harvard University Press.

(1996). *Female control: sexual selection by cryptic female choice*. Princeton, NJ: Princeton University Press.

Folstad, I. & Skarstein, F. (1997). Is male germ line control creating avenues for female choice? *Behavioral Ecology*, **8**, 109–12.

Foltz, D. W. (1981). Genetic evidence for long-term monogamy in a small rodent, *Peromyscus polionotus*. *American Naturalist*, **117**, 665–75.

Fowler, K. & Partridge, L. (1989). A cost of mating in female fruitflies. *Nature*, **338**, 760–1.

Freeman, S. (1990). The evolution of the scrotum: a new hypothesis. *Journal of Theoretical Biology*, **145**, 429–45.

Gibson, R. M. & Jewell, P. A. (1982). Semen quality, female choice and multiple mating in domestic sheep: a test of Trivers' sexual competence hypothesis. *Behavior*, **80**, 9–31.

Glover, T. D. (1960). Spermatozoa from the isolated cauda epididymis of rabbits and some effects of artificial cryptorchidism. *Jounal of Reproduction and Fertility*. **1**, 121–9.

(1973). Aspects of sperm production in some East African mammals. *Journal of Reproduction and Fertility*, **35**, 45–53.

Glover, T. D. & Sale, J. B. (1968). The reproductive system of the male rock hyrax (*Procavia* and *Heterohyrax*). *Journal of Zoology, London*, **156**, 351–62.

Gomendio, M. & Roldan, E. R. S. (1991). Sperm competition influences sperm size in mammals. *Proceedings of the Royal Society of London, B*, **243**, 181–5.

Gomendio, M., Harcourt, A. H. & Roldan, E. R. S. (1998). Sperm competition in mammals. In *Sperm competition and sexual selection*, ed. T. R. Birkhead & A. P. Møller. London: Academic Press (in press).

Harcourt, A. H. (1989). Deformed sperm are probably not adaptive. *Animal Behavior*, **37**, 863–5.

(1991). Sperm competition and the evolution of nonfertilizing sperm in mammals. *Evolution*, **45**, 314–28.

Harcourt, A. H. & Gardiner, J. (1994). Sexual selection and genital anatomy of male primates. *Proceedings of the Royal Society of London, B*, **255**, 47–53.

Harcourt, A. H., Purvis, A. & Liles, L. (1995). Sperm competition: mating system, not breeding season, affects testes size of primates. *Functional Ecology*, **9**, 468–76.

Harshman, L. G. & Prout, T. (1994). Sperm displacement without sperm transfer in *Drosophila melanogaster*. *Evolution*, **48**, 758–66.

Hartung, T. G. & Dewsbury, D. A. (1978). A comparative analysis of copulatory plugs in muroid mammals and their relationship to copulatory behaviour. *Journal of Mammalogy*, **59**, 717–23.

Harvey, P. H. & Pagel, M. D. (1991). *The comparative method in evolutionary biology*. Oxford: Oxford University Press.

Hillgarth, N., Ramenofsky, M. & Wingfield, J. (1997). Testosterone and sexual selection. *Behavioral Ecology*, **8**, 108–12.

Huck, U. W., Tonias, B. A. & Lisk, R. D. (1989). The effectiveness of competitive male inseminations in golden hamsters, *Mesocricetus auratus*, depends on an interaction of mating order, time delay between males and the time of mating relative to ovulation. *Animal Behavior*, **37**, 674–80.

Hunter, R. H. F. (1995). *The fallopian tubes*. Berlin: Springer Verlag.

Kelly, R. W., Taylor, P. L., Hearn, J. P., Short, R. V., Martin, D. E. & Marston J. H. (1976). 19-Hydroxyprostaglandin E, as a major component of the semen of primates. *Nature*, **260**, 544–5.

Knobil, E. & Neil, J. D. (eds.). (1994). *The physiology of reproduction*. New York: Raven Press.

Krebs, J. R. & Davies, N. B. (1997). *Behavioural ecology: an evolutionary approach*. Oxford: Blackwell.

Lindsay, D. R. (1991). Reproduction in the sheep and goat. In *Reproduction in domestic animals*, ed. P. T. Cupps, pp. 491–515. San Diego, LA: Academic Press.

Loher, W. I., Ganjian, I., Kubo, I., Stanley-Samuelson, D. & Tobe, S. S. (1981). Prostaglandins: their role in egg-laying of the cricket *Teleogryllus commodus*. *Proceedings of the National Academy of Sciences, USA*, **78**, 7835–8.

MacIntyre, S. & Sooman, A. (1991). Non-paternity and prenatal genetic screening. *Lancet*, **338**, 869–71.

Martin, P. A. & Dziuk, P. J. (1977). Assessment of relative fertility of males (cockrels and boars) by competitive mating. *Journal of Reproduction and Fertility*, **49**, 323–9.

Møller, A. P. (1988). Ejaculate quality, testis size and sperm competition in primates. *Journal of Human Evolution*, **17**, 479–88.

(1989). Ejaculate quality, testis size and sperm production in mammals. *Functional Ecology*, **3**, 91–6.

(1994). *Sexual selection and the barn swallow*. Oxford: Oxford University Press.

Møller, A. P. & Briskie, J. V. (1995). Extra-pair paternity, sperm competition and the evolution of testis size in birds. *Behaviour, Ecology and Sociobiology*, **36**, 357–65.

Mortimer, D. (1994). *Practical laboratory andrology*. New York: Oxford University Press.

Parker, G. A. (1970). Sperm competition and its evolutionary consequences in the insects. *Biological Reviews*, **45**, 525–67.

Reimann, J. G., Moen, D. O. & Thorson, B. J. (1967). Female monogamy and its control in the housefly, *Musca domestica* L. *Journal of Insect Physiology*, **13**, 407–18.

Rice, W. R. (1996). Sexually antagonistic male adaptation triggered by experimental arrest of female evolution. *Nature*, **381**, 232–43.

Roldan, E. R. S., Gomendio, M. & Vitullo, A. D. (1992). The evolution of eutherian spermatozoa and underlying selective forces: female selection and sperm competition. *Biological Reviews*, **67**, 1–43.

Salamon, S. (1962). Studies on the artificial insemination of merino sheep. *Australian Journal of Agricultural Science*, **13**, 1237–50.

Schierwater, B., Streit, B., Wagner, G. P. & DeSalle, R. (eds.) (1994). *Molecular ecology and evolution: approaches and application*. Basel: Birkhauser Verlag.

Short, R. V. (1979). Sexual selection and its component parts, somatic and genital selection as illustrated by man and the great apes. *Advances in Studies of Behavior*, **9**, 131–58.

(1981). Sexual selection in man and great apes. In *Reproductive biology of the great apes*, ed. C. E. Graham, pp. 319–41. London: Academic Press.

Sillén-Tulberg, B. & Møller, A. P. (1993). The relationship between concealed ovulation and mating systems in anthropoid primates: a phylogenetic analysis. *American Naturalist*, **141**, 1–25.

Smith, R. L. (ed.) (1984*a*). *Sperm competition and the evolution of animal mating systems*. Orlando, FL: Academic Press.

(1984*b*). Human sperm competition. In *Sperm competition and the evolution of animal mating systems*, ed. R. L. Smith, pp. 601–59. Orlando, FL: Academic Press.

Travis, S. E., Slobodchikoff, C. N. & Keim, P. (1996). Social assemblages and mating relationships in praire dogs: a DNA fingerprint analysis. *Behavioral Ecology*, **7**, 95–100.

Verrell, P. A. (1992). Primate penile morphologies and social systems: further evidence for an association. *Folia Primatologia*, **59**, 114–20.

Waberski, D., Claasen, R., Hahn, T., Jungblut, P. W., Parvizi, N., Kallweit, E. & Weitze, K. F. (1997). LH profile and advancement of ovulation after trans-cervical infusion of seminal plasma at different stages of oestrus in gilts. *Journal of Reproduction and Fertility*, **109**, 29–34.

Wickler, W. (1967). Socio-sexual signals and their intraspecific imitation among primates. In *Primate ethology*, ed. D. Morris, pp. 69–147. London: Weidenfeld and Nicholson.

Williams, G. C. (1966). *Adaptation and natural selection*, Princeton, NJ: Princeton University Press.

Wolfson, A. (1954). Sperm storage at lower-than-body temperature outside the body cavity in some passerine birds. *Science*, **120**, 68–71.

3 Sperm production and delivery in mammals, including man

HECTOR DOTT AND TIM GLOVER

Introduction

At a time of rapid technological advance such as we have seen over the past few years in the field of human reproduction, the basic principles of mammalian male reproductive biology can easily be obscured or overlooked. Chapter 3 has been written with this in mind and is intended to be a simple reminder of fundamentals.

The function of a spermatozoon is to deposit a haploid set of chromosomes in the cytoplasm of the oocyte and to contribute to the first cleavage division. To enable it to do this, it is produced from a diploid gonium with enough cytoplasmic components to propel it for a limited distance and to survive its passage from the testis to the site of fertilization. It also contains pro-enzymes which, in the presence of an oocyte, are activated to prepare the spermatozoon for penetration of the zona pellucida, passage through the vitelline membrane and entry into the ooplasm.

The production and delivery of the spermatozoon is the sole biological *raison d'être* of the male mammal. Production is the province of the testis, whilst delivery involves the epididymis, seminal emission, an ejaculatory reflex (following penile erection) and coordination of the rest of the body with external events. These processes together constitute male sexual behaviour.

The effect of mammalian male sexual behaviour is to deposit semen in a suitable part of the female tract at a time propitious for the spermatozoa to reach the site of fertilization and fertilize an oocyte. In all mammalian species so far investigated, some ejaculated spermatozoa are sequestered for a few hours (or months in some species of bats) in a part of the female tract from which they emerge in a steady or intermittent stream. In the absence of an oocyte, they are carried past the site of fertilization into the peritoneal cavity. As the spermatozoa pass through the utero-tubal junction, they become hyperactive. This increases the probability of contact with an oocyte and the ability of the spermatozoa to penetrate the cumulus. To achieve this, the male must ensure that spermatozoa are produced and matured in sufficient numbers to maintain a reservoir in the male tract, from which the sperm component of the ejaculate can be drawn. In addition, if a male is to be most effective, he must be able to detect the optimum time to bring courtship to a climax. Some seminal plasma is absorbed at the site of deposition (vagina, cervix or uterus) and the rest, and those spermatozoa not sequestered, are extruded from the vagina.

As a prerequisite of its existence, each species of mammal has developed a combination of semen production and delivery that is consistent with its social structure. This enables the highest proportion of offspring to reach maturity in the selected habitat. However, social structures may themselves be influenced by sexual behaviour.

This combination of sperm production and delivery is influenced by a variety of factors. These include the significance of mating as part of the social structure, the anatomy of the female tract and stimulation required by the female to initiate a pregnancy in addition to a fertilized egg. The vulnerability of the mating couple to predators is also a factor.

Mating and social structure

Some adult mammals such as the leopard and the aardvark meet other adults of the same species only to mate. Others live in groups except during the mating season, at which time an adult male will seek to mate with as many females as possible and prevent others from mating with 'his' females. Prevention may be achieved by threatening subordinate males, but, in some species, subordinate males are inhibited from producing spermatozoa while they are subordinate, a sort of behavioural castration. The springbok is an example. Other mammalian species live in groups, either in hierarchical packs, or where there is a dominant male or female. Among these species, mating is often unrelated to breeding and associated with keeping the family together. This situation is seen in porcupines.

There are a few monogamous animals too, some of which cohabit for life and rear successive litters. Primates provide a number of examples, including the gibbon, the tamarin and some of the lemurids.

These are just a few examples of the many social structures that occur in mammals, with each species having its own appropriately tailored system of sperm production and delivery.

Anatomy of the female tract

Most animal species deposit both male and female gametes into water and rely on precise timing and physical proximity to achieve fertilization. When fertilization is internal, as in the mammalian female, the tract is adapted to nurture the embryo and fewer oocytes are produced. The mammalian female tract provides a duct for the gametes to meet and the male gametes retain their ability to fertilize for a longer period than those that are released into water. However, the timing of the release of oocytes and spermatozoa from the gonads tends to be less precise in mammals and a reduction of the number of spermatozoa could be a distinct disadvantage. For example, the bucktooth parrotfish uses about 16 000 spermatozoa per egg (Marcanato & Shapiro, 1996), whereas the reindeer uses about 230 million (Dott & Utsi, 1971).

The need for induced ovulation

In most mammalian species, ovulation can occur without the presence of a male, but some species have retained (or developed or redeveloped) an ovulatory mechanism that is dependent on the presence of a sexually active male. For example, all wild ruminants ovulate spontaneously and many, such as the reindeer cow, mate only once during an oestrous cycle. In contrast, female lions mate every 15 or 20 min for 24 to 48 h. The composition of the semen at these matings is unknown, but the frequent matings appear to be necessary if the females are to ovulate. Similarly, other felids such as the domestic cat, and also lagomorphs, are induced ovulators, and coitus in rats provides a signal for the corpora lutea to be established as corpora lutea of pregnancy.

Vulnerability to predators

Lions and wild ruminants illustrate a difference between those species that are essentially predators and those that are usually preyed upon. Generally, the time spent in mating is greater among predatory animals than among prey species.

Production of spermatozoa in mammals (incorporating epididymal function)

In mammals, the term 'testicle' strictly refers to both the testis and the epididymis. However, the two components might have been subject to different evolutionary pressures in different species, so it is appropriate to discuss each organ separately. (Strictly, the epididymis is part of the sperm delivery system, but it is appropriate to include it under this heading, because of its close topographical association with the testis and because it plays a major part in what is delivered. In other words, it can also be regarded as part of the production mechanism.)

The testis produces spermatozoa and secretes androgens. The spermatozoa are produced in the seminiferous tubules and androgens are synthesized and secreted by the Leydig cells of the intertubular tissue. The relative proportion of the testis occupied by these two compartments varies from species to species and may vary from season to season within a species. Body size, season and the demand for spermatozoa can all affect the volume of the testis.

Overall, there is an inverse allometric relationship between testis size and body mass (Cummins & Woodall, 1985). But since the body is merely the vehicle for carrying the testis, it might be instructive to express the relationship inversely, namely as grams of body weight per gram of testis. The testes of oriental men are usually smaller than those of caucasians and their body mass is also usually smaller. Moreover, there is no evidence that sperm output differs significantly between the two races, so in man the relationship between body size, testis size and sperm output is not precise.

The testis size of sexually active rock hyraxes is up to four times that of sexually quiescent animals and this is due to an increase both in the diameter of the seminiferous tubules and the volume of intertubular tissue. This striking increase in testicular size and weight (see Miller & Glover, 1970) is facilitated by the testes being situated in the abdomen. Changes in testicular size are much less marked in scrotal mammals. Nevertheless, the testes volume of springbok (a scrotal mammal) is greater in territorial males than in bachelor males and smaller in the hot dry summer than in other seasons (Skinner *et al.*, 1996) and the testes of larger antelopes are bigger in the breeding season than in the non-breeding season (Glover *et al.*, 1990). The breeding season of many antelopes and also the rock hyrax is short and regular, but by contrast, the springbok of the Kalahari can produce spermatozoa and breed at any time of the year.

The number of spermatozoa produced by a given volume of testicular tissue in a given time depends on the proportion of testis occupied by the seminiferous tissue and the rate of spermatogenesis. Boyd & Vandemark (1957) showed, for example, that bulls produce 2.8×10^6 spermatozoa per day. The rate can be assessed from the length of the spermatogenic cycle (cyclic re-entry of a spermatogonium into spermatogenesis). In humans, this is twice as long as in pigs (see Clermont, 1963, and Swierstra, 1968, respectively). Thus, there is considerable variation in sperm production between different mammalian species.

Genetic composition of spermatozoa

Spermatozoa do not have the same genetic composition as somatic cells. Because of the chiasmata, each spermatozoon has it own set of genes, although, as a result of the non-pairing segments of sex chromosomes, half of them carry the X chromosome and half of them the Y chromosome. Except for rather crude differences in morphology, which might arise when reduction division or spermatid maturation has been faulty, spermatozoa do not normally express their genotype phenotypically. Therefore, they could be said to carry these chromosomes rather than possess them.

Sperm transport in the male tract

In 'primitive' vertebrates such as the cyclostomes (e.g. the lamprey), no duct is available for the transport of spermatozoa to the exterior; they are simply deposited in the coelomic cavity. In most vertebrates, however, the seminiferous tissue is arranged in tubular form and a duct is provided to transport the spermatozoa out of the body. Teleosts, for example, typically have a short sperm duct (vas deferens) leading from the testis. This means that storage and maturation of spermatozoa in these fishes must take place within the testis (Van der Horst, 1976; Billard, 1990).

Amniotes (including mammals) have evolved rather differently and like some elasmobranchs, amphibians, reptiles and birds, the mesonephric (wolffian) duct has been modified to transport spermatozoa. In some sharks and urodeles the mesonephric duct is used for the transport of both urine and spermatozoa, but in mammals, as in all amniotes, urine is conducted through a ureter to the bladder and thence to the urethra. The mesonephric duct is relatively long, however, and thus the maturation and storage of spermatozoa in mammals have both become extra-testicular events and the mesonephric duct, now recognized as the epididymis and ductus (vas) deferens, has had to take responsibility for both. The efferent ductules, derived as they are from the wolffian body, are also essentially kidney tubules and they attach the testis to the upper part of the epididymis in a variable fashion according to species. The cytology of the epididymis itself also differs at different levels and between species (Glover & Nicander, 1971).

The speed of sperm flow through the epididymis is not likely to be constant at all levels of the duct, because of the tubular secretion and absorption which is typical of what is essentially a kidney duct. In most mammals (with humans as an exception) spermatozoa are quickly transported through the initial segment of the epididymis, where fluid is added, but in many species they become concentrated in the lower end of the head, and upper part of the body, of the epididymis, where fluid is absorbed. This occurs before they are flushed into the sperm store (tail of the epididymis) by more fluid being added at lower levels of the body of the epididymis. These events occur at slightly different levels of the duct in different species (Glover & Nicander, 1971). In man, because the efferent ductules extend from the testis in a fan-like form, there is no typical initial segment and spermatozoa may sometimes be seen concentrated even in the efferent ductules (Glover, 1982).

Maturation of spermatozoa in the epididymis

When a spermatozoon is released from the germinal tissue of the testis, remnants of spermatid Golgi material (most of which has contributed to the formation of the acrosome) are found in the region of the proximal centriole. This forms the cytoplasmic droplet which has the same enzymic composition as the acrosome (Dott & Dingle, 1968). In most species, the droplet migrates down the flagellum to the end of the midpiece whilst the spermatozoa are passing through the epididymis. It is discarded at ejaculation. The presence in an ejaculate of a large proportion of spermatozoa with a proximal droplet indicates that sperm maturation is deficient. In man, however, the situation is not quite so clear cut, because invariably, the cytoplasmic droplet is more diffuse and does not migrate along the midpiece in quite such a defined and regular manner as in other mammalian species. Nevertheless, the presence of a droplet on an ejaculated human spermatozoon suggests that it has failed to mature properly.

Mammalian spermatozoa undergo other important changes during their passage through the epididymis, many of which are the result of changes in the nature and composition of the plasma membrane, for example, the tightening of S–S linkages (Calvin & Bedford, 1971). These changes, which constitute epididymal sperm maturation, ensure that the spermatozoon can traverse the female tract and, after capacitation, can fertilize an oocyte. Some of the changes, however, cannot be identified without prior destruction of the spermatozoa.

Work on this subject has lacked quantification, so that the relative numbers of mature and immature spermatozoa at different levels of the epididymis have not been assessed. Furthermore, we do not know how long the process takes, whether it is a change that is initiated from within the spermatozoa, whether each stage of maturation requires a different and special milieu, or what triggers the process in the first place. The removal and addition of fluid at different levels of the epididymis certainly indicates that the environment within the duct is critical to the process. Schoysman (1969) showed that, in epididymovasostomy in humans, best results are obtained when the anastomosis is made low down in the epididymis. This suggests that some sperm maturation is taking place in human spermatozoa during epididymal transit. However, it has been shown in the rabbit that occlusion of the epididymis allows some maturation changes to occur higher up in the duct (Gaddum & Glover, 1965). In man, if the presence of a cytoplasmic droplet is used as a criterion of immaturity, the number of immature spermatozoa found in the head of the epididymis when the duct is blocked may be as low as 45% (T. D. Glover, unpublished results).

If, under the conditions of epididymal occlusion, it is possible for some spermatozoa to mature without the need to pass through the entire epididymis, then some pregnancies following epididymovasostomy are to be expected. But where do most spermatozoa mature in the intact duct? In man, this remains uncertain. It would seem that some sperm maturation might occur high up in the epididymis; otherwise, taking into account the relatively rapid transport through the human duct, the process might not be completed in some spermatozoa by the time they reach the tail of the epididymis. To some extent, this depends on the degree of mixing at different levels of the epididymis. In rabbits there is probably less mixing than in man and a much greater proportion of mature spermatozoa are to be found in the lower body of the epididymis than in its head (Bedford, 1966). This finding has led to widespread acceptance of sperm maturation being completed at this level of the duct. The result could also be interpreted, however, as an accumulation of mature forms in the lower epididymal body rather than the process actually being completed there. Indeed, evolutionary evidence indicates that most sperm maturation takes place in the head and upper body of the epididymis. So it is important to establish, both in man and in other species, precisely the level of the epididymis at which sperm maturation occurs in the majority of spermatozoa. Currently, we are unable to say with any certainty, but the issue is examined thoroughly in Chapter 5.

A number of substances in epididymal fluid are, it is claimed, associated with sperm maturation and, in recent years, the distribution of various gene proteins has been described in the epididymis of experimental animals (Orgebin-Crist, 1996; Kirchhoff, 1997). Both androgen and temperature appear to act synergistically, at least in regulating CD52 (the main maturation antigen), and this leads us some way to understanding how endocrine and other factors might act in influencing sperm maturation. It is important now to translate the distribution of epididymal genes into functional terms and it would be interesting to assess it in a wider variety of species against a backdrop of different sexual strategies and mating systems.

Sperm storage in the epididymis

In the past, interest has focused particularly on sperm maturation and the all-important role of the epididymis in sperm storage has received less attention. The storage of spermatozoa occurs in a terminal region of the epididymis that is usually referred to as the tail of the epididymis. A sperm reservoir is formed here, but its capacity varies widely between species. Males of species that copulate in quick succession with different females are likely have a large sperm store. Thus, the tail of the epididymis in polygynous and promiscuous ruminants is characteristically voluminous. In sharp contrast, the region is diminutive both in size and capacity in most species that do not have a restricted breeding season and tend to be monogamous. The human is a good example (Glover & Young, 1963; Amman & Howards, 1980).

The reservoir is created by a widening of the epididymal lumen towards its distal end, with a sharp reduction in luminal diameter in the ductus (vas) deferens. In essence, this morphological arrangement acts like a valve, causing some damming back of the sperm stream and thus drastically slowing sperm flow through the tail of the epididymis. In the absence of coitus (or masturbation), pressure increases due to the continuous production of spermatozoa and secretions, causing the oldest spermatozoa to pass into the ductus deferens. These spermatozoa reach the ampulla and are voided in the urine. Other spermatozoa may be absorbed, but the number that is absorbed probably differs from species to species.

Mechanisms for sperm absorption by the lining cells of the epididymis are found in laboratory animals and spermiophagy by epididymal cells can also occur in man (Glover, 1982). What stimulates this absorption or how significant it is in normal individuals is not clear. It is certainly not sufficient to match sperm output in high sperm producers (Amman, 1987), but it might be connected to the speed of sperm flow through the duct and to the degree of sperm disintegration within the duct. In a seasonally breeding mammal such as the rock hyrax, for instance, it has been reported that epididymal spermatozoa swell and lose their acrosomes prior to their evanescence in the duct at the end of the season (Millar, 1972).

Temperature and sperm storage

The greater the capacity of the sperm store, the longer most of the contained spermatozoa are likely to remain there. This is because only a small fraction of the sperm population is released with each emission (Amman & Almquist, 1962). The environment within the tail of the epididymis must ensure that it contains viable spermatozoa throughout a mating season. Although breeding seasons are usually short, most species start to produce spermatozoa well in advance of the season and before male dominance is established. Furthermore, there might be a passing female in oestrus after the season has officially closed. Some spermatozoa will, therefore, remain in the tail of the epididymis for quite a long period. This has been demonstrated most strikingly in the bat (Racey, 1974), but also occurs in red deer and probably holds true for other wild ruminants also. Temperature is likely to be a factor in preserving viability there. In the rabbit, for example, spermatozoa remain viable in the tail of the epididymis for at least 28 days (Tesh & Glover, 1969). In contrast, they are only viable for 35 h in the female tract, where they are subjected to body temperature (Tesh, 1966).

It is interesting to find, therefore, that the sperm store in, for example, the rock hyrax, is situated close to the surface of the body in the pelvic cavity (where it is likely to be cooler), in spite of its testes lying deep in the abdomen adjacent to the kidney (Glover & Sale, 1968). This finding suggests that stored spermatozoa might need to be kept relatively cool and this is confirmed in the North American swamp sparrow, in which the sperm store resides in its own scrotal sack, whilst the testes remain typically abdominal. It is confirmed also in the rodent *Apodemus sylvaticus* mentioned in Chapter 2, in which the testis and epididymis have separate scrotal sacks.

It has long been known that the testes of scrotal mammals are temperature sensitive, but it was not recognized until much later that epididymal spermatozoa (including mature spermatozoa) in scrotal mammals are themselves temperature sensitive (Glover, 1955a, 1959, 1960), or succumb to a changed environment within the epididymis occasioned by increased temperature.

On the basis of this accumulated evidence, Glover (1973) suggested that the evolutionary descent of the sperm store into a scrotum might well have preceded that of the testis and that testicular descent could have been secondary to this. Bedford (1977) produced some experimental data in rabbits, which lent some support to this hypothesis and he expanded on the theme.

He also claimed that sperm maturation was not temperature sensitive. This is true for testiconid mammals (those with abdominal testes), but not for scrotal mammals in which immature spermatozoa are especially vulnerable to increased temperature (Glover, 1955b, 1962). Attention is focused here, however, on stored spermatozoa and these are already mature. It is also possible that the testes descended for reasons that are unrelated to epididymal spermatozoa. For example, the frequency of spermatogenic mutations could be reduced at a lower temperature (see Short, 1997).

The abdomino-testicular temperature difference in rams and bulls is 6–8 deg.C, but in man it is only about 2.8 deg.C. This raises the possibility of variations between species, not only in the temperature sensitivity of the testes, but also in the vulnerability of spermatozoa in the tail of the epididymis to increased temperature. As yet, this has not been examined comprehensively.

If such variation between species exists, it could be related to the evolution of different mating systems. Seasonal animals, especially promiscuous or polygynous ones, have large testes (adapted to the scrotal environment) capable of creating a capacious, relatively static sperm reservoir. In these circumstances, a lower temperature would be an advantage. This picture is typical of sheep and to a lesser extent of antelopes and other wild ruminants, although here the picture is blurred by additional cursorial demands (big testes must hamper a quick getaway). Non-seasonal breeders such as humans, are likely to have a slow and steady stream of spermatozoa through the rather confined tail of the epididymis. The need for cooling might thus be reduced.

Available evidence strongly suggests that the human testis and epididymal spermatozoa are less sensitive to the effects of elevated temperature than those of the sheep or rabbit, since sperm cooling will be less necessary. Experimental evidence confirms this.

The effects of insulation of the scrotum in a man and in rams is compared in Fig. 3.1. Admittedly, data from only a single man are hardly statistically valid, but the results are nevetheless instructive. Two weeks' insulation of the scrotum of a human subject resulted in nothing more than an insignificant dip in sperm count with no effect on sperm morphology or motility. In rams and male rabbits, the same sort of treatment results in massive sperm degradation and virtual azoospermia.

Only 24 h of scrotal insulation are needed in rams to yield almost total decapitation of spermatozoa ejaculated two to three weeks later (Glover, 1955b), although the number of spermatozoa is unaffected. Therefore, these decapitate spermatozoa must have been immature at the time of scrotal insulation. In man, by contrast, this treatment has no effect whatsoever (T. D. Glover, unpublished results). Recently, B. P. Setchell et al., (personal communication) have also shown in rams that only 8 h of insulation of the scrotum are sufficient to exert an effect. Moreover, following vasectomy in man, spermatozoa may in some cases remain in a viable state in the ampulla (where they must be subjected to body temperature), for a longer period

Fig. 3.1. The effect of abdominal temperature on semen characteristics in three mammalian species. Note: the arrowed lines denote onset and end of treatment. (a) Effects of experimental cryptorchidism (Glover, 1960). Mean data from 14 rabbits. Insulation of the scrotum with acrylite sheeting lined with expanded polystyrene elicits a similar response. Treatment continued until complete azoospermia. (b) Effects of scrotal insulation (Glover, 1955b). Mean data from four rams. Scrotum insulated with Kapok and a rubber pack. Treatment continued until complete azoospermia. (c) Effects of scrotal insulation (T. D. Glover, unpublished results). Data from one man. Scrotum insulated by bandage, cotton wool and a plastic pack. Treatment ended after two weeks.

(a) RABBIT

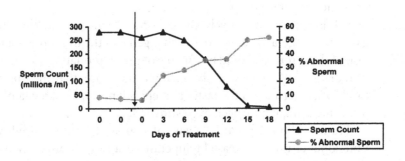

(b) RAM

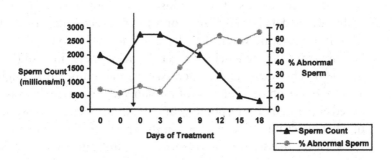

(c) MAN

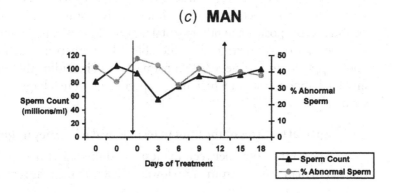

than would be possible in rams or rabbits. Some clinicians have found this out to their cost!

Brindley (1982) showed that deep scrotal temperatures were 5 deg.C lower in men wearing boxer shorts than in those wearing Y-front underpants, and he pointed out that scrotal temperatures in paraplegic men, who often have a poor semen quality, are elevated. However, Brindley (1982) also conceded that temperature might not be the only factor contributing to deficient semen quality in these cases and, if the human testis is relatively insensitive to heat, even long-term elevation of scrotal temperature would not matter. Any effect of Y-fronts is not to be compared to that caused by deliberate scrotal insulation as referred to in Fig. 3.1.

Whilst radiation is likely to be curtailed in men wearing briefs, the garment is regularly removed and changed and the thermoregulatory function of the scrotum should be capable of accommodating a slight reduction in radiation. We suggest in this chapter, therefore, that the importance of local hyperthermia on the testes and epididymal spermatozoa of normally fertile men might have been overestimated.

From a clinical point of view, of course, extrasusceptibility of subfunctional testes to increased temperature cannot be discounted (Lynch *et al.*, 1986; Mieusset *et al.*, 1987; Mieusset & Bujan, 1995), nor can the effects of special occupational conditions (Thonneau *et al.*, 1996). There might also be individual variation in the sensitivity of testes to temperature, just as there are breed differences in sheep. Suffolk rams, for example, are slightly more resistant to the effects of scrotal insulation than Romney Marsh rams. In addition, the data in Fig. 3.1 refer only to relatively acute temperature elevation. It appears, however, that decreased testicular temperature (induced hypothermia) can beneficially affect pregnancy rates in man (Zorgniotti *et al.*, 1986). This suggests that increased scrotal temperature might elicit an adverse effect on the function of human spermatozoa which is not manifested either in their morphology or in their number. So far, we are unaware of what effect might be incurred in the sperm nucleus under these conditions. Nevertheless, overall evidence to date indicates that testicular and epididymal temperatures are not important factors in the fertility of most humans. The cautious approach adopted by the RCOG Infertility Guidelines Group on this subject, is, to our mind, entirely justified. This is in marked contrast to the position in other scrotal mammals, whose testes and epididymal spermatozoa are extremely vulnerable to hyperthermia. Such sensitivity could apply to the testicles of other primates also, including the chimpanzee and the baboon, both of which have a sperm store much larger than that of man.

Special features of the human testicle and what they might mean

Sperm transport between the testis and the tail of the epididymis is quicker in man (3 days; Amman & Howards, 1980) than in the rabbit (14 days;

Orgebin-Crist, 1965; Amman *et al.*, 1965) or in the ram (20 days; Ortavant, 1954) and it looks as if the passage of spermatozoa through the tail of the epididymis is also quicker. Both these factors may contribute to the apparent invulnerability of human spermatozoa to elevated temperature in the testicle. Moreover, in man, sperm output by the testes is relatively low (based on ejaculated sperm numbers) and there may be an extra facility for sperm absorption within the epididymis, especially if sperm flow is obstructed (vasectomy does not result in the initial ballooning of the epididymis that is seen in rabbits). It looks, therefore, as if there is little need for long-term sperm storage in the human epididymis and the structure of the duct suggests a monogamous or polygynous history rather than one of promiscuity.

Delivery of spermatozoa

The reproductive fitness of a male can be measured by the number of functional spermatozoa he is capable of delivering. This is a more important consideration than the size of testes, even though large testes usually signify a high rate of sperm production. However, sperm delivery also involves storage capacity (already discussed under the heading of sperm production) and the efficiency of seminal discharge. Not only this, but a variety of neural, vascular and hormonal factors come into the equation. These were admirably summarized by Bishop & Walton (1960) and there has been little serious advance in our knowledge of this subject since then. This arises largely from the fact that a proper assessment of male fertility in animals is time consuming and expensive. A worthwhile investigation would demand that up to a 100 females in oestrus be inseminated with each ejaculate to be tested and that each would have to be collected using a different female as a teaser. This would be a major undertaking. It is, however, necessary, because, in laboratory animals, when the same female is used as a teaser, the concentration of spermatozoa decreases markedly and progressively after the second ejaculate. Ultimately, the male either will fail to mate, or appear to be aspermic or azoospermic. Azoospermia under these circumstances may occur either because there are insufficient spermatozoa in the tail of the epididymis or because there is a failure of the emission reflex.

Transfer to the female tract

Mammalian spermatozoa, suspended in seminal plasma, are transferred to the female at coitus through an erect penis. But the structure of the penis varies between species and so does the composition and quantity of the seminal plasma.

Structure of the penis

The elaborate structure of the penis in mammals suggests that it is more than a mere tube for the delivery of semen to the female. In primates, it

Table 3.1. Species differences in semen characteristics relative to differences in their mating habits

Species	Ejac. volume (ml)	Total sperm number (×10)	Gel	Ejaculation Time	Site	Type of ovulation	Type of penis	Mating system
Boar	250	25	+	800	IC	S?	1	Pg?
Horse	70	8.4	+	120	IC	S?	2	Pg
Ass	40	12	+	120	IC	S	2	Pg?
Dog	9	2.7	−	600	IC*	S	2	Pg
Cattle	4	4	−	<10	IV	S	1	Pg
Red deer	4	0.8	−	<10	IV	S	1	Pg
Human	3	0.24	+	<10	IV	S?	2	Mg
Buffalo	2.5	1.5	−	<10	IV	S	1	Pg
Goat	1	3	−	<10	IV	S	1	Pg
Sheep	1	3	−	<10	IV	S	1	Pg
Rabbit	1	0.15	+	<10	IV	I	2	Pm
Reindeer	0.5	0.23	−	<10	IV	S	1	Pg
Cat	0.03	0.051	−	<10	IV	I	2	Pm?

IC, intracervical; IV< intravaginal; S, spontaneous ovulation; I, Induced ovulation; 1, fibro-elastic; 2, vascular; Pg, polygynous; Mg, monogamous; Pm, promiscuous; ?(ovulation), male may influence ovulation; ?(mating), probably.

Polygynous: male mates with >1 female and attempts to prevent other males from mating with them.

Monogamous: male mates with 1 female which does not usually mate with any other male during the breeding season.

Promiscuous: male mates with any receptive female it encounters; that is, it usually mates with >1 female, but does not prevent other males from mating with them.

Modified from Mann, 1964.

might well serve an epigamic function, but the ornate nature of the glans in many non-primate mammals indicates that the penis might have a role in stimulating, and thereby encouraging, ovulation. This we know to be true in non-spontaneous ovulators and the principle might not have been discarded totally in all spontaneously ovulating species (Glover, 1994). In other words, even in these animals, a male might help the female to ovulate.

All mammalian penes erect by means of vascular engorgement, but whereas truly vascular ones swell, as in stallions, dogs and man (and stiffness is aided in many such species by much of the corpus cavernosum penis becoming ossified into a baculum or os penis), fibro-elastic penes such as those of ruminants and pigs are protruded when erect by extension of a sigmoid flexure in the shaft. The length or size of a penis in a given species (and even its basic structure) is consistent with the anatomy of the female tract and with the mating system, which includes the mode of insemination. But the evolutionary path by which this was developed is obscure. The same can be said of the volume of ejaculates. Table 3.1 illustrates that, although coitus is prolonged when the semen volume is large, the structure of the penis is unrelated to the volume of ejaculate.

The erect penis of ruminants is long, but semen is deposited on the vaginal floor during a short coitus. This contrasts with the boar, whose equally long penis penetrates and is thrust high up into the cervix in a prolonged coitus. The stallion has a vascular penis of much greater diameter, but also deposits semen into the cervix without cervical penetration by anything other than a small urethral process.

Man has a vascular penis and is an intravaginal inseminator, but although his semen volume is small, the length of human coitus is long. It has been suggested that this prolonged mating process in man is related to bonding. This is probably true and underscores the importance of evolution in the fashioning of different mating systems. Clearly, for instance, these systems are closely related to the level to which a species is exposed to predation. Prey animals mate briefly, for obvious reasons, whilst predators can afford the luxury of more prolonged and leisurely coitus.

Changes in the female tract

Spermatozoa undergo a number of changes in the female tract, particularly as the site of fertilization is approached. These changes involve the flagellum and outer membranes, particularly the outer acrosomal membrane. The flagellar changes cause the sperm head to move vigorously in a circular or side to side manner, but slow down forward progression of the whole spermatozoon. This maximizes the chance of contact with an oocyte in the vicinity. The first acrosomal change (capacitation) takes several hours to complete and begins when the spermatozoon is deposited in the female. The second (the acrosome reaction) involves the activation of enzymes which enable the spermatozoon to penetrate the zona and pass into the oocyte. This can only happen in a capacitated spermatozoon (see Brown *et al.*, Chapter 6).

In many species, it is well known that mating and/or the deposition of seminal plasma in the female tract, initiates peristaltic contractions of the myometrium, which accelerate sperm transport. Spermatozoa that are already *in situ* may then be swept through the site of fertilization into the peritoneal cavity.

Seminal plasma and its constituents

Mann (1964) provided a comprehensive account of the constituents of seminal plasma, which vary between species. In most (with the notable exception of canids), the mixture contains a glycolysable sugar (fructose) and has a pH of between 6.5 and 7. But it is not particularly supportive of spermatozoa. For example, semen collected from bulls or rams immediately before slaughter typically contains 15–25% of eosinophilic (dead) spermatozoa, but < 5% of epididymal spermatozoa collected after slaughter are eosinophilic (H. M. Dott, unpublished results). It is possible that older spermatozoa are unable to adapt to the conditions prevailing in unadulterated semen. At coitus, the various portions of the semen (e.g. the sperm-rich fraction) are ejaculated sequentially and mix with secretions from the female tract.

'Gel' in semen

Across the mammalian spectrum, the sperm-rich fraction of semen has a low viscosity, but in several species subsequent fractions have a high viscosity when they are mixed at ejaculation and may form gelatinous lumps, which coalesce and constitute the 'gel'. The gel, which is hygroscopic, prevents the sperm-rich fraction of the semen from being expelled from the female tract following coitus. Intrauterine inseminators with voluminous ejaculates, such as boars and stallions, yield a great deal of gel (although it is variable in amount in stallions), whilst the semen of intravaginal inseminators such as ruminants contains no gel. In rabbits, the seminal gel blocks outflow, not from the cervix, but from the anterior chamber of the vagina and the *bouchon vaginale* of rodents may plug the whole of the vagina. Dogs produce quite a large volume of semen and yet have no gel, but backflow here is prevented by the 'tie'. The clot in freshly ejaculated human semen is transient and probably prevents backflow until spermatozoa have been adequately sequestered in the cervical mucus.

It has been suggested that the gel may prevent the spermatozoa of competing males from reaching the site of fertilization in the female tract rather than preventing backflow. In some species it may do both. The possibility of competition within the female tract between spermatozoa from different males is discussed by Birkhead (Chapter 2), but it must be viewed in relation to the social and mating system operating in each species. For example, most polygynous ruminants have little or no male competition, once they have acquired a territory and females; indeed, females in some species mate only once in an oestrous period. Thus, it could be argued that they need no gel in their semen and, when frequent ejaculation is demanded, gel would be an inconvenience. In a promiscuous breeder such as the rabbit, gel is often found in the first few ejaculates only.

Semen characteristics

A rough guide to the volume of semen, number of spermatozoa and time of ejaculation in a number of mammalian species is presented in Table 3.1, together with the site of deposition in the female tract and the type of ovulation stimulus. The species are listed in order of semen volume ejaculated. A large volume usually coincides with intracervical insemination, but the corollary is not necessarily true.

Semen volume

In simple terms, semen volume is governed by whether or not insemination is intravaginal or intracervical. When whole semen is deposited directly into the uterus, the volume is large, as against the semen of intravaginal inseminators, which is not (see Table 3.1). There is a great deal of variation in semen volume between and within individuals. This variation may partly reflect ejaculation frequency, but it can also be the result of inflammatory or fibrotic conditions of the accessory organs. These appear to be more common in humans than in other mammalian species. For example, the high incidence of leukocytes and other cells with their attendant reactive oxygen species is characteristic of human semen.

Sperm numbers

The importance of how many spermatozoa are delivered at coitus is difficult to judge. If fertilization is a statistical random chance phenomenon, then the more functionally sound spermatozoa that are deposited at coitus, the more likely fertilization is to occur. But we are not sure that it is random and, if not, the total number of spermatozoa is irrevelant, provided there are sufficient live, motile, morphologically normal spermatozoa present. The difficulty in estimating this has been a major stumbling block in assessing human male fertility by means of semen analysis.

In conventional semen analysis some of the parameters being measured, in addition to sperm concentration, might be irrelevant (especially since they are based mostly on semen tests for animals of much higher fertility). A totally inaccurate assessment of the fertilizing capacity of a semen sample could be the result. This brings us to the all-important subjects of sperm motility and sperm morphology.

Sperm motility

It is not within the ambit of this chapter to discuss details of sperm motility, but it is a prerequisite of sexual reproduction in all vertebrates. In mammals, immotile spermatozoa are unable to overcome the barriers of the female tract or to penetrate the cumulus. The main question, however, is whether in cases of human asthenozoospermia the nuclei of immotile or poorly motile spermatozoa carry damaged DNA in addition to having flagellar dysfunction. The question has not yet been answered. But, from the point of view of sperm delivery, sluggish spermatozoa may never reach the site of fertilization and are simply selected out.

Sperm morphology

We do not yet know for certain whether, after their delivery into the vagina or cervix, most morphologically abnormal spermatozoa also fail to reach the site of fertilization through the barriers of the female tract, or whether, if they do, which of them is capable of fertilization and which, if they fertilize, will yield a viable zygote.

Bishop *et al.* (1954) found in cattle that the correlation between sperm morphology and fertility was low, but the bulls they studied had been selected for high fertility, partly on the basis of the proportion of abnormal spermatozoa in the semen. Nevertheless, other characteristics provided a better correlation with fertility, in particular motility and the incidence of live spermatozoa in the sample. A high incidence of dead spermatozoa is probably not important in itself, but it may be an indicator of the condition of the live spermatozoa in the same sample.

The spermatozoa of most mammals, with rodents being a notable exception, are similar in general appearance, although between species, they differ greatly in head area and the proportion of the flagellum that is occupied by the midpiece. The difference in head area also suggests that they differ in thickness or the degree of condensation of the nuclear content. The extent of the area covered by the acrosome also differs between species. In most of them, the dimensions of the head of a spermatozoon that is considered to be morphologically normal have a coefficient of variation of approximately 10%. In the human it is markedly higher than this.

It is worth noting that two mammalian species which have not been rigorously selected for fertility are the human and the thoroughbred racehorse. In both these species, the range of sizes and shapes of ejaculated spermatozoa are greater than in most other mammals. Other species with a high degree of sperm pleiomorphism are among those which are not subject to predation or in which the female mates with only one male during an oestrous period. The gorilla, some of the lemurs, the cheetah and probably the Australian hopping mouse (*Notomys*) (Breed, 1980) fall into this category. In man, therefore, even those spermatozoa that are classified on the basis of head shape to be normal show much more variation in head size that those of domestic ruminants.

Thus, in routine light microscopy, a morphologically 'normal' human spermatozoon is particularly elusive (Freund, 1967); its definition is usually a matter of personal interpretation and is bound to be arbitrary. It is unlikely though that a primary (testicular) abnormality carries a single predisposing gene, otherwise half the spermatozoa produced by the individual would have the abnormality. Nevertheless, individuals, be they men or other male animals, tend to produce a predominance of a paritcular abnormality on a regular basis and the possibility that these spermatozoa might be carrying a genomic disorder cannot be discounted.

The particular spermatozoon in an ejaculate which penetrates and fertilizes an egg is unknown and consequently only one primary abnormality has been definitely associated with infertility. This is an abnormality of the acrosome referred to as being 'knobbed'. It was first described by Donald & Hancock (1953) in the bull and subsequently, in diverse species (Cran & Dott, 1976; Dott & Skinner, 1989). But the inheritance of primary abnormalities is otherwise a matter of conjecture. The inheritance of a tendency to produce a high proportion of spermatozoa with a secondary (post-testicular) abnormality has only been established in one breed of cattle in which bulls bearing a double recessive gene produce decapitate spermatozoa and in a group of Landrace boars that produced semen containing up to 90% of spermatozoa with proximal cytoplasmic droplets. Animals in both groups were infertile. However, Glover (1988) has shown that exceptionally high levels of morphological sperm abnormalities in human ejaculates are usually accompanied by other seminal deficiencies. But, with human spermatozoa being characteristically pleiomorphic, it is difficult to know what incidence of sperm abnormalities can be regarded as normal. A high level of abnormalities in the semen of any one individual may simply reflect a wide spectrum of normality.

In brief, it would seem imprudent deliberately to insert a spermatozoon into an egg if the former has either a primary or secondary abnormality. The abnormality might be signalling faulty meiotic division. However, animal studies indicate that sperm motility and the incidence of live spermatozoa provide a better correlation with fertility than does sperm morphology.

Conclusion

In conclusion, it looks as if the overall theme of sperm production and delivery is common to all mammals including humans, but there are species differences. Nevertheless, work on animals provides a sound and valuable basis for understanding the nuances of human male fertility, largely because it illustrates how different social and mating systems have come to influence semen quality. This is important to know if semen pictures in man are to be interpreted meaningfully.

In this context, it is helpful to be aware of how behavioural factors can influence semen quality and much is being made today of the significance of sperm competition. We should not shrink from asking, however, how far it applies among mammals.

It should be borne in mind that, when spermatozoa are deposited in the female tract, they are not all in the same condition (some are already eosinophilic). Even the best ones then undergo changes (such as capacitation) that render them more susceptible to environmental conditions. Such susceptibility is particularly important following any convulsive contractions of the myometrium, which must disturb those spematozoa that are already established in a sperm reservoir. Thus, some of the circumstances which are suggestive of sperm competition can be explained on the grounds of a differential susceptibility of spermatozoa to the environment within the female tract. Competition between mammalian males is not in dispute and cryptic female choice need not be sperm led. In our view, it is important to look at both sides of the coin.

It can sometimes be instructive to go back to basics. For example, a spermatozoon may or may not reach the site of fertilization or penetrate the cytoplasm of an oocyte. Its nuclear material may or may not decondense and its chromosomes may or may not combine with those of the egg to give rise to a viable two-cell entity. If a spermatozoon accomplished all these steps unaided, then it was fully functional, but if at any stage it was assisted there is no sure way as yet of predicting its functional status. But we first need to define a 'normal' spermatozoon. In any species, a normal spermatozoon must have all the characteristics that are close to the mean for the species. Many of these characteristics, which are the expression of a particular genetic composition, may need to be confined to certain numerical limits, if fertility is to be achieved unaided. Sperm motility is an example, although in man these limits appear to be very wide. Therefore, if a spermatozoon that falls outside these limits is assisted by artificial means, it is unlikely to be in the best long-term interests of the species.

Fundamental considerations such as have been outlined in this chapter require particular attention in a scientific and technological climate that is becoming increasingly reductionist. In spite of the advent of ICSI in human patients and the ensuing use of testicular spermatozoa for fertilization in some cases, semen analysis will continue to play a role as an initial guide to both clinician and patient in examining infertile couples. The problem lies in knowing whether or not we are using the most appropriate parameters. This, we believe, can be judged finally only by looking at the wider picture of mammalian reproduction in general.

References

Amman, R. P. (1987). Function of the epididymis in bulls and rams. *Journal of Reproduction and Fertility, Suppl.*, **34**, 115–31.

Amman, R. P. & Almquist, J. O. (1962). Reproductive capacity of dairy bulls. VI. Effects of unilateral vasectomy and ejaculation frequency on sperm reserves; aspects of epididymal physiology. *Journal of Reproduction and Fertility*, **3**, 260–8.

Amman, R. P. & Howards, S. S. (1980). Daily spermatozoal production and epididymal spermatozoal reserves of the human male. *Journal of Urology*, **124**, 211–15.

Amman, R. P. Koefoed-Johsen, H. H. & Levi, H. (1965). Excretion pattern of labelled spermatozoa and the timing of spermatozoa formation and epididymal transit in rabbits injected with thymidine-^{3}H. *Journal of Reproduction and Fertility*, **10**, 169–83.

Bedford, J. M. (1966). Development of fertilizing ability of spermatozoa in the epididymis of the rabbit. *Journal of Experimental Zoology*, **163**, 319.

(1977). Evolution of the scrotum: the epididymis as the prime mover? In *Reproduction and evolution*, ed. J. H. Calaby & C. H. Tynale-Biscoe, pp. 171–82. Canberra: Australian Academy of Sciences.

Billard, R. (1990). Spermatogenesis in teleost fish. In *Marshall's physiology of reproduction*, 4th edn, ed. G.E. Lamming, vol. 2, pp. 183–212. Edinburgh: Churchill Livingstone.

Bishop, M. W. H. & Walton, A. (1960). Spermatogenesis and the structure of mammalian spermatozoa. In *Marshall's physiology of reproduction*, 3rd edn, ed. A. S. Parkes. vol. 1, part 2, pp. 1–129. London: Longmans Green.

Bishop, M. W. H., Campbell, R. C., Hancock, J. L. & Walton, A. (1954). Semen characteristics and fertility in the bull. *Journal of Agricultural Science, Cambridge*, **44**, 227–48.

Boyd, J. L. & Vandemark, N. L. (1957). Spermatogenic capacity of the male bovine: a measurement technique. *Journal of Dairy Science*, **40**, 689–97.

Breed, W. G. (1980). Further observations on spermatozoa morphology and male reproductive tract anatomy of *Pseudomys* and *Notomys* species (Mammalia: Rodentia). *Transactions of the Royal Society of South Australia*, **104**, 51–5.

Brindley, G. S. (1982). Deep scrotal temperature and the effect on it of clothing, air temperature, activity, posture and paraplegia. *British Journal of Urology*, **54**, 49–55.

Calvin, H. I. & Bedford, J. M. (1971). Formation of disulphide bonds in the nucleus and accessory structures of mammalian spermatozoa during maturation in the epididymis. *Journal of Reproduction and Fertility, Suppl.*, **13**, 65–75.

Clermont, Y. (1963). The cycle of the seminiferous epithelium in man. *American Journal of Anatomy*, **112**, 35–51.

Cran, D. G. & Dott, H. M. (1976). The ultrastructure of knobbed bull spermatozoa. *Journal of Reproduction and Fertility*, **47**, 407–8.

Cummins, J. M. & Woodall, P. F. (1985). On mammalian sperm dimensions. *Journal of Reproduction and Fertility*, **75**, 153–75.

Donald, H. P. & Hancock, J. L. (1953). Evidence of gene controlled sterility in bulls. *Journal of Agricultural Science*, **43**, 178–81.

Dott, H. M. & Dingle, J. T. (1968). Distribution of lysosomal enzymes in spermatozoa and cytoplasmic droplets of bull and ram. *Experimental Cell Research*, **58**, 528–40.

Dott, H. M. & Skinner, J. D. (1989). Collection, examination and storage of spermatozoa from some South African mammals. *African Journal of Zoology*, **23**, 151–60.

Dott, H. M. & Utsi, M. N. P. (1971). The collection and examination of reindeer semen. *Journal of Zoology, London*, **164**, 419–24.

Freund, M. (1967) Standards for the ratings of human sperm morphology. *International Journal of Fertility*, **11**, 97–180.

Gaddum, P. & Glover, T. D. (1965). Some reactions of rabbit spermatozoa to ligation of the epididymis. *Journal of Reproduction and Fertility*. **9**, 119–30.

Glover, T. D. (1955a). Some effects of scrotal insulation on the semen of the ram. *Proceedings of the Society for the Study of Fertility*, **7**, 66–75.

(1955b). The effect of a short period of scrotal insulation on the semen of the ram. *Journal of Physiology*, **128**, 22P.

(1959). Experimental induction of seminal degeneration in rabbits. *Studies in Fertility*, **10**, 80–94.

(1960). Spermatozoa from the isolated cauda epididymidis of rabbits and some effects of artificial cryptorchidism. *Journal of Reproduction and Fertility*, **1**, 121–9.

(1962). The response of rabbit spermatozoa to artificial cryptorchidism and ligation of the epididymis. *Journal of Endocrinology*, **23**, 317–28.

(1973). Aspects of sperm production in some East African mammals. *Journal of Reproduction and Fertility*, **35**, 45–53.

(1982). The epididymis. In *Scientific foundations of urology*, 2nd edn, ed. G. D. Chisholm, pp. 544–55. London: Heinemann.

(1988). Semen analysis. In *Advances in clinical andrology*, ed. C. L. R. Barratt & L. I. D. Cooke, pp. 15–29. Lancaster: MTP Press.

(1994). Some facts and phalluses. *Australian Biologist*, **7**(4), 169–74.

Glover, T. D. & Nicander, L. (1971). Some aspects of structure and function in the mammalian epididymis. *Journal of Reproduction and Fertility, Suppl.*, **13**, 39–50.

Glover, T. D. & Sale, J. B. (1968). The reproductive system of male rock hyrax (*Procavia* and *Heterohyrax*). *Journal of Zoology, London*, **156**, 351–62.

Glover, T. D. & Young, D. H. (1963). Temperature and the production of spermatozoa. *Fertility and Sterility*, **14**, 441–50.

Glover, T. D., d'Occhio, M. J. & Millar, R. P. (1990). Male life cycle and seasonality. In *Marshall's physiology of reproduction*, 4th edn, ed. G. E. Lamming, vol. 2, pp. 213–379. Edinburgh: Churchill Livingstone.

Kirchhoff, C. (1997). Molecular aspects of epididymal function. *International Journal of Andrology*, **20**, *Suppl.* 1, 78 (no. 312).

Lynch, R., Lewis Jones, D. I. Machin, D. I. Machin, D. G. & Desmond, A. D. (1986). Improved seminal characteristics in infertile men after a conservative treatment regimen based on the avoidance of testicular hyperthermia. *Fertility and Sterility*, **46**, 476–97.

Mann, T. (1964). *The biochemistry of semen and the male reproductive tract.* London: Methuen.

Marcanato, A. & Shapiro, D. Y. (1996). Sperm activation, sperm production and fertilization rates in the bucktooth parrotfish. *Animal Behaviour*, **52**, 971–80.

Mieusset, R. & Bujan, L. (1995). Testicular heating and its possible contributions to male infertility. *International Journal of Andrology*, **18**, 169–84.

Mieusset, R. Bujan, L., Mondinat, C., Mansat, A. Pontinnier, F. & Grandjean, H. (1987). Association of scrotal hyperthermia with impaired spermatogenesis in infertile men. *Fertility and Sterility*, **48**, 1006–11.

Millar, R. P. (1972). Degradation of spermatozoa in the epididymis of a seasonally breeding mammal, the rock hyrax (*Procavia capensis*). *Journal of Reproduction and Fertility*, **30**, 447–50.

Millar, R. P. & Glover, T. D. (1970). Seasonal changes in the reproductive tract of the male rock hyrax. *Journal of Reproduction and Fertility*, **23**, 497–9.

Orgebin-Crist, M.-C. (1965). Passage of spermatozoa labelled with thymidine-^{3}H through the ductus epididymidis of the rabbit. *Journal of Reproduction and Fertility*, **10**, 241–51.

(1996). Androgens and epididymal function. In *Pharmacology, biology; and clinical applications of androgens*, ed. S. Bhasin, C. R. Drew, H. L. Gabelnick, J. M. Spieler, R. S. Swerdloft & C. Wang, pp. 27–38. New York: Wiley-Liss.

Ortavant, R. (1954). Détermination de la vitesse de transfert des spermatozoides dans l'épididyme du bélier à l'aide du ³²P. *Compte Rendue du Société Biologique, Paris,* **148**, 866–8.

Racey, P. A. (1974). The reproductive cycle in male noctule bats *Nyctalus noctula. Journal of Reproduction and Fertility,* **41**, 169–82.

Schoysman, R. (1969). Surgical treatment of male sterility. *Andrologie,* 1 33–39.

Short, R. V. (1997). The testis: the witness of the mating system, the site of mutation and the engine of desire. *Acta Paediatrica,* Suppl., **322**, 3–7.

Skinner, J. D., van Aaarde, R. J. Knight, M. H. & Dott, H. M. (1996). Morphometrics and reproduction in a population of springbok (*Antidorcus marsupialis*) in the southern Kalahari. *African Journal of Ecology,* **34**, 312–30.

Swierstra, E. E. (1968). Cytology and duration of the seminiferous epithelium of the boar. Duration of spermatozoon transit through the epididymis. *Anatomical Record,* **161**, 171–86.

Tesh, J. M. (1966). Effect of time of insemination and superovulation on fertilization in the rabbit. *Journal of Endocrinology,* **35**, 28–9.

Tesh, J. M. & Glover, T. D. (1969). Ageing of rabbit spermatozoa in the male tract and its effect on fertility. *Journal of Reproduction and Fertility,* **20**, 287–97.

Thonneau, P., Ducot, B., Bujan, L., Mieusset, R. & Spira, A. (1996). Heat exposure as a hazard to male fertility. *Lancet,* **347**, 204–5.

Van der Horst, G. (1976). Aspects of the reproductive biology of *Liza dumerili* (Steindachner, 1869) (Teleostei: Mugilidae) with special reference to sperm. Ph.D. thesis. University of Port Elizabeth, SouthAfrica.

Zorgniotti, A. W., Cohen, M. S. & Sealfon, A. I. (1986). Chronic scrotal hypothermia: results in 90 infertile couples. *Journal of Urology,* **135**, 944.

4 The local control of spermatogenesis

KATE LAKOSKI LOVELAND AND DAVID DE KRETSER

The major features of spermatogenesis

It is not possible to undertake a discussion of the regulation of spermatogenesis without properly understanding the key steps in sperm production, and details of this process have been extensively reviewed (de Kretser & Kerr, 1994: Sharpe, 1994). In the adult mammal, spermatogenesis, when fully established, can be subdivided into three essential phases: (1) the replication of stem cells, (2) the meiotic process, and (3) spermiogenesis.

Detailed understanding of the precise cell type(s) that constitutes the core stem in the testis is poor. In most species, it is recognized that one of the spermatogonial subclasses constitutes the basic stem cells, which, after certain treatments, can repopulate the seminiferous epithelium provided they are left physiologically intact. These spermatogonia, the cell types which must replace themselves and give rise to cohorts of germ cells that commence the meiotic process, divide by mitosis. The number of differing spermatogonial subtypes that have been identified varies between species as does the nature of the cytological classification that has been employed in their definition. In general, three spermatogonial subtypes can be identified – spermatogonia A, intermediate spermatogonia and type B spermatogonia – which appear to form a hierachical lineage, with the type B spermatogonia forming the cell type that will progress into meiosis.

The cytological criteria that are used to classify spermatogonia are very dependent on the type of fixation, which does not make identification and quantification easy. There is a great need to develop alternative markers, such as antibodies that bind to discrete germ cell types; this will enable the identification of these cell types and greatly add to our understanding of spermatogonial biology. The importance of this information has dramatically increased following the experiments of Brinster & Zimmerman (1994), which demonstrated that it is possible to transplant spermatogonial populations into tubules devoid of germ cells and fully re-establish the process of spermatogenesis. Such methods have important implications for biotechnology, for example in the creation of transgenic models, and for the future in clinical practice.

Through ill-defined mechanisms, cohorts of spermatogonia commence the meiotic process by entering the leptotene stage of the first meiotic prophase. These cells are classified as primary spermatocytes, and they progressively show the characteristic nuclear features used to identify the leptotene, zygotene, pachytene and diplotene stages of meiosis before entering the metaphase stage and dividing to form secondary spermatocytes. (It is not possible in this review to provide details of the cytological criteria used to define the individual stages of the first prophase of meiosis and readers are referred to de Kretser & Kerr, 1994.) The secondary spermatocytes in most species have a relatively short lifespan before dividing to form spermatids and thus they are represented less frequently than other cell types within the seminiferous epithelium.

The final phase of spermatogenesis involves no further cell division but represents a complex series of cytological changes that result in the transformation of a round cell (the round spermatid) into the complex structure of the spermatozoon (Fig. 4.1). This process involves the following:

1 Changes in the position of the nucleus from a central to an eccentric location, together with a progressive decrease in size of the nucleus. This is accompanied by alterations in the DNA and nuclear proteins such that the DNA is rendered stable by a cross-linking process.

2 The formation of a structure called the acrosome, which arises initially as a vesicle from the Golgi complex and takes up a position apposed to the nucleus and interposed between the nucleus and cell membrane. This

Fig. 4.1. The stages of spermatid development (Sa, Sb1, Sb2, Sc, Sd1, Sd2) during spermatogenesis according to the terminology used by Clermont (1963). (Reproduced by permission from de Kretser (1986). In *Male reproductive dysfunction*, ed. R. J. Santen & R. S. Swerdloff, pp. 3–28. Marcel Dekker Inc., New York.

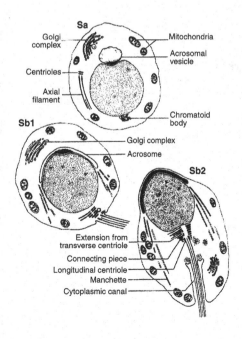
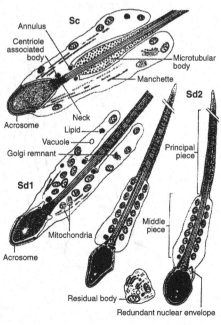

structure is a modified lysosome which contains hydrolytic enzymes essential for the process of penetration of the zona pellucida.

3 The initiation of tail formation from a pair of centrioles that lie adjacent to the Golgi complex. One of these centrioles sends a microtubular extension known as the axonemal complex or axial filament, which forms the core of the sperm tail. Subsequently, the core is surounded by a number of accessory structures called the outer dense fibres, found in the region of the middle piece of the sperm, and the fibrous sheath, which surrounds the axial filament in the region of the principal piece of the sperm. The final modification of the tail occurs late in spermiogenesis with the aggregation of mitochondria, previously peripherally placed in the spermatid, to form a helical arrangement around the axoneme in the region of the midpiece.

4 A progressive redistribution of the cytoplasm of the spermatid, which is finally lost in this process as residual bodies or residual cytoplasm, large amounts of which are phagacytosed by the Sertoli cells.

The seminiferous cycle

Studies in a range of mammalian species have shown that spermatogenesis is highly organized and coordinated. The complex epithelium is arranged in such a manner that specific cell types are always found together in the epithelium, forming cell associations also called stages of the spermatogenic cycle (Fig. 4.2). The number of stages into which spermatogenesis can be subdivided varies between species, and similarly the length of tubule

Fig. 4.2. The arrangement of stages of the seminiferous cycle along the seminiferous tubule in the rat testis. Arrows indicate the ends of one complete cycle. (From de Kretser & Kerr, 1994, reproduced with permission.)

Proximal

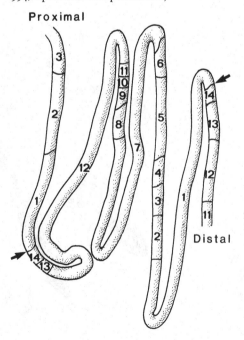

Distal

occupied by such stages is also variable (Clermont, 1972). In man, spermatogenesis appears to be quite disorganized, but the studies of Clermont (1963)
described the stages and showed that they occupied only irregular quadrants
of the tubule. When these cell associations are arranged in progressive order
they form what is known as the spermatogenic cycle. In many species these
stages are found to be linearly arranged along the length of the seminiferous
tubule, producing the appearance of a 'spermatogenic wave' (Perey *et al.*,
1961). The testis, therefore, is not a homogeneous structure and in effect each
length of seminiferous tubule at a particular stage of the cycle should be considered as a specific environment with unique molecular requirements.

The hormonal control of spermatogenesis

There is general agreement that for quantitatively normal spermatogenesis to occur, the testis requires stimulation by the pituitary gonadotrophins follicle-stimulating hormone (FSH) and luternizing hormone (LH).
While FSH acts directly on the seminiferous epithelium, LH exerts its
influence on spermatogenesis by stimulating testosterone secretion from the
Leydig cells, which lie adjacent to the seminiferous tubules (for review, see
Sharpe, 1994). This action of LH in stimulating the local production of testosterone is one example of the local control of spermatogenesis.

There is still considerable debate regarding the relative roles of FSH and
testosterone in the control of spermatogenesis and it serves as a topic on its
own for a review. The controversy concerning the requirement of FSH for
spermatogenesis has been fuelled by recent studies which showed that: (1)
spermatogenesis progresses to completion in mice wherein the gene encoding the β subunit of FSH had been 'knocked out' (Kumar *et al.*, 1997); (2)
testosterone restored spermatogenesis to completion in the hpg mouse
which lacks FSH and LH due to a genetically based lack of gonadotrophin-
releasing hormone (Singh et al. 1995); and (3) spermatogenesis was present
in patients with inactivating mutations of the FSH receptor (Tapanainen *et
al.*, 1997). All of these studies suggest that FSH is not required for spermatogenesis. However, there is evidence emerging to indicate that in all of these
states the sperm output from the testis is subnormal, indicating that, whilst
each of the steps in spermatogenesis can be completed in the absence of FSH,
this hormone plays a crucial role in ensuring optimal sperm production.

The actions of both FSH and testosterone involve local control mechanisms, as receptors for these two hormones cannot be found on germ cells.
Receptors for both hormones can be found on the Sertoli cells and testosterone receptors are also found on the peritubular cells (Grootegoed *et al.*,
1977; Sanborn *et al.*, 1977; Bremner *et al.*, 1994). Transduction of these hormonal signals to the germ cells must, therefore, involve the production of
molecules by the Sertoli and peritubular cells but as yet the nature of these
substances remains largely unknown. Some years ago, a substance termed

P-Mod-S, secreted by the peritubular cells and stimulated by testosterone, was described and shown to stimulate Sertoli cell function (Skinner *et al.*, 1988, 1989). Unfortunately, there has been little progress in the characterization of the nature of the molecule and its actions.

Why consider local control?

As discussed earlier, each segment of the seminiferous tubule at a specific stage of the spermatogenic cycle is a unique environment. Also, the overall hormonal regulation of the germ cells is not direct but must occur through the Leydig, Sertoli and peritubular cells. Both of these facts indicate that local control mechanisms must play an important role in the physiology of spermatogenesis.

It is also well established that the existence of the blood–testis barrier limits the entry of substances into the seminiferous tubules. The anatomical basis of this barrier is the tight junctions that occur between adjacent Sertoli cells, luminal to the location of spermatogonia (Dym & Fawcett, 1970). These tight junctions prevent intercellular transport and effectively subdivide the epithelium into two compartments, basal and adluminal (Fig. 4.3). The basal compartment contains the spermatogonia and the bases of the Sertoli cells, whilst the adluminal compartment contains all the other germ cell types. This arrangement means that all germ cells other than spermatogonia are dependent on the Sertoli cells and perhaps other neighbouring germ cells for maintenance of their environment, including the delivery of hormonal signals.

An additional anatomical feature of the testis, which makes local control mechanisms essential to our understanding of testicular function, is the location of the Leydig cells, the source of testosterone, outside the seminiferous tubules.

Evidence for local control

A considerable amount of evidence has accumulated to support the view that there are many examples of local regulatory mechanisms within the testis, between the tubule and intertubular compartments and between the cell types within those compartments (for reviews, see de Kretser, 1987, 1990; Parvinen *et al.*, 1987; Jégou, 1993; Kierszenbaum, 1994; Gnessi *et al.*, 1997). The major studies contributing to our understanding of local control mechanisms operative within the testis are discussed below.

Leydig cell–seminiferous tubule interaction

As dicussed earlier, the important role played by testosterone in the control of spermatogenesis is a clear example of a local control mechanism. Interference with the action of testosterone through a variety of mechanisms

Fig. 4.3. The arrangements of tight inter-Sertoli cell junctions forming the blood–testis barrier, including the manner in which these cell junctions 'open up' and re-form to allow the germ cells to process from the basal to the adluminal compartment as they mature from mitotic (a) to meiotic (b and c) cells. Arrows indicate points at which intercellular transport from the basal compartment is possible. (From de Kretser & Kerr, 1994, reproduced with permission.)

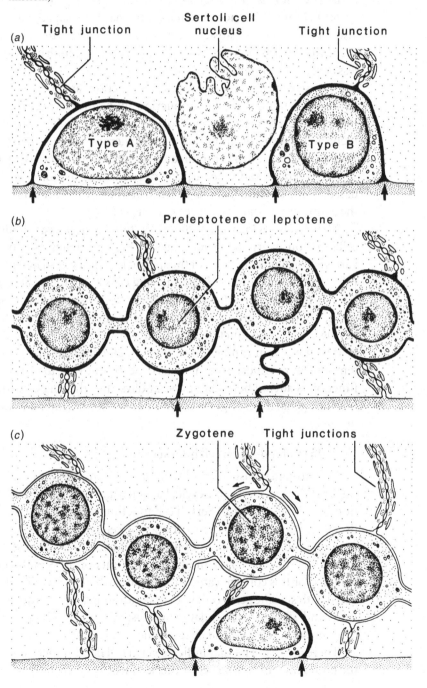

results in the disruption of spermatogenesis with particular stages of spermatogenesis being most sensitive (for a review, see Sharpe, 1994). Spermiogenesis is particularly dependent on testosterone and lowered levels of the hormone result in premature sloughing of the round spermatids from the epithelium, most likely due to the impairment of the production of certain cell adhesion molecules (Cameron & Muffly, 1991; Perryman et al., 1996; O'Donnell et al., 1996). Some studies have also suggested that meiosis is also very sensitive to testosterone deprivation, whereas there is general agreement that spermatogonial multiplication, while requiring testosterone, is less affected (Sun et al., 1989, 1990).

Testosterone also affects Sertoli cell function, as shown by a decrease in androgen-binding protein production and fluid secretion (Jégou et al., 1983). It is likely that other androgen-sensitive Sertoli cell proteins will be identified, given the influence of testosterone on spermatogenesis. The Leydig cells are known to produce a large number of proteins but their role in spermatogenesis and other aspects of testicular function is yet to be elucidated. Some of these include corticotrophin-releasing hormone, renin and the endorphins (for a review, see Gnessi et al., 1997).

There is also evidence that the seminiferous tubules can modulate Leydig cell function. Morphometric studies have shown that the size of Leydig cells varies according to the stage of the spermatogenic cycle in the adjacent seminiferous tubules, with the largest Leydig cells being found at stages VII and VIII (Bergh, 1982). In other studies, disruption of spermatogenesis by irradiation, chemotherapy or vitamin A deficiency resulted in alterations in Leydig cell size and function (Rich et al., 1979). A particularly good example of this interaction can be found if spermatogenesis in the rat is disrupted temporarily by exposure of the testis to heating at 43 °C for 15 min. Leydig cell function is altered between 14 and 21 days after the single heating episode, indicating that the changes in the tubule are affecting their function (Jégou et al., 1984).

Sertoli cell–germ cell interaction

Through the isolation of segments of seminiferous tubules at specific stages of the spermatogenic cycle, Parvinen and colleagues established that a number of parameters of Sertoli cell function changed at different stages of the cycle (Parvinen, 1982). Since the Sertoli cells at different stages of the cycle are surrounded by distinct populations of germ cells, these data suggested that the germ cells could modulate the function of Sertoli cells. Further support for this concept came from studies wherein Sertoli cells were incubated with specific germ cell types or conditioned media from germ cell cultures and shown to modulate some aspects of Sertoli cell secretion (Le Magueresse & Jégou, 1988a,b; Le Magueresse et al., 1988).

There are also data that indicate germ cell development is dependent on the production of substances by the Sertoli cells. There have been significant advances in our understanding of some of the molecular mechanisms which are the mediators of this cross-talk between Sertoli cells and germ cells and these are discussed in the subsequent sections of this chapter.

The Sertoli cell and initiation of testicular differentiation

The precursors of the Sertoli cells in the developing gonad arise from the somatic cells comprising the gonadal ridge and play an important role in differentiation of the testis, as they are the site of the expression of the gene *sry*, which represents the key element in testicular development (Koopman *et al.*, 1991). This gene, found on the Y chromosome, encodes the SRY protein, a transcription factor (Koopman *et al.*, 1991) produced by the mouse Sertoli cell, with *sry* transcripts first detected around 10.5 days postcoitum (dpc; Hacker *et al.*, 1995; Jeske *et al.*, 1995). It is into this environment that the primordial germ cells migrate from an extra-embryonic site adjacent to the yolk sac endoderm and are incorporated into the forming seminiferous cords, representing the first microscopically visible step of testicular development.

Sry expression is followed by the synthesis of müllerian inhibiting substance (MIS) in Sertoli cells, which mediates degeneration of the müllerian duct (the female reproductive tract precursor). This allows the normal development of the male reproductive tract from the wolffian (mesonephric) duct. The expression of MIS is regulated by the orphan nuclear receptor, SF-1 (steroidogeneic factor-1; Giuili *et al.*, 1997). In genetically modified mice which lack the *MIS* gene, the males have apparently normal testes and male reproductive tracts but are infertile (Berhringer *et al.*, 1994). Their infertility results from the presence of the female reproductive tract components (uterus, oviduct and vagina) that block sperm efflux during coitus. Thus, other factors apart from MIS are required to mediate development of the male reproductive tract.

The expression of another transcription factor, sox 9, is up-regulated by *sry* and the *sox 9* gene product regulates extracellular matrix synthesis through the *collagen 2* gene (Bell *et al.*, 1997; Ng *et al.*, 1997). Another Sertoli cell product expressed early in gonadal development is desert hedgehog (Dhh), which signals through the patched protein in Leydig cells, another male-specific gene product. Deletion of *Dhh* in mice results in male sterility, due to complete absence of spermatozoa (Bitgood *et al.*, 1996) and a broader understanding of the role of this protein in this and other mammals is awaited with interest. The SF-1 protein also interacts with DAX-1 (Ikeda *et al.*, 1996; Ito *et al.*, 1997) to regulate steroidogenesis in the Leydig cell through the steroidogenic acute regulatory protein gene (*StAR*) (Parker *et al.*, 1996), again emphasizing the importance of the intertubular compartment in the establishment of normal testicular function.

Sexual differentiation of the fetal testis is first morphologically apparent at 12.5 dpc in the mouse and at 13.5 dpc in the rat, with the appearance of Sertoli cells (Magre & Jost, 1991). These cells become polarized, forming intracellular adherens-type junctions and basal intercellular microfilament bundles, with the appearance of a continuous basal lamina evident by 15.5 dpc (Magre & Jost, 1991). The formation of the basal lamina appears to be a prerequisite for cord formation but not for Sertoli cell differentiation, as incubation of rat testicular primordia with an inhibitor of collagen synthesis prevents cord formation but not development of Sertoli cells and MIS synthesis (Jost et al., 1988). In many biological systems the basement membrane acts to store and regulate the action of growth factors. This paradigm is quite evident during early testis development and is likely to influence the function of the mature testis (Dym et al., 1991; for a review, see Dym, 1994).

Sertoli cell division establishes the framework for subsequent sperm production

The number of Sertoli cells in the testis is an important factor controlling the total testicular output of spermatozoa. This is based on increasing evidence indicating that each Sertoli cell in the mature testis can support only a fixed number of germ cells to maturity at any one time (Orth et al., 1988). Presumably this is due to a combination of structural and nutritive limitations. For this reason, the factors that influence Sertoli cell proliferation can exert a profound influence on the spermatogenic potential of the testis. The pattern of Sertoli cell division has been carefully described in the rat (Orth, 1982), with cell division active at 16 dpc, reaching a peak at 20 dpc, and ceasing by around 16 days post partum (dpp) in this species. In some mammals, Sertoli cell division stops relatively soon after birth. However, in other mammals with a prolonged period between birth and puberty, there is a further period of Sertoli cell multiplication during puberty. Data are available for the human and for cynomolgus monkey to show that Sertoli cell division continues into puberty (for a review, see Sharpe, 1994) and it is likely that other primates will exhibit a similar pattern. The relative importance of cell division during postnatal versus fetal life is yet to be established. It is unknown whether compensatory cell multiplication occurs in the postnatal period if division during the fetal period is abnormally reduced.

Sertoli cell division is regulated by the interplay of a variety of factors, and the relative influence of each factor appears to change as the testis matures. The primary importance of FSH has been established using a variety of approaches, although, as mentioned earlier, deletion from the mouse of the gene encoding the FSH β subunit results in mice that are fertile but have smaller testes (Kumar et al., 1997). This observation is at odds with the perception of FSH as the master controller of Sertoli cell division, but it is in accord with the concept of FSH as a modulator of the extent of Sertoli cell division. It will be interesting to uncover the pattern of Sertoli cell proliferation during development in these FSH knock-out animals, though the problem of discriminating between the direct and indirect effects of FSH on testis development in this model must be considered. Compensatory cell division may take place in later stages of development if factors other than FSH are able to stimulate Sertoli cell multiplication. It appears that the action of FSH on Sertoli cell proliferation may be mediated through the stimulation of cyclin D2, since deletion of this gene in mice results in small testes with qualitatively normal spermatogenesis (Sicinski *et al.*, 1996).

Elimination of the gene encoding the α subunit of inhibin (Matsuk *et al.*, 1992) results in mice which develop stromal cell tumours after birth, implicating inhibin, and indirectly activin, as modulators of Sertoli cell growth. Members of the transforming growth factor family, inhibin is formed as a disulphide-linked dimer of α and β subunits, and activin forms from dimers of β subunits. To date, there have been five distinct β subunit genes and one α subunit gene identified (Hotten *et al.*, 1995; Oda *et al.*, 1995; Fang *et al.*, 1996). The absence of the inhibin α subunit results in the formation of elevated levels of activin in those cells that normally produce inhibin. As inhibin is known to antagonize some of the actions of activin in a wide variety of developmental systems (for reviews, see de Paolo, 1997; Mather *et al.*, 1997; Ying *et al.*, 1997), by interfering with the binding of activin to its cell surface receptors (Martens *et al.*, 1997), deletion of the α subunit could lead to unregulated proliferation of those cells in which activin can stimulate division. Interference of the actions of activins by disruption of the activin type 2 receptor gene results in the formation of a small testis, albeit with qualitatively normal spermatogenesis (Matzuk *et al.*, 1995). However, it is difficult to interpret whether this effect is due to the interruption of the action of activin, or if it results from the lower FSH levels that are caused by the absence of activin's action at the pituitary. In addition, the binding of follistatin can reduce activin binding to its receptor (de Winter *et al.*, 1996), and recent evidence for its production within the seminiferous epithelium (Meinhardt *et al.*, 1998) suggests that it may influence the functions of both Sertoli and germ cells that are regulated by activin. α2-Macroglobulin also binds to activin and inhibin, but it does not appear to alter its bioactivity (Vaughn & Vale, 1993; Mather, 1996), but it is not present in the seminiferous epithelium until after Sertoli cell division is complete (Zhu *et al.*, 1994).

Several *in vitro* studies have provided evidence for important roles for activin and inhibin in Sertoli cell development. The level of activin βB mRNA is developmentally regulated in the rat Sertoli cell (Bunick *et al.*, 1994), being lower at birth and rising during testicular maturation. This correlates with measurements showing that the intratesticular level of inhibin in the postnatal testis appears to be highest in the first five days of life, coincident with the period of most active division for Sertoli cells (Maddocks & Sharpe, 1990; Sharpe, 1994). A culture of testis fragments from rats of increasing ages was used to examine the influence of activin on Sertoli cell multiplication in the presence and absence of FSH (Boitani *et al.*, 1995). Sertoli cells from newborn animals (3 dpp) showed enhanced proliferation in the presence of FSH but did not respond to exogenous activin. In contrast, Sertoli cells from 9-day-old animals were stimulated to divide only in the combined presence of activin and FSH, while neither factor stimulated division in the 18-day-old Sertoli cells, which would normally have stopped dividing. If inhibin is synthesized by Sertoli cells in high amounts in the early postnatal testis and acts in an autocrine manner, then the supply of exogenous activin in this experiment may not have been sufficient to reveal a stimulatory effect of this factor on Sertoli cell division until the testis reached a stage when inhibin production was reduced. The reduction in Sertoli cell responsiveness to FSH over time has been suggested to result from an increase in phosphodiesterase activity in these cells (Ritzén *et al.*, 1989). The addition of germ cells to Sertoli cells in culture has a similar effect on FSH responsiveness (Le Magueresse & Jégou, 1988*a*,*b*), suggesting that the expansion of the germ cell population in the developing testis impacts on Sertoli cell division through the production of growth factors. The identity of these factors is unknown, but a list of candidates can be derived from recent data concerning the production of cytokines and growth factors by germ cells (see next section).

A key role for thyroxine in regulating Sertoli cell division has been demonstrated through *in vivo* studies in which rat pups are rendered hypothyroid through the administration of propylthiouracil to the drinking water of their nursing mothers. The testes of these rats initially show a reduced weight, but by adulthood double their mass relative to their littermate controls (Francavilla *et al.* 1991). Histological analysis has revealed that the period of Sertoli cell division is prolonged to about 30 dpp, even if the period of hypothyroidism is extended up to 60 days (Van Haaster *et al.*, 1992). Germ cell maturation is grossly impaired, with very few germ cells completing meiosis and with markedly reduced numbers of round spermatids present in the 30-day rat testis (Simorangkir *et al.*, 1995). The means by which thyroxine regulates Sertoli cell division is currently unclear but modulation of growth factor and basement membrane production have each been implicated. In the hypothyroid rat testis, Sertoli cells show prolonged synthesis of mRNAs characteristic of their immature phenotype (e.g. MIS) and delayed onset of expression of mRNAs upregulated in the postmitotic differentiated cell (inhibin βB and androgen-binding protein; Bunick *et al.*, 1994). In addition, maturation of the basement membrane is delayed, and this is likely to reflect an influence of thyroxine on both Sertoli and peritubular cells (Loveland *et al.*, 1998). This model highlights the coordinated regulation of development that occurs between the different cell types in the testis, and indicates that the mitotic, immature Sertoli cell is incapable of supporting germ cell maturation. It is interesting that in germ cell-depleted rats, produced through X-irradiation *in utero*, the formation of tight junctions between Sertoli cells is similarly delayed until 30 dpp (Maddocks *et al.*, 1992), data that support the concept of bidirectional control of cell maturation within the seminiferous epithelium.

Interactions between stem cell factor and c-kit are critical for several processes in testicular development

The importance of local regulation is well illustrated by the production of stem cell factor (SCF) by the Sertoli cell and its action on germ cells through the SCF receptor c-kit. SCF is synthesized as a membrane-anchored protein in two isoforms, which are distinguished by the presence or absence of exon 6, as a result of alternative splicing of the SCF mRNA (for reviews, see Galli *et al.*, 1994; Loveland & Schlatt, 1997). Encoded within exon 6 is a site which is recognized, and readily cleaved by, a cell surface protease to release a soluble SCF protein (Huang *et al.*, 1992). Both soluble and membrane-bound forms bind to and activate the receptor protein, c-kit, but each appears to produce a different effect on the target cell (Miyazawa *et al.*, 1995). The c-kit protein contains an intracellular tyrosine kinase domain that is activated upon SCF binding to produce a variety of cellular responses, including proliferation, survival, migration and adhesion (Reith & Bernstein, 1991). While both proteins show a widespread tissue distribution, it is their influence on stem cell development that has received the most attention (for a review, see Donovan, 1994). The initial recognition that each of these proteins is critical for stem cell development came from observations of mice, which developed white fur patches as the result of genetic lesions at two distinct loci. The *W* locus (subsequently shown to encode c-kit) and the *Sl* locus (encoding SCF) mice were found to have deficient migration and proliferation of melanocytes, haematopoietic stem cells, and primordial germ cells, and both exhibited a phenotype of white fur patches, anaemia and infertility. To date, a large number of *W* and *Sl* mutants have been described, with heterogeneity in each of these phenotypes (Silvers, 1979; Dubreuil *et al.*, 1990; Reith & Bernstein, 1991).

The impact of these proteins on testicular development was recognized in analyses of primordial germ cells (Mintz & Russell, 1957; McCoshen & McCallion, 1975), in which the number of primordial germ cells reaching the gonadal ridge was reduced to 6–10% of normal, whilst migration of these cells to ectopic sites was also increased. Migration of primordial germ cells to the gonadal ridge involves a progressive change in the strength of their binding to the extracellular matrix components, fibronectin and laminin (de Felici & Dolci, 1989; Garcio-Castro *et al.*, 1997). The distribution of these molecules along the path of migration and within the developing gonadal ridge implicates these interactions as key to establishing the normal complement of germ cells within the fetal gonad (Garcia-Castro *et al.*, 1997), and c-kit has been directly implicated in primordial germ cell adhesion to somatic cells *in vitro* (Pesce *et al.*, 1997). A link between stem cell factor and integrin-mediated events (which are translated to the target cell via binding to fibronectin) has been demonstrated with a mast cell line in which a transient binding of cells to fibronectin via an integrin receptor was stimulated by the presence of SCF and dependent upon c-kit tyrosine kinase activity in the target cell (Kinashi & Springer, 1994). The interaction between these molecules has not been explored in the testis, but it is clear that both SCF and extracellular matrix components are key local regulators of primordial germ cell migration and viabililty. Several other locally produced factors have been tested for their influence on primordial germ cell survival and proliferation using *in vitro* culture systems. While SCF and leukaemia-inhibitory factor (LIF) have been shown to support primordial germ cell survival (Dolci *et al.*, 1991; Godin *et al.*, 1991; Matsui *et al.*, 1991; Pesce *et al.*, 1993), LIF (Dolci *et al.*, 1993), Gas 6 (Matsubara *et al.*, 1996) and fibroblast growth factor (FGF) (Kawase *et al.*, 1996) have all been shown to enhance proliferation of these cells. A culture system that can support development of primordial germ cells employs undergrowing feeder layers that synthesize the larger, membrane-bound form of SCF (Kawase *et al.*, 1996). In this system, proliferation continues past the normal *in vivo* time point, but does stop, which suggests that some aspect of normal development has been sustained. In addition, the proliferative response to Gas 6 was observed only when cells were grown on these feeder layers containing SCF (Matsubara *et al.*, 1996).

A role for SCF and c-kit in postnatal testis development was surmised from the pattern of expression of these proteins in wild-type animals and from the use of an antibody which blocks binding between SCF and c-kit. Within the seminiferous tubule, c-kit receptor expression has been described in gonocytes (Orth et al., 1996, 1997) and spermatogonia (Manova *et al.*, 1990; Yoshinaga *et al.*, 1991; Dym *et al.*, 1995). In meiotic and haploid germ cells, a truncated c-*kit* transcript is produced which encodes an intracellular protein, containing only the extreme carboxy-terminus of the full length receptor (Rossi *et al.*, 1992; Albanesi *et al.*, 1996). This protein has been implicated in activation of the oocyte: microinjection of mouse eggs with a recombinant form of the protein increases the rate of oocyte progression through meiosis *in vivo* (Sette *et al.*, 1997). Other recent immunological analyses have suggested that the acrosome of rodent and human spermatozoa contain c-kit isoforms that are yet to be fully characterized (Feng *et al.*, 1997; Sandlow *et al.*, 1997).

While c-kit expression has been localized exclusively to germ cells within the seminiferous tubule, several studies have demonstrated stem cell factor expression in Sertoli cells (Rossi *et al.*, 1993; Tajima *et al.*, 1993; Munsie *et al.*, 1997). The potential for FSH to elevate SCF mRNA levels and to influence the pattern of SCF mRNA splicing has been noted using *in vitro* systems (Rossi *et al.*, 1991, 1993; Tajima *et al.*, 1993). It is interesting that the total level of SCF mRNA in the rat testis increases dramatically at 5 dpp, coincident with the onset of spermatogonial differentiation (Munsie *et al.*, 1997) and contemporaneous with the change in SCF mRNA splicing from o dpp to 9 dpp to favour production of the membrane-association isoform, as documented in the mouse using a ribonuclease protection assay (Huang *et al.*, 1992). These data correlate with *in vivo* data obtained from wild-type mice that implicate SCF as a key component in regulating the onset of spermatogonial differentiation. Injection of adult and immature mice with a monoclonal antibody to c-kit (ACK2) led to the specific loss of type A_{2-4} and type B spermatogonia, whilst both less and more mature germ cell types were unaffected (Yoshinaga *et al.*, 1991; Tajima *et al.*, 1994). In a separate analysis, this type of protocol was noted to result in higher levels of apoptotic germ cells, both at mitotic and meiotic stages of development (Packer *et al.*, 1995). These findings are consistent with a role for SCF in mediating survival and/or proliferation of the germ cells first entering the committed pathway of differentiation; that is, the four divisions of the type A spermatogonia in the rodent. Further support has been gained from a model in which administration of a Sertoli cell toxicant, 2,5-hexanedione, causes loss of all germ cells (except for stem cells) and some type A spermatogonia. Recovery of germ cell proliferation is increased following continuous intratesticular administration of SCF for two weeks after 2,5-hexanedione exposure (Allard *et al.*, 1996).

Local factors influencing gonocyte development

The commencement of the spermatogenic process in all mammalian species involves activation of the gonocytes to begin their transformation to spermatogonia, the stem cells for spermatogenesis. The gonocytes, centrally placed within the seminiferous cords, migrate to the basement membrane and commence a period of mitotic division. In the rat, this process occurs at 3 days after birth (Orth, 1993) and migration and division can occur independently, with some cells dividing before making contact with the basement membrane and other cells in mitosis at the basement membrane (McGuiness & Orth, 1992). The delay in this process in the hypothyroid rat suggests that it is influenced, at least in part by the continued proliferation and 'immaturity' of the Sertoli cells in this experimental model (Simorangkir *et al.*, 1995). Adhesion between gonocytes and Sertoli cells at the time of birth is mediated at least partially through the neural cell adhesion molecule (NCAM) in the rat testis, and the function of this NCAM-mediated interaction appears to change as the testis matures (Orth & Jester, 1995).

Locally produced factors which appear to influence gonocyte proliferation include platelet-derived growth factor (PDGF; Li *et al.*, 1997); oestradiol (Li *et al.*, 1997), basic fibroblast growth factor (FGF-2; van Dissel-Emiliani, 1996), LIF (de Miguel *et al.*, 1996) and oncostatin M (de Miguel *et al.*, 1997), while both LIF and ciliary neurotropic factor (CNTF) both enhance gono-cyte and Sertoli cell survival in co-cultures (de Miguel et al., 1996). In con-trast, the addition of MIS to testes from newborn mice decreases progression of gonocytes to type A spermatogonia when cultured in the presence of 10% (v/v) fetal calf serum for up to a week (Zhou et al., 1993).

Local factors affecting spermatogonial progression

The number of postnatal mitotic divisions which the committed male germ cell undergoes before entering meiosis differs between species. During this process of spermatogonial proliferation, a proportion of the cells undergo apoptosis (Allan et al., 1987, 1992). The balance between cell multi-plication and death is likely to be critical for maintaining the ratio of Sertoli cells to germ cells that will support full maturation of the maximum number of spermatozoa per testis, as described above (Orth et al., 1988). Maintenance of this balance in many developmental systems is known to be regulated through the equilibrium of expression of the 'cell survival' and the 'cell death' genes in the bcl2 family (Boise et al., 1993; for a review, see Schwartzman & Cidlowski, 1993).

In the testis, expression of the bak (Krajewski et al., 1996), bclxL (Krajewski et al., 1994; Rodriguez et al., 1997) and bclw genes has been docu-mented (Gibson et al., 1996), while an absence of bcl2 has been reported (Hockenbery et al., 1991; Rodriguez et al., 1997). Ectopic expression of the bcl2 gene in spermatogonia was achieved following the production of a trans-genic mouse bearing this gene under the transcriptional control of a small 3' region of the EF-1α promoter (Furuchi et al., 1996). The resulting ultimate phenotype was sterile, owing to a huge accumulation of spermatogonia, and degeneration of the few, often multinucleated, spermatocytes that did develop. Deletion of the bax gene from mice resulted in a similar phenotype, with the appearance of multinucleated spermatocytes, and an absence of elongated spermatids and spermatozoa (Knudson et al., 1995). Another report describes the disruption of spermatogenesis by misexpression of bcl2 and overexpression of bclxL (Rodrigeuz et al., 1997), which also results in the appearance of multinucleated spermatocytes within the seminiferous tubule (see also p. 84n). These data have been interpreted as reinforcing the concept that regulated germ cell death is essential for achieving full spermatogenic potential. It remains to be determined what factors influence the expression of bcl2 family members in the testis and at what sites they act.

It is important to note that the p53 gene, known to regulate bax expression (Miyashita & Reed, 1995), is present in relatively higher levels in the imma-ture testis, and is found in spermatocytes of the adult. Reduction of the p53 protein levels in the testis can also produce a moderate testis phenotype, with some appearance of abnormally large germ cells, as described above (Rotter et al., 1993).

In addition to the role for stem cell factor illustrated with the *in vivo* administration of the ACK2 antibody, several other factors have been shown to influence the rate of DNA synthesis of mitotic male germ cells. Inhibin has been postulated to decrease the numbers of all spermatogonial types in mice and Chinese hamsters following intratesticular or interperitoneal injection with bovine follicular fluid (containing high levels of inhibin) with partially purified inhibin preparations (van Dissel-Emilliani *et al.*, 1989). The addition of activin A to co-cultures of dissociated germ cells and Sertoli cells from immature rats increased the rate of germ cell proliferation over 3 days in culture (Mather *et al.*, 1990, 1993). When follistatin was added to neutralize the action of activin, it prevented the activin-stimulated reaggregation of Sertoli cells, but did not reduce the activin-mediated increase in germ cell DNA synthesis (Mather *et al.*, 1993). The latter result may be due to the production of follistatin in germ cells (Meinhardt *et al.*, 1998), which could diminish the influence of exogenous follistatin on these cells. The use of an alternative *in vitro* system to test the effects of FSH and activin involved culturing fragments of 9 dpp rat testes for three days on an agar support (Boitani *et al.*, 1995). The presence of FSH-stimulated spermatogonial division approximately six-fold, while activin on its own had no effect relative to medium-only controls. However, in the presence of FSH, a negative effect of activin on spermatogonial proliferation was seen. The influence of these factors was observed only on differentiated, or committed, spermatogonia, and proliferation of the undifferentiated spermatogonia was unaffected. Whether activin blocks spermatogonial proliferation through a direct influence on germ cell activin receptors, or indirectly by affecting Sertoli cell function, is currently unknown. It will be interesting to determine whether it is related to the contrasting stimulatory influence that activin has been shown to have on DNA synthesis in preleptotene male germ cells during culture of tubule segments from adult rats (Hakovirta *et al.*, 1993).

Several factors have been investigated as potential regulators of spermatogonial function, often using models of testis recovery following testicular damage in the adult. Fragments of testes from mice rendered cryptorchid to eliminate meiotic and postmeiotic germ cells were cultured for 9 days in the presence of PDGF, FGF, transforming growth factor-α (TGF-α) and insulin-like growth factor-1 (IGF-1). Only the latter two substances were seen to increase the differentiation and proliferation of germ cells (Tajima *et al.*, 1995). One model that is of particular clinical relevance is spermatogenic recovery following radiation and chemotherapy. In this approach, the testis is depleted of meiotic and postmeiotic germ cells as the mitotic and meitotic precursor cells are destroyed. Recovery, if it occurs, results from the repopulation of the tubule by mitosis of remaining stem cells. Meistrich & Kangasniemi (1997) showed that the degree of recovery of spermatogenesis after irradiation could be significantly improved in rats if they were treated with a gonadotrophin-releasing hormone agonist and testosterone for ten weeks after irradiation. This period of treatment could be delayed for up to 18 weeks following irradiation. The manner in which this treatment acts to stimulate the recovery is unclear but the observations are clearly of importance to patients undergoing radiation and chemotherapy for cancer. By means of this model, interleukin 11 (IL-11) has also been identified as a candidate for regulating spermatogonial progression. Its expression in the testis has been reported as being restricted to germ cells and, in mice rendered infertile through exposure to radiation and chemotherapeutic agents, the administration of IL-11 results in a significant acceleration of spermatogonial recovery (Du *et al.*, 1996).

Local factors regulating development of the postmitotic germ cell

As described above, the dysfunctional regulation of spermatogonial proliferation and survival will impact on the subsequent steps of spermatogenesis, and this may be due either to a direct influence of germ cell-derived products on their adjacent siblings, or to indirect effects mediated through the enveloping Sertoli cells. Germ cells at the same stage of development can communicate with each other through intercellular bridges that persist after cell division, as a result of incomplete cytokinesis (Dym & Fawcett, 1971). The number of germ cells linked in this manner are substantial and probably form the basis of symplast formation and multinuculeate giant cells, which can appear after exposure of the testis to a variety of agents capable of damaging spermatogenesis. There is no clear picture of how adjacent germ cell populations at different stages of development influence each other, though this understanding will emerge as the identification of the local factors produced and the sites of their receptors becomes more complete.

As mentioned above, activin can stimulate DNA synthesis in spermatogonia and in preleptotene spermatocytes in cultured tubule fragments, whereas inhibin has an inhibitory effect and transforming growth factor-β (TGF-β) has a more modest stimulatory effect (Hakovirta *et al.*, 1993). It is apparent that Sertoli cells and germ cells can produce TGF-β proteins and receptors (Mullaney & Skinner, 1993; Teerds & Dorrington, 1993; Caussanel *et al.*, 1997), while receptors for activin have been found on both somatic and germ cells of the testis (de Winter *et al.*, 1992; Kaipia *et al.*, 1993; Krummen *et al.*, 1994; Majdic *et al.*, 1997). Similarly, IL-6 has been found to inhibit the onset of DNA synthesis in preleptotene spermatocytes in adult tubule segment cultures (Hakovirta *et al.*, 1995), and the synthesis of IL-6 has been reported in Sertoli cells in culture (Syed *et al.*, 1993). In contrast, nerve growth factor (NGF) is produced by meiotic germ cells and its receptor has been identified on Sertoli cells (Parvinen *et al.*, 1992). The addition of NGF to tubule fragments *in vivo* also stimulated DNA synthesis in meiotic cells, but, in this case, the effect is presumed to be indirect, with NGF acting on Sertoli cells to affect production of a different local factor to which the germ cells are responsive.

The bone morphogenic proteins Bmp 8a and Bmp 8b, also members of the TGF-β superfamily, have recently been implicated as regulators of germ cell development (Zhao & Hogan, 1996; Zhao *et al.*, 1996). In immature mice (up to 3.5 weeks postpartum) the *Bmp8a* and *8b* mRNAs are expressed in spermatogonia and spermatocytes at low levels, but, in older animals, strong expression is evident in round spermatids and the spermatogonial expression is lost. Deletion of the *Bmp8b* gene results in mice that are infertile due to the lack of germ cell proliferation (Zhao *et al.*, 1996). In the first few weeks postpartum, there is an obvious absence of proliferating germ cells, which accounts for the reduced testis weight and absence of maturing germ cells in the *Bmp8b* homozygous mutant animals. An increase in spermatocyte apoptosis was recorded in the adult animals, resulting ultimately in sterility. These data imply that the Bmp8b protein may function separately in initiation and then in maintenance of spermatogenesis, and it will be important to consider whether there are distinct signalling mechanisms used by cells responding to Bmp8 proteins at different stages of testis development.

The influence of local factors on germ cell protein synthesis is a reflection of their ability to regulate germ cell differentiation. A stimulatory influence on postmitotic germ cell RNA synthesis was measured at 2 h after addition of FGF-2, TGF-β, or somatomedin C, indicating the presence of receptors for these components on spermatids (Fradin *et al.*, 1989). Proteins secreted by cultured Sertoli cells were shown to inhibit the affect of FGF-2, while in contrast, the effect of TGF-β was amplified. These data indicate that germ cells contain several simultaneously active receptor systems which are modulated by the local production of factors from Sertoli cells (Fradin *et al.*, 1989).

A primary influence of testosterone on spermatid maturation has been documented (McLachlan *et al.*, 1994; O'Donnell *et al.*, 1994), and knowledge of the local factors that mediate this is now emerging. As indicated earlier, this effect of testosterone must be exerted through the Sertoli cell, since the spermatid does not contain receptors for this hormone. This intermediary effect may well be through the action of both testosterone and FSH on the production of specific adhesion molecules that enable cell junctions to form between spermatids and the Sertoli cell (Cameron & Muffly, 1991; Perryman *et al.*, 1996). This observation may echo the earlier paradigm of primordial germ cell adhesion to stem cell factor and extracellular matrix components that is essential for normal migration and development.

The mechanisms that regulate spermiogenesis are clearly complex. Significant progress in defining some of the molecular mechanisms in some of these processes has recently been achieved and the regulation of the genes involved is under active investigation. It seems likely that transcription factors, growth factors and possibly testosterone are involved in modulating a complex metamorphosis from the round spermatid to the spermatozoon.

Acknowledgement

The authors thank Dr Cris Print for his helpful comments and acknowledge support from the NH&MRC of Australia.

References

Albanesi, C., Geremia, R., Giorgio, M., Dolci, S., Sette, C. & Rossi, P. (1996). A cell- and developmental stage-specific promoter drives the expression of a truncated c-*kit* protein during mouse spermatid elongation. *Development*, **122**, 1291–302.

Allan, D. J., Harmon, B. V. & Kerr, J. F. R. (1987). Cell death in spermatogenesis. In *Perspectives on mammalian cell death*, ed. C. S. Potten, pp. 229–58. London: Oxford University Press.

Allan, D. J., Harmon, B. V. & Roberts, S. A. (1992). Spermatogonial apoptosis has three morphologically recognizable phases and shows no circadian rhythm during normal spermatogenesis in the rat. *Cell Proliferation*, **25**, 241–50.

Allard, E. K., Blanchard, K. T. & Boekelheide, K. (1996). Exogenous stem cell factor (SCF) compensates for altered endogenous SCF expression in 2,5-hexane-dione-induced testicular atrophy in rats. *Biology of Reproduction*, **55**, 185–93.

Behringer, R. R., Finegold, M. J. & Cate, R. L. (1994). Müllerian-inhibiting substance function during mammalian sexual development. *Cell*, **79**, 415–25.

Bell, D. M., Leung, K. K., Wheatley, S. C., Ng, L. J., Zhou, S., Ling, K. W., Sham, M. H., Koopman, P., Tam, P. P. & Cheah. K. S. (1997). SOX9 directly regulates the type-II collagen gene. *Nature Genetics*, **16**(2), 174–8.

Bergh, A. (1982). Local differences in Leydig cell morphology in the adult rat testis: evidence for a local control of Leydig cells by adjacent seminiferous tubules. *International Journal of Andrology*, **5**, 325–30.

Bitgood, M. J., Shen, L. & McMahon, A. P. (1996). Sertoli cell signaling by desert hedgehog regulates the male germline. *Current Biology*, **6**(3), 298–304.

Boise, L. H., Gonzalez-Garcia, M., Postema, C. E., Ding, L., Lindsten, T., Turka, L. A., Mao, X., Nunez, G. & Thompson, C. B. (1993). *bcl-x*, a *bcl-2* related gene that functions as a dominant regulator of apoptotic cell death. *Cell*, **74**, 597–608.

Boitani, C., Stefanini, M., Fragale, A. & Morena, A. R. (1995). Activin stimulates Sertoli cell proliferation in a defined period of rat testis development. *Endocrinology*, **136**, 5438–4.

Bremner, W. J., Millar, M. R. & Sharpe, R. M. (1994). Immunohistochemical localization of androgen receptors in the rat testis: evidence of a stage dependent expression and regulation by androgens. *Endocrinology*, **135**, 1227–34.

Brinster, R. L. & Zimmerman, J. W. (1994). Spermatogenesis following male germ cell transplantation. *Proceedings of the National Academy of Sciences, USA*, **91**, 11298–302.

Bunick, D., Kirby, J., Hess, R. A. & Cooke, P. S. (1994). Developmental expression of testis messenger ribonucleic acids in the rat following propylthiouracil-induced neonatal hypothyroidism. *Biology of Reproduction*, **51**, 706–13.

Cameron, D. F. & Muffly, K. E. (1991). Hormonal regulation of spermatid binding. *Journal of Cell Science*, **100**, 623–33.

Caussanel, V., Tabone, E., Hendrick, J. C., Dacheux, F. & Benahmed, M. (1997). Cellular distribution of transforming growth factor betas 1, 2, and 3 and their types I and II receptors during postnatal development and spermatogenesis in the boar testis. *Biology of Reproduction*, **56**, 357–67.

Clermont, Y. (1963). The cycle of the seminiferous epithelium in man. *American Journal of Anatomy*, **112**, 35–51.

(1972). Kinetics of spermatogenesis in mammals: seminiferous, epithelium cycle and spermatogonial renewal. *Physiological Review*, **52**, 198–236.

de Felici, M. & Dolci, S. (1989). *In vitro* adhesion of mouse fetal germ cells to extracellular matrix components. Cell *Differentiation and Development*, **26**, 87–96.

de Kretser, D. M. (1986). Light and electron microscopic anatomy of the normal human testis. In *Male reproductive dysfunction*, ed. R. J. Sauten & R. S. Swerdloft, pp. 3–28. New York: Marcel Dekker Inc.

(1987). Local regulation of testicular function. *International Review of Cytology*, **10**, 89–112.

(1990). Germ cell–Sertoli cell interactions. *Reproduction, Fertility and Development*, **2**, 225–35.

de Kretser, D. M. & Kerr, J. B. (1994). The cytology of the testis. In *The physiology of reproduction*, 2nd edn, ed. E. Knobil & J. D. Neill, pp. 1177–290. New York: Raven Press.

de Miguel, M. P., de Boer-Brouwer, M., Paniagua, R., van den Hurk, R., de Rooij, D. G. & Dissel-Emiliani, F. M. F. (1996). Leukemia inhibitory factor and ciliary neurotropic factor promote the survival of Sertoli cells and gonocytes in a coculture system. *Endocrinology*, **137**, 1885–93.

de Miguel, M. P., de Boer-Brouwer, M., de Rooij, D. G., Paniagua, R. & van Dissel-Emiliani, F. M. F. (1997). Ontogeny and localization of an oncostatin M-like protein in the rat testis: its possible role at the start of spermatogenesis. Cell *Growth and Differentiation*, **8**, 611–18.

de Paolo, L. V. (1997). Inhibins, activins, and follistatins: the saga continues. *Proceedings of the Society for Experimental Biology and Medicine*, **214**, 328–30.

de Winter, J. P., Themmen, A. P. N., Hoogerbrugge, J. W., Klaij, I. A., Grootegoed, J. A. & de Jong, F. H. (1992). Activin receptor mRNA expression in rat testicular cell types. *Molecular and Cellular Endocrinology*, **83**, R1–R8.

de Winter, J. P., ten Dijke, P., de Vries, C. J. M., van Achterberg, T. A. E., Sugino, H., de Waele, P., Huylebroeck, D., Verschueren, K. & van den Eijnden-van Raajj, A. J. M. (1996). Follistatins neutralize activin bioactivity by inhibition of activin binding to its type II receptors. *Molecular and Cellular Endocrinology*, **116**, 105–14.

Dolci, S., Williams, D. E., Ernst, M. K., Resnick, J. L., Brannan, C. I., Fock, L. F., Lyman, S. D., Boswell, S. H. & Donovan, P. J. (1991). Requirements for mast cell growth factor for primordial germ cell survival in culture. *Nature*, **352**, 809–11.

Dolci, S., Pesce, M. & de Felici, M. (1993). Combined action of stem cell factor, leukemia inhibitory factor and cAMP on *in vitro* proliferation of mouse primordial germ cells. *Molecular Reproduction and Development*, **35**, 134–9.

Donovan, P. J. (1994). Growth factor regulation of mouse primodial germ cell development. *Current Topics in Developmental Biology*, **29**, 189–225.

Du, X., Everett, E. T., Wang, G., Lee, W.-H., Yang, Z. & Williams, D. A. (1996). Murine interleukin-11 (IL-11) is expressed at high levels in the hippocampus and expression is developmentally regulated in the testis. *Journal of Cellular Physiology*, **168**, 362–72.

Dubreuil, P., Rottapel, R., Reith, A., Forrester, L. & Bernstein, A. (1990). The mouse W/c-*kit* locus: a mammalian gene that controls the development of three distinct cell lineages. *Annals of the NY Academy of Sciences*, **599**, 58–65.

Dym, M. (1994). Basement membrane regulation of Sertoli cells. *Endocrine Reviews*, **15**(10), 102–15.

Dym, M. & Fawcett, D. W. (1970). The blood–testis barrier in the rat and the physiological compartmentation of the seminiferous epithelium. *Biology of Reproduction*, **3**, 308–26.

(1971). Further observations on the numbers of spermatogonia, spermatocytes and spermatids connected by bridges in the mammalian testis. *Biology of Reproduction*, **4**, 195–215.

Dym, M., Lamsam-Casalotti, S., Jia, M.-C., Kleinman, H. K. & Papadopoulos, V. (1991). Basement membrane increases G-protein levels and follicle-stimulating hormone responsiveness of Sertoli cell adenylyl cyclase activity. *Endocrinology*, **128**, 1167–76.

Dym, M., Jia, M.-C., Dirama, G., Price, J. M., Rabin, S. J., Mocchetti, I. & Ravindranath, N. (1995). Expression of c-*kit* receptor and its autophosphorylation in immature rat type A spermatogonia. *Biology of Reproduction*, **52**, 8–19.

Fang, J., Yin, W., Smiley, E., Wang, S. Q. & Bonadio, J. (1996). Molecular cloning of the mouse activin β_E subunit gene. *Biochemical and Biophysical Research Communications*, **228**, 669–74.

Feng, H., Sandlow, J. I. & Sandra, A. (1997). Expression and function of the c-*kit* proto-oncogene protein in mouse sperm. *Biology of Reproduction*, **57**, 194–203.

Fradin, S., Barbey, P. & Drosdowsky, M. A. (1989). *In vitro* effects of growth factors on rat germ cell RNA synthesis and their modulation by Sertoli cell-secreted proteins. *Molecular Reproduction and Development*, **1**, 122–8.

Francavilla, S., Cordeschi, G., Properzi, G., Di Cicco, L., Jannini, E. A., Palmero, S., Fugassa, E., Loras, B. & D'Armiento, M. (1991). Effect of thyroid hormone on the pre- and post-natal development of the rat testis. *Journal of Endocrinology*, **129**, 35–42.

Furuchi, T., Masuko, K., Nishimune, Y., Obinata, M. & Matsui, Y. (1996). Inhibition of testicular germ cell apoptosis and differentiation in mice misexpressing Bcl-2 in spermatogonia. *Development*, **122**, 1703–9.

Galli, S. J., Zsebo, K. M. & Geissler, E. N. (1994). The kit ligand: stem cell factor. *Advances in Immunology*, **55**, 1–96.

Garcia-Castro, M. I., Anderson, R., Heasman, J. & Wylie, C. (1997). Interactions between germ cells and extracellular matrix glycoproteins during migration and gonad assembly in the mouse embryo. *Journal of Cell Biology*, **138**, 471–80.

Gibson, L., Holmgreen, S. P., Huang, D. C. S., Bernard, O., Copeland, N. G., Jenkins, N. A., Sutherland, G. R., Baker, E., Adams, J. M. & Cory, S. (1996). bcl-w, a novel member of the bcl-2 family, promotes cell survival. *Oncogene*, **13**, 665–75.

Giuili, G., Shen, W. H. & Ingraham, H. A. (1997). The nuclear receptor SF-1 mediates sexually dimorphic expression of müllerian inhibiting substance, *in vivo*. *Development*, **124**, 1799–807.

Gnessi, L., Fabbri, A. & Spera, G. (1997). Gonadal peptides as mediators of development and functional control of the testis: an integrated system with hormones and local environment. *Endocrine Reviews*, **18**, 541–609.

Godin, I., Deed, R., Cooke, J., Zsebo, K., Dexter, M. & Wylie, C. C. (1991). Effects of the *Steel* gene product on mouse primordial germ cells in culture. *Nature*, **352**, 807–9.

Grootegoed, J. A., Peters, M. J., Mulder, E., Rommerts, F. F. G. & van der Molen, H. J. (1977). Absence of nuclear androgen receptor in isolated germinal cells of rat testis. *Molecular and Cellular Endocrinology*, **9**, 159–67.

Hacker, A., Capel, B., Goodfellow, P. & Lovell-Badge, R. (1995). Expression of Sry, the mouse sex determining gene. *Development*, **121**, 1603–14.

Hakovirta, H., Kaipia, A., Söder, O. & Parvinen, M. (1993). Effects of activin-A, inhibin-A, and transforming growth factor-β1 on stage-specific deoxyribonucleic acid syntheses during rat seminiferous epithelial cycle. *Endocrinology*, **133**, 1664–8.

Hakovirta, H., Syed, V., Jégou, B. & Parvinen, M. (1995). Function of interleukin-6 as an inhibitor of meiotic DNA synthesis in the rat seminiferous epithelium. *Molecular and Cellular Endocrinology*, **108**, 193–8.

Hockenbery, D. M., Zutter, M., Hickey, W., Nahm, M. & Korsmeyer, S. J. (1991). BCL2 protein is topographically restricted in tissues characterized by apoptotic cell death. *Proceedings of the National Academy of Sciences, USA*, **88**, 6961–5.

Hotten, G., Neidhardt, H., Schneider, C. & Pohl, J. (1995). Cloning of a new member of the TGF-β family: a putative new activin βC chain. *Biochemical and Biophysical Research Communications*, **206**, 608–13.

Huang, E., Nocka, K., Buck, J. & Besmer, P. (1992). Differential expression and processing of two cell associated forms of the kit-ligand: KL-1 and KL-2. *Molecular Biology of the Cell*, **3**, 349–62.

Ikeda, Y., Swain, A., Weber, T. J., Hentges, K. E., Zanaria, E., Lalli, E., Tamai, K. T., Sassone-Corsi, P., Lovell-Badge, R., Camerino, G. & Parker, K. L. (1996). Steroidogenic factor 1 and Dax-1 colocalize in multiple cell lineages: potential links in endocrine development. *Molecular Endocrinology*, **10**, 1261–72.

Ito, M., Yu, R. & Jameson, J. L. (1997). DAX-1 inhibits SF-1-mediated transactivation via a carboxy-terminal domain that is deleted in adrenal hypoplasia congenita. *Molecular and Cellular Biology*, **117** 1476–83.

Jégou, B. (1993). The Sertoli–germ cell communication network in mammals. *International Review of Cytology*, **147**, 25–96.

Jégou, B., Le Gac, F., Irby, D. & de Kretser, D. M. (1983). Studies on seminiferous tubule fluid production in the adult rat: effect of hypophysectomy and treatment with FSH, LH and testosterone. *International Journal of Andrology*, **6**, 249–60.

Jégou, B., Laws, A. O. & de Kretser, D. M. (1984). Changes in testicular function induced by short-term exposure of the rat testis to heat: further evidence for interaction of germ cells, Sertoli cells and Leydig cells. *International Journal of Andrology*, **7**, 244–57.

Jeske, Y. W., Bowles, J., Greenfield, A. & Koopman, P. (1995). Expression of a linear Sry transcript in the mouse genital ridge. *Nature Genetics*, **10**, 480–2.

Jost, A., Perlman, S., Valentino, O., Castanier, M., Scholler, R. & Magre, S. (1998). Experimental control of the differentiation of Leydig cells in the fetal rat testis. *Proceedings of the National Academy of Sciences, USA*, **85**, 8094–7.

Kaipia, A., Parvinen, M. & Toppari, J. (1993). Localization of activin receptor (ActR-11B) mRNA in the rat seminiferous epithelium. *Endocrinology*, **132**, 477–80.

Kawase, E., Shirayoshi, Y., Hashimoto, K. & Nakatsuji, N. (1996). A combination of buffalo rat liver cell-conditioned medium, forskolin and membrane-bound stem cell factor stimulates rapid proliferation of mouse primordial germ cells *in vitro* similar to that *in vivo*. *Development, Growth and Differentiation*, **38**, 315–22.

Kierszenbaum, A. L. (1994). Mammalian spermatogenesis *in vivo*, and *in vitro*: a partnership of spermatogenic and somatic cell lineages. *Endocrine Reviews*, **15** 116–34.

Kinashi, T. & Springer, T. (1994). Steel factor and c-*kit* regulate cell matrix adhesion. *Blood*, **83**, 1033–8.

Knudson, C. M., Tung, K. S. K., Tourtellotte, W. G., Brown, G. A. J. & Korsmeyer, S. J. (1995). Bax-deficient mice with lymphoid hyperplasia and male germ cell death. *Science*, **270**, 96–9.

Koopman, P., Gubbay, J., Vivian, N., Goodfellow, P. & Lovell-Badge, R. (1991). Male development of chromosomally female mice transgenic for Sry. *Nature*, **351**, 117–21.

Krajewski, S., Krajewski, M., Shabaik, A., Wang, H. G., Irie, S., Fong, L. & Reed, J. C. (1994). Immunohistochemical analysis of *in vivo* patterns of Bcl-X expression. *Cancer Research*, **54**, 5501–7.

Krajewski, S., Krajewska, M. & Reed, J. C. (1996). Immunohistochemical analysis of *in vivo* patterns of Bak expression, a proapoptotic member of the Bcl-2 protein family. *Cancer Research*, **56**, 2849–55.

Krummen, L. A., Moore, A., Woodruss, T. K., Covello, R., Taylor, R., Working, P. & Mather, J. P. (1994). Localization of inhibin and activin binding sites in the testis during development by *in situ* ligand binding. *Biology of Reproduction*, **50**, 734–44.

Kumar, T. R., Wang, Y., Lu, N. & Matzuk, M. (1997). Follicle stimulating hormone is required for ovarian follicle maturation but not male fertility. *Nature Genetics*, **15**, 201–4.

Le Magueresse, B. & Jégou, B. (1988*a*). Paracrine control of immature Sertoli cells by adult germ cells in the rat (an *in vitro* study). Cell–cell interactions within the testis. *Molecular and Cellular Endocrinology*, **58**, 65–72.

(1988*b*). *In vitro* effects of germ cells on the secretory activity of Sertoli cells recovered from rats of different ages. *Endocrinology*, **122**, 1672–80.

Le Magueresse, B., Pineau, C., Guillou, F. & Jégou, B. (1988). Influence of germ cells upon transferrin secretion by rat Sertoli cells *in vitro*. *Journal of Endocrinology*, **118**, R13–R16.

Li, H., Papadopoulos, V., Vidic, B., Dym, M. & Culty, M. (1997). Regulation of rat testis gonocyte proliferation by platelet-derived growth factor and estradiol: identification of signaling mechanisms involved. *Endocrinology*, **138**, 1289–98.

Loveland, K. L. & Schlatt, S. (1997). Stem cell factor and c-*kit* in the mammalian testis: lessons originating from Mother Nature's gene knockouts. *Journal of Endocrinology*, **153**, 337–44.

Loveland, K., Schlatt, S., Sasaki, T., Chu, M.-L., Timpl, R. & Dziadek, M. (1998). Developmental changes in the basement membrane of the normal and hypothyroid postnatal rat testis: segmental localization of fibulin-2 and fibronectin. *Biology of Reproduction*, **58**, 1123–30.

Maddocks, S. & Sharpe, R. M. (1990). The effects of sexual maturation and altered steroid synthesis on the production and route of secretion of inhibin-α from the rat testis. *Endocrinology*, **126**, 1541–50.

Maddocks, S., Kerr, J. B., Allenby, G. & Sharpe, R. M. (1992). Evaluation of the role of germ cells in regulating the route of secretion of immunoactive inhibin from the rat testis. *Journal of Endocrinology*, **132**, 439–48.

Magre, S. & Jost, A. (1991). Sertoli cells and testicular differentiation in the rat fetus. *Journal of Electron Microscopy Techniques*, **19**, 172–88.

Majdic, G., McNeilly, A. S., Sharpe, R. M., Evans, L. R., Groome, N. P. & Saunders, P. T. K. (1997). Testicular expression of inhibin and activin subunits and follistatin in the rat and human fetus and neonate and during postnatal development in the rat. *Endocrinology*, **138**, 2136–47.

Manova, K., Nocka, K., Besmer, P. & Bachvarova, R. F. (1990). Gonadal expression of c-*kit* encoded at the W locus of the mouse. *Development*, **110** 1057–69.

Martens, J. W. M., de Winter, J. P., Timmerman, M. A., McLuskey, A., van Schaik, R. H. N. Themmen, A. P. N. & de Jong, F. H. (1997). Inhibin interferes with activin signaling at the level of the activin receptor complex in Chinese hamster ovary cells. *Endocrinology*, **138**, 2928–36.

Mather, J. P. (1996). Follistatins and alpha 2-macroglobulin are soluble binding proteins for inhibin and activin. *Hormone Research*, **45**(3–5), 207–10.

Mather, J. P., Attie, K. M., Woodruff, T. K., Rice, G. C. & Phillips, D. M. (1990). Activin stimulates spermatogonial proliferation in germ–Sertoli cell cocultures from immature rat testis. *Endocrinology*, **127**, 3206–14.

Mather, J. P., Roberts, P. E. & Krummen, L. A. (1993). Follistatin modulates activin activity in a cell- and tissue-specific manner. *Endocrinology*, **132**, 2732–4.

Mather, J. P., Moore, A. & Rong-Hao, L. (1997). Activins, inhibins, and follistatins: further thoughts on a growing family of regulators. *Proceedings of the Society for Experimental Biology and Medicine*, **215**, 209–22.

Matsubara, N., Takahashi, Y., Nishina, Y., Mukouyama, Y., Yanagisawa, M., Watanabe, T., Nakano, T., Nomura, K., Arita, H., Nishimune, Y., Obinata, M. & Matsui, Y. (1996). A receptor tyrosine kinase, sky, and its ligand gas 6 are expressed in gonads and support primordial germ cell growth or survival in culture. *Developmental Biology*, **180**, 499–510.

Matsui, Y., Toksoz, D., Nishikawa, S., Nishikawa, S. I., Williams, D., Zsebo, K. & Hogan, B. (1991). Effect of Steel factor and leukaemia inhibitory factor on murine primordial germ cells in culture. *Nature*, **353**, 750–1.

Matsuk, M.M., Finegold, M. J., Su, J. J-G., Hsueh, A. J. W. & Bradley, A. (1992). α-Inhibin is a tumour-suppressor gene with gonadal specificty in mice. *Nature*, **360**, 313–19.

Matzuk, M. M., Kumar, T. R. & Bradley, A. (1995). Different phenotypes for mice deficient for either activins or activin receptor type II. *Nature*, **374**, 356–60.

McCoshen, J. A. & McCallion, D. J. (1975). A study of the primodial germ cells during migratory phase in steel mutant mice. *Experientia*, **31**, 589–90.

McGuiness, M. P. & Orth, J. M. (1992). Reinitiation of gonocyte mitosis and movement of gonocytes to the basement membrane in testes of newborn rats *in vivo* and *in vitro*. *Anatomical Record*, **233**, 527–37.

McLachlan, R. I., Wreford, N. G., Meachem, S. J., de Kretser, D. M. & Robertson, D. M. (1994). Effects of testosterone on spermatogenic cell populations in the adult rat. *Biology of Reproduction*, **51**, 945–55.

Meinhardt, A., O'Bryan, M. K., Mc Farlane, J. R., Loveland, K. L., Mallidis, C., Foulds, L. M., Phillips, D. J. & de Kretser, D. M. (1998). Localisation of follistatin in the rat testis. *Journal of Reproduction and Fertility*, **112**, 233–41.

Meistrich, M. L. & Kangasniemi, M. (1997). Hormone treatment after irradiation stimulates recovery of rat spermatogenesis from surviving spermatogonia. *Journal of Andrology*, **18**, 80–7.

Mintz, B. & Russell, E. S. (1957). Gene-induced embryological modifications of primordial germ cells in the mouse. *Journal of Experimental Zoology*, **134**, 207–37.

Miyashita, T. & Reed, J. C. (1995). Tumor suppressor p53 is a direct transcriptional activator of the human *bax* gene. *Cell*, **80**, 293–99.

Miyazawa, K., Williams, D. A., Gotoh, A., Nishimaki, J., Broxmeyer, H. E. & Toyama, K. (1995). Membrane bound Steel factor induces more persistent tyrosine kinase activation and longer life span c-*kit* gene-encoded protein than its soluble form. *Blood*, **85**, 641–9.

Mullaney, B. P. & Skinner, M. K. (1993). Transforming growth factor-beta 1, beta 2, and beta 3 gene expression and action during pubertal development of the seminiferous tubule: potential role at the onset of spermatogenesis. *Molecular Endocrinology*, **7**, 67–76.

Munsie, M., Schlatt, S., de Kretser, D. M. & Loveland, K. L. (1997). Expression of stem cell factor in the postnatal rat testis. *Molecular Reproduction and Development*, **47**, 19–25.

Ng, L. J., Wheatley, S., Muscat, G. E., Conway-Campbell, J., Bowles, J., Wright, E., Bell, D. M., Tam, P. P., Cheah, K. S. & Koopman, P. (1997). SOX9 binds DNA, activates transcription, and coexpresses with type II collagen during chondrogenesis in the mouse. *Developmental Biology*, **183**, 108–21.

Oda, S., Nishimatsu, S.-I., Murakami, K. & Ueno, N. (1995). Molecular cloning and functional analysis of a new activin β subunit: a dorsal mesoderm-inducing activity in *Xenopus*. *Biochemical and Biophysical Research Communications*, **210**, 581–8.

O'Donnell, L., McLachlan, R. I., Wreford, N. G. & Robertson, D. M. (1994). Testosterone promotes the conversion of round spermatids between stages VII and VIII of the rat spermatogenic cycle. *Endocrinology*, **135**, 2608–14.

O'Donnell, L., McLachlan, R. I., Wreford, N., de Kretser, D. M. & Robertson, D. M. (1996). Testosterone withdrawal promotes stage-specific detachment of round spermatids from the rat seminiferous epithelium. *Biology of Reproduction*, **55**, 895–901.

Orth, J. M. (1982). Proliferation of Sertoli cells in fetal and postnatal rats: a quantitative autoradiographic study. *Anatomical Record*, **203**, 485–92.

(1993). Cell biology of testicular development in the fetus and neonate. In *Cell and molecular biology of the testis*, ed. C. Desjardins & L. Ewing, pp. 3–42. New York: Oxford University Press.

Orth, J. M. & Jester, W. F. (1995). NCAM mediates adhesion between gonocytes and Sertoli cells in cocultures from testes of neonatal rats. *Journal of Andrology*, **16**, 389–99.

Orth, J.M., Gunsalus, G. L. & Lamperti, A. A. (1988). Evidence from Sertoli cell-depleted rats indicates that spermatid number in adults depends on numbers of Sertoli cells produced during perinatal development. *Endocrinology*, **122**, 787–94.

Orth, J. M., Jester, W. F. Jr, & Qiu, J. (1996). Gonocytes in testes of neonatal rats express the c-*kit* gene. *Molecular Reproduction and Development*, **45**, 123–31.

Orth, J. M., Qiu, J., Jester, W. F. Jr & Pilder, S. (1997). Expression of the c-*kit* gene is critical for migration of neonatal rat gonocytes *in vitro*. *Biology of Reproduction*, **57**, 676–83.

Packer, A. I., Besmer, P. & Bachvarova, R. F. (1995). Kit ligand mediates survival of type A spermatogonia and dividing spermatocytes in postnatal mouse testes. *Molecular Reproduction and Development*, **42**, 303–10.

Parker, K. L., Ikeda, Y. & Luo, X. (1996). The roles of the cell-selective nuclear receptor SF-1 in reproductive function. In *Signal transduction in testicular cells*, ed. V. Hansson, F. O. Levy & K. Tasken, pp. 1–12. Heidelberg: Springer Verlag.

Parvinen, M. (1982). Regulation of the seminferous epithelium. *Endocrine Reviews*, **3**, 404–17.

Parvinen, M., Vihko, K. K. Vihko, K. K., & Toppari, J. (1987). Cell interactions during the seminiferous epithelial cycle. *International Review of Cytology*, **104**, 115–51.

Parvinen, M., Pelto-Huikko, M., Söder, O., Schultz, R., Kaipia, A., Mali, P., Toppari, J., Hakovirta, H., Lönnerberg, P., Ritzén, E. M., Ebendal, T., Olson, L., Hökfelt, T. & Persson, H. (1992). Expression of β-nerve growth factor and its receptor in rat seminiferous epithelium: specific function at the onset of meiosis. *Journal of Cell Biology*, **117**, 629–41.

Perey, B., Clermont, Y. & Le Blond, C. P. (1961). The wave of the seminiferous epithelium in the rat. *American Journal of Anatomy*, **108**, 47–77.

Perryman, K. J., Stanton, P. G., Loveland, K. L., McLachlan, R. I. & Robertson, D. (1996). Hormonal dependency of neural cadherin in the binding of round spermatids to Sertoli cells *in vitro*. *Endocrinology*, **137**, 3877–83.

Pesce, M., Farrace, M. G., Piacentini, M., Dolci, S. & de Felici, M. (1993). Stem cell factor and leukemia inhibitory factor promote primordial germ cell survival by suppressing programmed cell death (apoptosis). *Development*, **118**, 1089–94.

Pesce, M., di Carlo, A. & de Felici, M. (1997). The c-*kit* receptor is involved in the adhesion of mouse primordial germ cells to somatic cells in culture. *Mechanisms of Development*, **68**, 37–44.

Reith, A. D. & Bernstein, A. (1991). Molecular biology of the *W* and *Steel* loci. In *Genome analysis*, vol. 3 *Genes and phenotypes* ed. R. E. Davies & S. M. Tilghman, pp. 105–31. Cold Spring Harbor, NY: Cold Spring Harbor Laboratory Press.

Rich, K. A., Kerr, J. B. & de Kretser, D. M. (1979). Evidence for Leydig cell dysfunction in rats with seminiferous tubule damage. *Molecular and Cellular Endocrinology*, **13**, 123–35.

Ritzén, E. M., Hansson, V. & French, F. S. (1989). The Sertoli cell. In *The Testis*, 2nd edn, ed. H. Burger & D. M. de Kretser, pp. 269–302. New York: Raven Press.

Rodriguez, I., Ody, C., Araki, K., Garcia, I. & Vassailli, P. (1997). An early and massive wave of germinal cell apoptosis is required for the development of functional spermatogenesis. *EMBO Journal*, **16**, 2262–70.

Rossi, P., Albanesi, C., Grimaldi, P. & Geremia, R. (1991). Expression of the mRNA for the ligand of c-*kit* in mouse Sertoli cells. *Biochemical and Biophysical Research Communications*, **176**, 910–14.

Rossi, P., Marziali, G., Alanesi, C., Charlesworth, A., Geremia, R. & Sorrentino, V. (1992). A novel c-*kit* transcript, potentially encoding a truncated receptor, originates within a *kit* gene intron in mouse spermatids. *Developmental Biology*, **152**, 203–7.

Rossi, P., Dolci, S., Albanesi, C., Grimaldi, P., Ricca, R. & Geremia, R. (1993). Follicle-stimulating hormone induction of steel factor (SLF) mRNA in mouse Sertoli cells and stimulation of DNA synthesis in spermatogonia by soluble SLF. *Developmental Biology*, **155**, 68–74.

Rotter, V., Schwartz, D., Almon, E., Goldfinger, N., Kapon, A., Meshover, A., Donehower, L. A. & Levine, A. J. (1993). Mice with reduced levels of p53 protein exhibit the testicular giant-cell degenerative syndrome. *Proceedings of the National Academy of Sciences, USA*, **90**, 9075–9.

Sanborn, B. M., Steinberger, A., Tcholakian, R. K. & Steinberger, E. (1977). Direct measurement of androgen receptors in cultured Sertoli cells. *Steroids*, **29**, 493–502.

Sandlow, J. I., Feng, H.-L. & Sandra, A. (1997). Localization and expression of the c-*kit* receptor protein in human and rodent testis and sperm. *Urology*, **49**, 494–500.

Schwartzman, R. A. & Cidlowski, J. A. (1993). Apoptosis: the biochemistry and molecular biology of programmed cell death. *Endocrine Reviews*, **14**, 133–51.

Sette, C., Bevilacqua, A., Bianchini, A., Mangia, F., Geremia, R. & Rossi, P. (1997). Parthenogenetic activation of mouse eggs by microinjection of a truncated c-*kit* tyrosine kinase present in spermatozoa. *Development*, **124**, 2267–74.

Sharpe, R. M. (1994). Regulation of spermatogenesis. In *Physiology of reproduction*, vol. 1, ed. E. Knobil, pp. 1363–434. New York: Raven Press.

Sicinski, P., Donaher, J. L., Geng, Y., Parker, S. B., Gardner, H., Park, M. Y., Robker, R. L., Richards, J. S., McGinnis, L. K., Biggers, J. D., Eppig, J. J., Bronson, R.

T., Elledge, S. J. & Weinberg, R. A. (1996). Cyclin D2 is an FSH-responsive gene involved in gonadal cell proliferation and oncogenesis. *Nature*, **384**, 470–4.

Silvers, W. K. (1979). Dominant spotting, Patch and Rump-white. In *Coat colours of mice*, pp. 106–332. New York: Springer-Verlag.

Simorangkir, D. R., de Kretser, D. M. & Wreford, N. G. (1995). Increased numbers of Sertoli and germ cells in adult rat testes induced by synergistic action of transient neonatal hypothyroidism and neonatal hemicastration. *Journal of Reproduction and Fertility*, **104**, 207–13.

Singh, J., O'Neill, C. & Handelsman, D. J. (1995). Induction of spermatogenesis by androgens in gonadotrophin deficient (hpg) mice. *Endocrinology*, **136**, 5311–21.

Skinner, M. K., Fetterolf, P. M. & Anthony, C. T. (1988). Purification of a paracrine factor, P-Mod-S, produced by testicular peritubular cells that modulates Sertoli cell function. *Journal of Biology Chemistry*, **25**, 2884–90.

Skinner, M. K., McLachlan, R. I. & Bremner, W. J. (1989). Stimulation of Sertoli cell inhibin secretion by the testicular paracrine factor PModS. *Molecular and Cellular Endocrinology*, **66**, 239–49.

Sun, Y. T., Irby, D. C., Robertson, D. M. & de Kretser, D. M. (1989). The effects of exogenously administered testosterone on spermatogenesis in intact and hypophysectomized rats. *Endocrinology*, **125**, 1000–10.

Sun, Y. T., Wreford, N. G., Robertson, D. M. & de Kretser, D. M. (1990). Quantitative cytological studies of spermatogenesis in intact hypophysec-tomized rats: identification of androgen-dependent stages. *Endocrinology*, **127**, 1215–23.

Syed, V., Gerard, N., Kaipia, A., Bardin, C. W., Parvinen, M. & Jégou, B. (1993). Identification, ontogeny, and regulation of an interleukin-6-like factor in the rat seminiferous tubule. *Endocrinology*, **132**, 293–99.

Tajima, Y., Koshimizu, U., Jippo, T., Kitamura, Y. & Nishimune, Y. (1993). Effects of hormones, cyclic AMP analogues and growth factors on steel factor (SF) production in mouse Sertoli cell cultures. *Journal of Reproduction and Fertility*, **99**, 571–5.

Tajima, Y., Sawade, K., Morimoto, T. & Nishimune, Y. (1994). Switching of mouse spermatogonial proliferation from the c-*kit* receptor-independent type to the receptor-dependent type during differentiation. *Journal of Reproduction and Fertility*, **102**, 117–22.

Tajima, Y., Watanabe, D., Koshimizu, U., Matsuzawa, T. & Nishimune, Y. (1995). Insulin-like growth factor-1 and transforming growth factor-α stimulate differentiation of type A spermatogonia in organ culture of adult mouse cryptorchid testes. *International Journal of Andrology*, **18**, 8–12.

Tapanainen, J. S., Aittomaki, K., Min, J., Vaskvimo, T. & Huhtaniemi, I. (1997). Men homozygous for an inactivating mutation of the follicle stimulating hormone (FSH) receptor gene present variable suppression of spermato-genesis and fertility. *Nature Genetics*, **15**, 205–6.

Teerds, K. J. & Dorrington, J. H. (1993). Localization of transforming growth factor beta 1 and beta 2 during testicular development in the rat. *Biology of Reproduction*, **48**, 40–5.

Torney, A. H., Robertson, D. M. & de Kretser, D. M. (1992). Characterization of inhibin and related proteins in bovine fetal testicular and ovarian extracts: evidence for the presence of inhibin subunit products and FSH-suppressing protein. *Journal of Endocrinology*, **133**, 111–20.

van Dissel-Emiliani, F. M. F., Grootenhuis, A. J., de Jong, F. H. & Rooij, D. G. (1989). Inhibin reduces spermatogonial numbers in testes of adult mice and Chinese hamsters. *Endocrinology*, **125**, 1899–903.

van Dissel-Emiliani, F. M. F., de Boer-Brouwer, M. & de Rooij, D. G. (1996). Effect of fibroblast growth factor-2 on Sertoli cells and gonocytes in coculture during the perinatal period. *Endocrinology*, **137**, 647–54.

Van Haaster, L. H., de Jong, F. H., Docter, R. & de Rooij, D. G. (1992). The effect of hypothyroidism on Sertoli cell proliferation and differentiation and hormone levels during testicular development in the rat. *Endocrinology*, **131**, 1574–6.

Vaughn, J. M. & Vale, W. W. (1993). α2-Macroglobulin is a binding protein of activin and inhibin. *Endocrinology*, **132**, 2038–50.

Ying, S.-Y., Zhang, Z., Burst, B., Batres, Y., Huang, G. & Li, G. (1997). Activins and activin receptors in cell growth. *Proceedings of the Society for Experimental Biology and Medicine*, **214**, 114–12.

Yoshinaga, K., Nishikawa, S., Ogawa, M., Hayashi, S., Kunisada, T., Fujimoto, T. & Nishikawa, S. (1991). Role of c-*kit* in mouse spermatogenesis: identification of spermatogonia as a specific site of c-*kit* expression and function. *Development*, **113**, 689–99.

Zhao, G.-Q. & Hogan, B. L. M. (1996). Evidence that mouse *bmp8a* (*Op2*) and *bmp8b* are duplicated genes that play a role in spermatogenesis and placental development. *Mechanisms of Development*, **57**, 159–68.

Zhao, G.-Q., Deng, K., Labosky, P. A., Liaw, L. & Hogan, B. L. M. (1996). The gene encoding bone morphogenetic protein 8B is required for the initiation and maintenance of spermatogenesis in the mouse. *Genes and Development*, **10**, 1657–69.

Zhou, B., Watts, L. M. & Hutson, J. M. (1993). Germ cell development in neonatal mouse testes *in vitro* requires müllerian inhibiting substance. *Journal of Urology*, **150**, 613–16.

Zhu, L. J., Cheng, C. Y., Phillips, D. M. & Bardin, C. W. (1994). The immunohistochemical localization of alpha 2-macroglobulin in rat testis is consistent with its role in germ cell movement and spermiation. *Journal of Andrology*, **15**, 575–82.

Note added in proof:
Deletion of *bcl-w* disrupts spermatogenesis after the first wave has established apparently normal testis function (A. J. Ross *et al.* (1998), *Nature Genetics*, **18**, 251–6; C. G. Print *et al.* (1998), *Proceedings of the National Academy of Sciences* (in press)).

5   Some misconceptions of the human epididymis

ROY JONES

Introduction

The mammalian epididymis is part of the system of male accessory sex glands whose secretions constitute ejaculated seminal plasma (Mann & Lutwack-Mann, 1981). Unlike the other accessory glands, however, the epididymis is intimately involved with the development of spermatozoa from the moment they leave the testis to the point when they are ejaculated and deposited in the female tract. The basis for this statement is the large number of investigations carried out over many years on a wide variety of species, beginning with the pioneering experimental studies of Young (1929, 1931) on guinea pigs, which have enabled some basic principles to be established (Cooper, 1986; Orgebin-Crist, 1987). The molecular details of precisely how an infertile testicular spermatozoon is transformed into a fully fertile one in the epididymis are only slowly being unravelled and it is still not possible to pin-point any particular process or molecular component and say unequivocally that this is the crucial difference between fertility and infertility. The factors involved are almost certainly complex and interactive but there are enough experimental data to indicate that they exist and that the epididymis has an important regulatory role to play.

Despite the evidence alluded to above, and described in more detail below, a notion has arisen in recent years that in man the epididymis is relatively non-functional. This view seems to be based on a failure to appreciate the variation in the structure and physiology of the epididymis between different species and reflects an overreliance on clinical data derived from reports of congenital malformations (e.g. absence of the vas deferens) or unusual aberrant conditions (e.g. blockage of the epididymal duct through injury or infection). This chapter attempts to provide an understanding of why some of these misconceptions have arisen and to explain why concepts developed in animal models still apply to the human epididymis.

Comparative morphology and physiology of the mammalian epididymis

In all mammalian species the epididymis consists of a single highly convoluted duct that varies in length from approx. 6 m in rats (Jiang *et al.*, 1994) to over 40 m in large domestic animals such as the bull, boar and ram (Bishop, 1961). In man the length has been estimated as 6–7 m although the source of this observation is rarely, if at all, quoted. However, it is not an unreasonable figure given the gross size and morphology of the human epididymis. Despite these substantial differences in length, estimates of the time of sperm transit through the epididymis from efferent ductules to the vas deferens consistently give figures of between 8 and 12 days in most species (Robaire & Hermio, 1988). This implies that, in those species with a very long epididymis (e.g. boar), peristaltic activity of the smooth musculature surrounding the duct must be greater than in those with a shorter duct (e.g. rat). However, other relevant variables are the viscosity of the fluid (which in the rat is very high and may impede intraluminal flow) and the extent to which spermatozoa are refluxed back and forth within different sections of the duct. This refluxing would obviously delay sperm passage but it may have an important function in facilitating mixing of spermatozoa to ensure that they all gain access to newly secreted glycoproteins from the epithelium. Intraluminal flow rates have been measured in the rat epididymis and are faster in the caput (18.5–32 mm/h) than in the cauda (2.5–13 mm/h) (Jaakkola, 1983; Turner *et al.*, 1990). In each of these studies oscillatory movements of oil droplets injected into the lumen of the duct were observed, supporting the idea of reflux mixing. In the human, estimates of sperm transit time through the epididymis vary from 1 to 12 days (Rowley *et al.*, 1970; Amann & Howards, 1980; Johnson & Varner, 1988). This range is due largely to the obvious difficulties of obtaining normal human material and having to rely on indirect methods of estimation but suggests, at the very least, that some spermatozoa may pass through the epididymis very rapidly, resulting in considerable heterogeneity in the cauda/vas deferens with respect to age.

Whether 'fast-moving' spermatozoa are fully mature and fertile is not known but the phenomenon raises questions about the overall morphology and organization of the human epididymal duct. In the human, the part of the epididymis that overlies the dorsal pole of the testis (and which in other species would be called the initial segment and the proximal caput) actually consists of an extensive network of efferent ductules (Holstein, 1969; Yeung *et al.*, 1991; Fig. 5.1). As a consequence, the initial segment and areas equivalent to the caput and the corpus extend along the lateral aspect of the testis and, superficially at least, are indistinguishable from each other.

A second noteworthy feature of the human epididymis is that the cauda region does not have the characteristic bulbous appearance it assumes in most animal species. Instead, the duct in the distal regions gradually increases in width until it becomes part of the vas deferens (sometimes referred to as the epididymal vas). This departure from the usual arrangement typified by the rat has somehow given rise to the view that the human epididymis is exceptional and that this arrangement is incompatible with concepts of sperm maturation and storage derived from animal models. In fact, it merely represents a variation on a general theme. A precedent for such variation is found in the guinea pig, in which the efferent ductules are very short and the initial segment of the epididymis becomes so attenuated that it overlies the whole dorsal and lateral aspects of the testis (Glover & Nicander, 1971; Hoffer & Greenberg, 1978). The regions equivalent to caput, corpus and cauda are, in turn, foreshortened into the bulbous area at the ventral pole of the testis and the proximal vas deferens becomes a major site for sperm storage. Although this peculiar morphology of the guinea pig epididymis was described in detail some time ago, it appears to have escaped widespread attention.

Explanations for apparent redundancy of the human epididymis in sperm maturation

Appreciation of species variation in morphology of the epididymis described above is important in the light of recent reports that human spermatozoa removed directly from the testis, or that have passed through only a very short segment of the epididymis, are fertile (Silber, 1980, 1988, 1989; Schoysman & Bedford, 1986; Schoysman, 1993). (It should be emphasized at the onset that this review does not refer to intracytoplasmic sperm injection (ICSI) techniques but only when the fertilizing capacity of the spermatozoa has been tested by *in vitro* fertilization, insemination or natural mating.)

Fig. 5.1. Comparative morphology of the mammalian epididymis. Schematic drawings (not to scale) of the testis and epididymis from rat, guinea pig and human to illustrate differences in the relative extent of the efferent ductules (ED, arrows), initial segment region (stippled) and cauda epididymidis/vas deferens (hatched). T, testis; VD, vas deferens. Drawings are based on photographs in publications by Hamilton (1975), Hoffer & Greenberg (1978), Holstein (1969) and Bedford (1994).

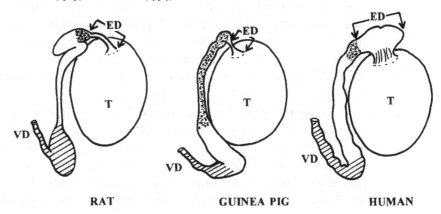

RAT   GUINEA PIG   HUMAN

This view is based largely on attempts to restore fertility in patients suffering from congenital absence of the vas deferens or a long-term blockage of the epididymal duct. The technique of epididymovasostomy, in which the vas deferens is reconnected to the epididymis above the blockage site, has been utilized by clinicians for approximately 40 years, with varying degrees of success. In a recent study involving over 100 such individuals, Schoysman & Bedford (1986) reported that it was possible to obtain approx. 40% pregnancies when the vas deferens was anastomosed to a site 10 mm or further away from 'the proximal border of the caput'. This implies that spermatozoa only have to pass through the efferent ductules, and possibly a very short region of the initial segment, to become fertile. The authors emphasized, however, that the further distal the site of anastomosis then the greater the incidence of pregnancy. Subsequently, Silber (1988, 1989; Silber *et al.*, 1990) reported that spermatozoa aspirated from the efferent ductules of patients with congenital absence of the vas deferens could fertilize eggs *in vitro* and give an approximately 31% pregnancy rate. Together these observations seemed to cast doubt on the entrenched belief, established from work on animal models, that it is obligatory for spermatozoa to pass through the caput and corpus epididymidis in order to acquire their fertilizing capacity and that this process is regulated by specific secretions and/or the general intraluminal milieu created by the principal cells lining the duct.

Although the above results are important from the clinical standpoint of correcting infertility, there is currently an unfortunate trend for them to be overinterpreted. A major problem is the validity of using an epididymis (and testis) that has been subjected to very long-term obstruction, either from birth or for 10–30 years postpuberty, for predicting the physiology of the 'normal' condition. The first point of concern is the response of the epididymis to blockage and the extent to which spermatozoa and luminal fluid are refluxed in a proximal direction (i.e. towards the testis) from the site of obstruction. It is known from experiments in animals that a ligature placed on the corpus epididymidis rapidly causes distention of the duct above it and eventually swelling of the testis due to back pressure from accumulation of spermatozoa (Bedford, 1967; Glover, 1969). In rabbits subjected to this experiment, the fertilization rate of spermatozoa removed from the caput flexure 4 days after ligation was > 80% whereas in the contralateral control it remained < 5%. Thus, even with these acute experiments it is possible to create a situation where spermatozoa mature without physically passing through the corpus and cauda regions.

It is not known to what extent retrograde mixing of luminal contents takes place above the site of obstruction but there are indications that it can become significant over long periods of time. In the author's laboratory ram epididymides collected from abattoirs have occasionally been found to contain obstructions. In two particular cases a calcified nodule was present within the duct in the cauda epididymidis and clearly had been in place for several years. Granulomata had not formed. Spermatozoa were absent distal to the nodule but above it the epididymal duct was distended with fluid and contained large numbers of spermatozoa. The back pressure had extended as far as the testis so that when the efferent doctules were punctured, copious quantities of a viscous, yellowish fluid emerged containing large numbers of motile spermatozoa reminiscent of those from the cauda epididymidis of a normal animal. Furthermore, this 'testicular' fluid contained high concentrations of epididymal-specific secretory products such as carnitine and glycerylphosphorylcholine (R. Jones, unpublished observations). In a bull with unilateral congenital absence of the cauda epididymidis, motile spermatozoa with distal cytoplasmic droplets were present in testicular fluid, several millilitres of which flowed readily out of the rete testis without the application of external pressure. The contralateral side, in contrast, was normal, with immotile testicular spermatozoa carrying proximal cytoplasmic droplets. Thus, in experimentally induced and spontaneous cases of epididymal obstruction there is evidence that the physiological pattern of sperm development becomes so distorted that it is impossible to extrapolate from it to the situation in the normal epididymis. This, however, is what appears to have been done for the human.

A second point of concern is the misconception that all epididymal secretory products are completely region specific and that spermatozoa are exposed to them only if they pass through that particular area. It is more accurate to say that they are preferentially region specific rather than exclusively region specific. Northern blot analysis and sensitive reverse transcriptase – polymerase chain reaction (RT-PCR) assays show that approx. 50% of known epididymal glycoproteins are synthesized in low levels throughout the duct, although they are quantitatively more abundant in some regions than others (Cornwall & Hann, 1995; Syntin *et al.*, 1996). Interaction of many of these glycoproteins with the plasma membrane of spermatozoa is important for maturation (Jones, 1989) but it is not clear just how much (in terms of numbers of molecules) is quantitatively necessary. In an obstructed epididymis, even a low rate of secretion would allow glycoproteins to accumulate within the lumen over time and, once the critical amount on spermatozoa had been reached, the appropriate change in functionality would be induced. In this way spermatozoa in the efferent ductules and initial segment would gradually be exposed to a luminal environment more and more like that in the normal caput/corpus and consequently acquire a degree of fertility, thereby creating the impression that they have achieved this state without intervention from the epididymis.

A third factor is a change in the functionality of the human vas deferens following epididymovasostomy. In animal models such as the rabbit, the vas deferens has been shown to sustain the same luminal environment established earlier in the cauda, even under extreme conditions such as vasectomy when there is considerable distension of the duct (Jones, 1973). Given the size and extent of the epididymal vas in the human (Hoffer, 1976), it has a possible role as a site of sperm storage. The persistence of low amounts of carnitine and glycerylphosphorylcholine (classic markers of epididymal functionality) in human semen after long-term vasectomy suggests that the vas deferens is able to behave like the epididymis to a limited degree (Frenkel et al., 1974). This means that when anastomosed to the initial segment or efferent ductules, the vas would be able to absorb fluid, sodium and chloride ions, and secrete potassium, glycoproteins etc., especially if it came under the influence of factors in testicular fluid (see below). It is not inconceivable, therefore, that following epididymovasostomy the vas deferens could gradually assume some of the functions of the proximal regions of the epididymis and eventually provide a luminal microenvironment conducive to the maturation of spermatozoa. It has been suggested that this may be one of the reasons for the delay (1–2 years) in restoration of fertility following this operation (Cooper, 1990).

Current concepts of epididymal function in animal models and their applicability to the human epididymis

The role of the epididymis in the post-testicular development of spermatozoa has traditionally centred on three main functions. First, it absorbs testicular fluid and concentrates spermatozoa after they leave the testis. Secondly, it creates a specialized milieu or microenvironment within the lumen of the duct that is conducive to the development of motility and fertilizing capacity. Thirdly, it stores spermatozoa in a viable form before they are ejaculated. In the remainder of this chapter, current concepts on these areas will be reviewed and discussed in relation to the human epididymis.

Function of the initial segment in absorbing testicular fluid

The normal adult testis in the males of most species (ram, bull, boar, rat, rabbit and monkey) secretes a watery fluid containing between 10^7 and 10^8 spermatozoa/ml at a rate of 10–20 μl/g per h as measured by direct catheterization of the extratesticular rete testis (Setchell, 1978). In a rat this translates into approx. 240–480 μl/day and for a ram as much as approx. 140 ml/day. Clearly, this volume of fluid is not sustainable in the reproductive tract and from measurements of spermatocrits (packed cell volume) in luminal fluid collected by micropuncture from different levels of the duct it has been estimated that >95% of the fluid is reabsorbed in the efferent ductules and initial segment (Crabo, 1965: Levine & Marsh, 1971). Correspondingly, the principal cells lining the initial segment show extensive pinocytotic activity and accumulation of large multivesicular bodies in the apical cytoplasm, and they readily take up electron-dense particles introduced experimentally into the seminiferous tubules (Nicander, 1965;

Hamilton, 1975; Jones *et al.*, 1979). The flow rate of fluid from the normal human rete testis is not known but in macaque monkeys (which have a testis size comparable to that of man; approx. 15–20 g) it has been measured at 5–10 μl/g per h or approx. 2.4–4.8 ml/day (Waites & Einer-Jensen, 1974). In man, histological and ultrastructural analyses of the efferent ductules and initial segment region again show a concentrating effect on spermatozoa in the lumen coincident with extensive pinocytotic activity in the epithelial cells lining the duct, all features consistent with rapid fluid uptake (Holstein, 1969; Yeung *et al.*, 1991). It is reasonable to presume, therefore, that the efferent ductules and initial segment in the normal human epididymis function to absorb testicular fluid in a manner very similar to that in animal models.

There are also long-standing observations that factors in testicular fluid are required for the functionality of the initial segment and hence indirectly affect sperm maturation. Various secretory products of Sertoli cells (e.g. inhibin, androgen-binding protein, growth factors) are reabsorbed in the initial segment and are thought to be important, since occlusion of the efferent ductules by ligatures causes atrophy of the lining epithelium that cannot be reversed by exogenous androgens (Fawcett & Hoffer, 1979). It can be argued that such a response is to be expected if there is no fluid to absorb. However, there is now evidence that synthesis of several proteins in the initial segment and proximal caput epididymidis is stimulated specifically by factors in testicular fluid. In rats and mice, synthesis of 23 kDa and 27 kDa proteins, respectively, disappear following efferent ductule ligation, whereas major androgen-dependent proteins are relatively unaffected (Jones *et al.*, 1980; Holland *et al.*, 1992). Similarly, mRNAs encoding CRES and proenkephalin genes in the mouse caput epididymidis decrease to undetectable levels following castration and are not restored by testosterone replacement (Garrett *et al.*, 1990; Cornwall *et al.*, 1992).

Besides this stimulatory response, an inhibitory effect of testicular fluid on gene expression is apparent from studies on expression of a-*raf* oncogene (Winer & Wolgemuth, 1995). In the normal animal a-*raf* is not expressed in the initial segment, although it is present in the proximal and distal caput regions. Following efferent ductule ligation, however, a-*raf* expression suddenly appears in the principal cells of the initial segment, indicating that its synthesis is normally suppressed. Precisely what components of testicular fluid are responsible for these effects are not known. Perhaps the most direct demonstration of the importance of the initial segment region is provided by recent work with transgenic mice carrying a null mutation for c-*ros*, an oncogene encoding a tyrosine kinase receptor protein (Sonneberg-Reithmacher *et al.*, 1996). Males that are homozygous for this condition were sterile, not because of any defect in spermatogenesis or sperm motility, but because the initial segment failed to differentiate during neonatal development. For reasons that are as yet unknown, absence of the initial segment adversely affected sperm transport in the female reproductive tract, suggesting that exposure of spermatozoa to the epididymal microenvironment is important for subsequent developmental processes that occur in the female. Probably more than anything else, this single unexpected result highlights the importance of signalling processes between the epididymal epithelium and the spermatozoa. Together, these findings suggest that oncogene expression is involved in regulating signalling pathways within the principal cells of the initial segment and that these signals are ultimately translated to spermatozoa in the lumen of the duct. There are, as yet, no studies on c-*ros* or a-*raf* expression in the initial segment of the human epididymis but given the morphological similarity to its counterpart in animal models, it is to be expected that these oncogenes will be regulated in a comparable fashion and that passage of spermatozoa through the initial segment will be crucial for their ability to react to the female reproductive tract.

Sperm maturation in animal models and evidence for the phenomenon in the human epididymis

The debate over whether maturation is intrinsic to spermatozoa or whether the epididymis actively induces it, is overwhelmingly in favour of the latter, although details of the mechanisms involved remain frustratingly elusive. In animal models for which there are comparable data (rat, mouse, hamster, rabbit, boar), the two most widely used criteria for assessing the maturation status of a spermatozoon are progressive motility *in vitro* and fertilizing capacity. In all the aforementioned species, it is well established that these parameters are low in the initial segment and caput regions but increase rapidly by the time the spermatozoa reach the distal corpus epididymidis (summarized by Turner, 1995). Although the data for the human are less clear cut, there is acceptable evidence that a similar situation prevails. In epididymides collected from men aged 61–77 years who were undergoing surgery for prostatic carcinoma, but were otherwise untreated, the percentage motility and straight-line velocity of spermatozoa increased progressively from the efferent ductules to the corpus region (Yeung *et al.*, 1993). Paradoxically, it then decreased slightly in the cauda/vas deferens regions, probably because of the age-related heterogeneity of the stored sperm. In another report using the zona-free hamster egg penetration test, there was an increase in the incidence of sperm binding from 0% in the initial segment/proximal caput to approx. 60% in the cauda/vas deferens (Moore *et al.*, 1992). This is strongly indicative of a progressive increase in their fertilizing capacity with transport through the duct, and, allowing for the slightly unusual nature of the material (age, etc.), these results are entirely consistent with the situation found in animals.

Aside from these functional tests, human spermatozoa in the epididymis also conform with several other indirect assays that have been developed in animal models to assess *in vitro* the degree of sperm maturation. These include an increase in the −S–S–dependent stability of the nucleoprotein, migration of the cytoplasmic droplet from the neck to the principal piece of the tail and an increase in net negative charge as revealed by binding of cationic ferritin (Bedford *et al.*, 1973).

Secretion of glycoproteins by the epididymis and regulation of their synthesis by androgens have been areas of interest for many years. A considerable number of these secreted glycoproteins interact with spermatozoa and form part of the phenomenon of maturation antigens (i.e. antigens that are acquired during passage through the epididymis and are not present on testicular spermatozoa), which has been described using antibody probes. In theory, these new antigenic determinants may arise from uptake of epididymal secretory glycoproteins, modification and processing of pre-existing proteins, conformational changes brought about by migration to new surface domains or a combination of all three. The net result is that extensive remodelling of the plasma membrane takes place concomitantly with acquisition of fertilizing capacity (Jones, 1989). Many epididymal glycoproteins have now been sequenced and some of their homologues described in the human epididymis (Table 5.1). Although putative functions can be predicted for many of them, based on similarity to known sequences in data bases, this has been demonstrated on relatively few occasions. Two exceptions are retinoic acid binding protein MEP10 and superoxide dismutase (Rankin *et al.*, 1992; Perry *et al.*, 1993a).

As mentioned earlier, the expression of many of these glycoproteins is preferentially, rather than absolutely region specific. Region-specific expression, usually in response to androgens, suggests regulation at the level of the gene by transcription factors or specific DNA *cis*-regulatory elements. In this respect it is of interest that PEA3 response elements have been described for epididymal glutathione peroxidase (Ghyselinck *et al.*, 1993) and *cis*-regulatory DNA for proenkephalin genes (Borsook *et al.*, 1992). The synthesis, secretion and binding of HE5 (CD52) to human spermatozoa is typical of many maturation antigens that originate in the epididymis (Hale *et al.*, 1993; Kirchhoff, 1996; Yeung *et al.*, 1997). An intriguing aspect of these 'coating' antigens is that they frequently bind to a restricted region on the sperm surface rather than non-specifically all over the plasma membrane. This implies an asymmetric distribution of intrinsic 'receptors' or some special property of the antigen itself that leads to its incorporation into one domain and not another. As far as current concepts go on this topic, therefore, the human epididymis does not appear to be any different from that in other animal species.

Sperm storage in the epididymis

In most animals, approx. 60% of extragonadal sperm reserves are found in the cauda epididymidis (Amann, 1981). When cauda epididymidal sperm numbers are expressed as a ratio to the daily sperm production

Table 5.1. Epididymal glycoproteins identified and sequenced in animal models and their human homologues

Ref.	Epididymal glycoprotein	Putative activity	Species	Human homologue
1	AEG/DE	Carboxypeptidase Y	Rat	ARP/CRISP-1
2	BC/MEP10	Retinol binding	Rat/mouse	—
3	EAP-1	ADAM/MDC family	Rat	—
4	PBP/MEP9	Phospholipid-binding	Rat/monkey/mouse	—
5	GPX	Glutathione peroxidase	Rat/monkey	—
6	SOD	Superoxide dismutase	Rat/monkey	—
7	CDw52	Complement lysis	Rat	CAMPATH1/HE5
8	pmE-ATI	Acrosin inhibitor	Monkey	HUSI-II/HE4
9	ESP14.6	Cholesterol binding	Monkey	HE1
10	Clusterin/SG-2	Cell aggregation/apoptosis	Many	Clusterin
11	CRES	Cystatin-related	Mouse	—
12	GGT	γ-Glutamyl transpeptidase	Rat	—
13	OPN	Osteopontin	Rat	—
14	PEM	Transcription factor	Rat	—
15	PEA-3	Transcription factor	Mouse	—
16	PAX-2	Transcription factor	Mouse	—
17	A-raf	Serine/threonine kinase	Mouse	—

References: (1) Lea *et al.* (1978); Jones *et al.* 1980; Brooks *et al.* (1987); Hayashi *et al.* (1996). (2) Brooks *et al.* (1987); Rankin *et al.* (1992). (3) Perry *et al.* (1992*b*). (4) Perry *et al.* (1994); Vierula *et al.* (1992). (5) Perry *et al.* (1992*c*); Ghyselinck *et al.* (1993). (6) Perry *et al.* (1993*a*). (7) Perry *et al.* (1992*a*); Hale *et al.* (1993); Kirchhoff *et al.* (1993). (8) Kirchhoff *et al.* (1991); Moritz *et al.* (1991); Perry *et al.* (1993*b*). (9) Krull *et al.* (1993); Perry *et al.* (1995). (10) Sylvester *et al.* (1991); O'Bryan *et al.* (1994). (11) Cornwall *et al.* (1992). (12) Palladino *et al.* (1994). (13) Siiteri *et al.* (1995). (14) Lindsey & Wilkinson (1996). (15) Wasylyk *et al.* (1989). (16) Fickenscher *et al.* (1993). (17) Winer & Wolgemuth (1995).

(estimated from quantitative testicular histology), values vary between 13.0 in the ram to 5.0 in the rat (Amann, 1981). In contrast, the ratio for the human is only 3.0 (Bedford, 1994), meaning that the relative proportion of epididymal sperm stored in the cauda region is much less. This is consistent with the gross morphological appearance of the human epididymis, which lacks the bulbous cauda characteristic of most other animal species. Instead, the human vas deferens and ampulla appear to constitute a storage area, a prediction supported by the data of Freund & Davis (1969), who found that semen from healthy men collected soon after vasectomy, contained about half the number of spermatozoa in pre-vasectomy ejaculates from the same individuals. In animals, the vas deferens actively maintains the same luminal environment established earlier in the proximal cauda in terms of ionic composition, pH, etc., and is, therefore, a legitimate storage area. Indeed, in some species, typified by the rabbit, the vas deferens is very resistant to rupture following vasectomy and the composition of the luminal fluid remains remarkably stable over long periods of time, despite distention of the duct and accumulation of large numbers of dead spermatozoa (Jones, 1973). This suggests that, as long as the testis is producing adequate amounts of androgens, the epididymis retains some capacity to maintain functional activity and to accommodate a variety of insults. In the androgen-stimulated animal, spermatozoa can survive in a fertile state in the isolated cauda epididymidis for remarkably long periods of time (28 days in rabbits, Tesh & Glover, 1969; 10–14 days in mice, Snell, 1933; 18–21 days in hamsters, Lubicz-Nawrocki & Glover, 1973). They do not, of course, survive indefinitely and it is common to find that sexual abstinence lowers the quality of the ejaculate (although overall fertility may be maintained). This is because spermatozoa naturally age and degenerate and large numbers of dead and effete spermatozoa accumulate in the distal vas deferens of sexually rested animals. Regular, periodic ejaculation nearly always improves the quality of spermatozoa by reducing the time they spend in the cauda. This is also true in humans (Bedford, 1994). An ejaculate from a normal man preceded by 6 weeks of abstinence contained <10% motile spermatozoa but in an ejaculate from the same individual 3 days later the proportion had increased to approx. 45%.

The longevity of human spermatozoa in the cauda/vas deferens is not known to the same level of accuracy as in other animal models. Like many other aspects of human epididymal physiology, opinions are frequently formed on the basis of anecdotal evidence and/or poorly controlled experiments. Much has been written about the role of the epididymal microenvironment in sperm survival yet the crucial factors involved have still not been identified. Recent attention has centred on the need to prevent lipid peroxidation initiated by oxygen free radicals and the role of superoxide dismutase (SOD) and glutathione peroxidase (GPX) as anti-oxidants (Storey, 1995; Aitken, 1997). Hydrogen peroxide, produced as a consequence of superoxide dismutation, is well known to be spermicidal but, provided reduced glutathione (GSH) is present hydrogen peroxide is destroyed by glutathione peroxidase. Extracellular SOD, GPX and GSH have been detected in rat cauda epididymal plasma (CEP) and epididymal cytosols (Ghyselinck *et al.*, 1991; Perry *et al.*, 1992*c*, 1993*a*; Hinton *et al.*, 1996), along with GSH-regenerating enzymes such as glutathione reductase and γ-glutamyl transpeptidase (Hinton *et al.*, 1996). Given that GPX, SOD and GSH are also present intracellularly in spermatozoa, there should be adequate protection against free radicals. However, this does not seem to be the case in sperm granulomata that form after blockage of the epididymis. In four rams that had been vasectomized for 4–5 years and contained large granulomata on the vas deferens and cauda epididymidis, we detected very high levels of lipid peroxides (R. Jones *et al.*, unpublished observations). Such a consequence can only reflect inadequate anti-oxidant activity that may exacerbate the difficulties of vasectomy reversal and re-establishment of a patent duct.

Bedford (1994) has drawn attention to the adverse effects of heat on

increasing sperm transport through the cauda epididymidis using the cryptepididymal rat model. Like the testis, epididymal temperature in scrotal
mammals is between 30 °C and 33 °C. Elevating the temperature to 37 °C
reduces survival time of rabbit spermatozoa in the isolated cauda region
(Cummins & Glover, 1970) with an associated disturbance, albeit not
drastic, in the composition of the luminal fluid (Jones, 1974). Since these
effects were acute (and therefore unlikely to be related to disruption of spermatogenesis), it indicates that temperature either had a direct effect on spermatozoa or else it perturbed some aspect of epididymal functionality crucial
for preserving spermatozoa in a quiescent state. In support of the former
possibility, it has been shown that for a reduction in temperature from 37 °C
to 30 °C, the respiratory rate of spermatozoa (mouse, rat, bull) declines by a
factor of 2.1 (Djakiew & Cardullo, 1986). Thus, a sudden oxygen demand by
caudal spermatozoa following temperature elevation may lead to their premature exhaustion, especially if it should induce activation of their motility.
The latter is a particularly vexatious point since it is not definitely established
whether or not spermatozoa in the cauda epididymidis are motile (Jones &
Murdoch, 1996). The general consensus of opinion is that they are immotile.
In some species such as the rat, the viscosity of the luminal secretions is so
high that spermatozoa cannot generate sufficient force to overcome its latent
drag. Motile rabbit spermatozoa diluted into rat CEP are immobilized
immediately on contact. According to Usselman & Cone (1983), this is
caused by the presence in CEP of a high molecular weight mucin appropriately termed 'immobilin'. In the rabbit and ram, however, caudal spermatozoa are vigorously motile upon removal from the cauda and exposure to the
air; dilution is not necessary. Small increases in intracellular pH, caused by
rapid release of CO_2, may be sufficient to induce this motility by altering the
balance between cytosolic levels of Ca^{2+}, cyclic AMP, and activity of protein
kinases and phosphoprotein phosphatases within the flagellum
(Vijayaraghavan et al., 1996). Of particular significance is that the protein
phosphatase I inhibitors, okadaic acid and calyculin A were able to induce
forward motility in bull caput epididymidal spermatozoa to a level characteristic of cauda spermatozoa and that these signalling systems are present in
the human and monkey (Smith et al., 1996).

There is also evidence that increased temperature has a direct and specific
effect on the activity of epididymal cells. The stability of CD52 (HE5) mRNA
in dog epididymal cells cultured in vitro decreased sharply during incubation at 37 °C relative to 33 °C and, in the unilateral cryptorchid dog epididymis, CD52 mRNA transcripts were much reduced in amount compared to
the scrotal epididymis (Pera et al., 1996). In the rabbit, body temperature
specifically reduced the synthesis of two epididymal glycoproteins (Regalado
et al., 1993) and in the cryptepididymal rat transport of inorganic ions across
the epithelium was adversely affected (Wong et al., 1982). Thus, temperature
reduces specific aspects of epididymal activity that are potentially damaging

to sperm survival. In view of the damaging effects of oxygen free radicals and lipid peroxidation on spermatozoa referred to above, it would be of interest to investigate how the epididymal SOD/GPX/GSH system reacts to heat.

In man, warm clothing, sedentary lifestyle and hot climate have long been suggested as contributing to reduced fertility and poor semen quality, and, although one feels intuitively from work on animal models that even a few degrees above 30 °C would be detrimental to epididymal function, information on the problem is diffuse and contradictory. This is largely due to the problem of distinguishing between an effect of heat mediated through the testis and a direct effect on spermatozoa in the cauda epididymidis. One way of addressing this problem has been to measure specific markers for epididymal function (carnitine, glycosidases, specific glycoproteins, etc.) in ejaculated seminal plasma. The difficulty with this approach is that the levels of these markers in semen from normal individuals is so variable that accuracy of prediction is poor. Even the question of insulated clothing having a detrimental effect is not settled. In a recent investigation it was found that wearing polyester athletic supports elevated scrotal skin temperatures by <1 °C and that this was insufficient to affect sperm numbers on motility in the ejaculate (Wang *et al.*, 1997). Heat exchange in the pampiniform plexus supplying blood to the human scrotal testis and epididymis, therefore, may be more efficient than has been generally thought. Obviously this does not apply to clinical conditions of cryptorchidism or varicocoele.

Conclusions

In this overview of the functionality of the mammalian epididymis, emphasis has been placed on comparing and contrasting information gained from research on animal models with that available on the human epididymis. For obvious reasons, much of what is known about the latter is clinically based and, as a result of recent work using corrective surgery (known as epididymovasostomy) on patients with congenital absence of the vas deferens or long-term blockage of the epididymal duct, the view has arisen that, in man, passage of spermatozoa through the epididymis is not necessary for acquisition of their fertilizing capacity. This conclusion is contrary to all the established and current information on sperm maturation in animal species. Possible explanations for these clinical situations are suggested and caution is urged in using them as an interpretative basis for extrapolating directly to the situation in the normal fertile man. Appraisal of recent research on the processes involved in epididymal sperm maturation and storage in animals emphasizes the importance of the luminal milieu or microenvironment created and maintained by the epithelial cells lining the duct. This fluid mediates the signalling processes between spermatozoa and the epididymis and evidence indicates that it varies in nature and extent at different levels of the duct. Of particular interest are recent findings that some antigens on spermatozoa are 'processed' during epididymal passage and that events in the initial segment are important for sperm transport in the female tract. The limited information available on the normal human epididymis does not substantially disagree with these findings and should be given greater credence in any future discussion of the role of this accessory gland in the regulation of fertility in man.

Acknowledgements

I am grateful to Dr Liz Howes for preparation of Fig. 5.1 and for helpful comments on the manuscript.

References

Aitken, R. J. (1997). Molecular mechanisms regulating human sperm function. *Molecular Human Reproduction*, **3**, 169–73.

Amann, R. P. (1981). A critical review of methods for evaluation of spermatogenesis from seminal characteristics. *Journal of Andrology*, **2**, 37–58.

Amann, R. P. & Howards, S. S. (1980). Daily spermatozoal production and epididymal spermatozoal reserves of the human male. *Journal of Urology*, **124**, 211–15.

Bedford, J. M. (1967). Effects of duct ligation on the fertilizing ability of spermatozoa from different regions of the rabbit epididymis. *Journal of Experimental Zoology*, **166**, 271–82.

(1994). The status and the state of the human epididymis. *Human Reproduction Update*, **9**, 2187–99.

Bedford, J. M., Calvin, H. & Cooper, G. W. (1973). The maturation of spermatozoa in the human epididymis. *Journal of Reproduction and Fertility, Suppl.*, **18**, 199–213.

Bishop, D. W. (1961). Biology of spermatozoa. In *Sex and internal secretions*, 3rd edn, vol. 2, ed. W. C. Young, pp. 707–96. Baltimore: Williams & Wilkins.

Borsook, D., Rosen, H., Collard, M., Dressler, H., Herrup, K., Comb, M. J. & Hyman, S. E. (1992). Expression and regulation of a proenkephalin β-galactosidase gene in the reproductive system of transgenic mice. *Molecular Endocrinology*, **6**, 1502–12.

Brooks, D. E., Means, A. R., Wright, E. J., Singh, S. P. & Tiver, K. K. (1987). Isolation and use of cDNA clones to study the structure and regulation of androgen-dependent secretory proteins associated with sperm maturation in the epididymis. In *New horizons in sperm cell research*, ed. H. Mori, pp. 56–61. Tokyo: Japan Scientific Societies Press.

Cooper, T. G. (1986). *The epididymis, sperm maturation and fertilization*. Berlin: Springer Verlag.

(1990). In defence of the human epididymis. *Fertility and Sterility*, **54**, 965–75.

Cornwall, G. A. & Hann, S. R. (1995). Specialized gene expression in the epididymis. *Journal of Andrology*, **16**, 379–83.

Cornwall, G. A., Orgebin-Crist, M. C. & Hann, S. R. (1992). The CRES gene: a unique testis-regulated gene related to the cystatin family is highly restricted in its expression to the proximal region of the mouse epididymis. *Molecular Endocrinology,* **6**, 1653–64.

Crabo, B. (1965). Studies on the composition of epididymal content in bulls and boars. *Acta Veterinaria Scandinavica,* **6**, *Suppl.* 5, 1–94.

Cummins, J. M. & Glover, T. D. (1970). Artificial cryptorchidism and fertility in the rabbit. *Journal of Reproduction and Fertility,* **23**, 423–33.

Djakiew, D. & Cardullo, R. (1986). Lower temperature of the cauda epididymidis facilitates the storage of sperm by enhancing oxygen availability. *Gamete Research,* **15**, 237–45.

Fawcett, D. W. & Hoffer, A. P. (1979). Failure of exogenous androgen to prevent regression of the initial segment of the rat epididymis after efferent duct ligation or orchietomy. *Biology of Reproduction,* **20**, 162–81.

Fickenscher, H. R., Chalepakis, G. & Gruss, P. (1993). Murine Pax-2 protein is a sequence-specific transactivator with expression in the genital system. *DNA and Cell Biology,* **12**, 381–91.

Frenkel, G., Peterson, R. N. Davis, J. E. & Freund, M. (1974). Glycerylphosphorylcholine and carnitine in normal human semen and in postvasectomy semen: differences in concentration. *Fertility and Sterility,* **25**, 84–7.

Freund, M. & Davis, J. E. (1969). Disappearance rate of sperm from the ejaculate following vasectomy. *Fertility and Sterility,* **20**, 163–70.

Garrett, J. E., Garrett, S. H. & Douglass, J. (1990). A spermatozoa-associated factor regulates proenkephalin gene expression in the rat epididymis. *Molecular Endocrinology,* **4**, 108–18.

Ghyselinck, N. B., Jimenez, C. & Dufaure, J. P. (1991). Sequence homology of androgen-regulated epididymal proteins with glutathione peroxidase in mice. *Journal of Reproduction and Fertlity,* **93**, 461–66.

Ghyselinck, N. B., Dufaure, I., Lareyre, J.-J., Rigaudière, N., Mattei, M.-G. & Dufaure, J.-P. (1993). Structural organization and regulation of the gene for the androgen-dependent glutathione peroxidase-like protein specific for the mouse epididymis. *Molecular Endocrinology,* **7**, 258–72.

Glover, T. D. (1969). Some aspects of function in the epididymis. Experimental occlusion of the epididymis in the rabbit. *International Journal of Fertility,* **14**, 216–21.

Glover, T. D. & Nicander, L. (1971). Some aspects of structure and function in the mammalian epididymis. *Journal of Reproduction and Fertility, Suppl.,* **13**, 39–50.

Hale, G., Rye, P. D., Worford, A., Lauder, I. & Britobabapulle, A. (1993). The glyco-sylphosphatidylinositol-anchored lymphocyte antigen CD_w52 is associated with the epididymal maturation of human spermatozoa. *Journal of Reproductive Immunology,* **23**, 189–205.

Hamilton, D. W. (1975). Structure and function of the epithelium lining the ductuli efferentes, ductus epididymidis, and ductus deferens in the rat. In *Handbook of physiology,* 1st edn, vol. 5, ed. D. W. Hamilton & R. O. Greep, pp. 259–317. Baltimore, MD: Williams & Wilkins.

Hayashi, M., Fujimoto, S., Takano, H., Ushiki, T., Abe, K., Ishikura, H., Yoshida, M. C., Kirchhoff, C., Ishibashi, T. & Kasahara, M. (1996). Characterization of a human glycoprotein with a potential role in sperm–egg fusion: cDNA cloning, immuno-histochemical localization, and chromosomal assignment of the gene (AEGL1). *Genomics*, **32**, 367–74.

Hinton, B. T., Palladino, M. A., Rudolph, D., Lan, Z. J. & Labus, J. C. (1996). The role of the epididymis in the protection of spermatozoa. *Current Topics in Developmental Biology*, **33**, 61–102.

Hoffer, A. P. (1976). The ultrastructure of the ductus deferens in man. *Biology of Reproduction*, **14**, 425–45.

Hoffer, A. P. & Greenberg, J. (1978). The structure of the epididymis, efferent ductules and ductus deferens of the guinea pig: a light microscopic study. *Anatomical Record*, **190**, 659–78.

Holland, M. K., Vreeburg, J. T. M. & Orgebin-Crist, M.-C. (1992). Testicular regulation of epdidymal protein secretion. *Journal of Andrology*, **13**, 266–73.

Holstein, A. F. (1969). Morphologische Studien am Nebenhoden des Mensehen. In *Zwanglose Abhandlungen aus dem Gebiet der Normalen und Pathologishen Anatomie*, ed. W. Bargmann & W. Doerr, pp. 1–91. Stuttgart: Georg Thiem Verlag.

Jaakkola, U. M. (1983). Regional variations in transport of the luminal contents of the rat epididymis *in vivo*. *Journal of Reproduction and Fertility*, **68**, 465–70.

Jiang, F. X., Temple-Smith, P. D. & Wreford, N. G. (1994). Postnatal differentiation and development of the rat epididymis: a stereological study. *Anatomical Record*, **238**, 191–8.

Johnson, L. & Varner, D. D. (1988). Effect of daily sperm production but not age on transit time of spermatozoa through the human epididymis. *Biology of Reproduction*, **39**, 812–17.

Jones, R. (1973). Epididymal function in the vasectomised rabbit. *Journal of Reproduction and Fertility*, **36**, 199–202.

(1974). The effects of artificial cryptorchidism on the composition of epididymal plasma in the rabbit. *Fertility and Sterility*, **25**, 432–8.

(1989). Membrane remodelling during sperm maturation in the epididymis. *Oxford reviews of reproductive biology*, vol. 11, ed. S. R. Milligan, pp. 285–337. Oxford: Oxford University Press.

Jones, R. C. & Murdoch, R. N. (1996). Regulation of the motility and metabolism of spermatozoa for storage in the epididymis of eutherian and marsupial mammals. *Reproduction, Fertility and Development*, **8**, 553–68.

Jones, R., Hamilton, D. W. & Fawcett, D. W. (1979). Morphology of the epithelium of the extra-testicular rete testis, ductuli efferentes and ductus epididymidis of the adult male rabbit. *American Journal of Anatomy*, **156**, 531–7.

Jones, R., Brown, C. R., von Glos, K. I. & Parker, M. G. (1980). Hormonal regulation of protein synthesis in the rat epididymis. Characterization of androgen-dependent and testicular fluid-dependent proteins. *Biochemical Journal*, **188**, 667–76.

Kirchhoff, C. (1996). CD52 is the 'major maturation-associated' sperm membrane antigen. *Molecular Human Reproduction*, **2**, 9–17.

Kirchhoff, C., Habben, I., Ivell, R. & Krull. N. (1991). A major human epididymal-specific cDNA encodes a protein with sequence homology to extracellular proteinase inhibitors. *Biology of Reproduction*, **45**, 350–57.

Kirchhoff, C., Krull, N., Pera, I. & Ivell, R. (1993). A major mRNA of the human epididymal principal cells, HE5 encodes the leucoyte differentiation CD_w52 peptide backbone. *Molecular Reproduction and Development*, **34**, 8–15.

Krull, N., Ivell, R., Osterhoff, C. & Kirchhoff, C. (1993). Region-specific variation of gene expression in the human epididymis as revealed by *in situ* hybridization with tissue specific cDNAs. *Molecular Reproduction and Development*, **34**, 16–24.

Lea, O. A., Petrusz, P. & French, F. S. (1978). Purification and localization of acidic epididymal glycoprotein (AEG): a sperm coating protein secreted by the rat epididymis. *International Journal of Andrology, Suppl.*, **2**, 592–607.

Levine, N. & Marsh, D. J. (1971). Micropuncture studies of the electrochemical aspects of fluid and electrolyte transport in individual seminferous tubules, the epididymis and the vas deferens in rats. *Journal of Physiology*, **213**, 557–70.

Lindsey, J. S. & Wilkinson, M. F. (1996). An androgen-regulated homeobox gene expressed in rat testis and epididymis. *Biology of Reproduction*, **55**, 975–83.

Lubicz-Nawrocki, C. M. & Glover, T. D. (1973). The influence of the testis on the survival of spermatozoa in the epididymis of the golden hamster, *Mesocricetus auratus. Journal of Reproduction and Fertility*, **34**, 315–29.

Mann, T. & Lutwak-Mann, C. (1981). *Male reproductive function and semen.* Berlin: Springer-Verlag.

Moore, H. D. M., Curr, M. R., Penfold, L. M. & Pryor, J. P. (1992). The culture of human epididymal epithelium and *in vitro* maturation of epididymal spermatozoa. *Ferility and Sterility*, **58**, 776–83.

Moritz, A., Litja, H. & Fink, E. (1991). Molecular cloning and sequence analysis of the cDNA encoding the human acrosin-trypsin inhibitor (HUSI-II). *FEBS Letters*, **278**, 127–30.

Nicander, L. (1965). An electron microscopical study of absorbing cells in the posterior caput epididymidis of rabbits. *Zeitschrift für Zellforschung und Mikroskopische Anatomie*, **66**, 829–47.

O'Bryan, M. K., Mallidis, C., Murphy, B. F. & Baker, H. W. G. (1994). The immunohistological localization of clusterin in the male human and marmoset genital tract. *Biology of Reproduction*, **50**, 502–9.

Orgebin-Crist, M.-C. (1987). Post-testicular development of mammalian spermatozoa. In *Morphological basis of human reproductive function*, ed. D. M. de Kretser & G. Spera, pp. 155–74. Amsterdam: Acta Medica.

Palladino, M. A., Laperche, Y. & Hinton, B. L. (1994). Multiple forms of gamma-glutamyl transpeptidase messenger ribonucleic acid are expressed in the adult rat testis and epididymis. *Biology of Reproduction*, **50**, 320–8.

Pera, I., Ivell, R. & Kirchhoff, C. (1996). Body temperature (37 °C) specifically down-regulates the messenger ribonucleic acid for the major sperm surface antigen CD52 in epididymal cell culture. *Endocrinology*, **137**, 4451–9.

Perry, A. C. F., Jones, R. & Hall, L. (1992*a*). Identification of an abundant monkey epididymal transcript encoding a homologue of human CAMPATH-1 antigen precursor. *Biochimica et Biophysica Acta*, **1171**, 122–4.

Perry, A. C. F., Jones, R., Barker, H. & Hall, L. (1992*b*). A mammalian epididymal protein with remarkable sequence similarity to snake venom haemorrhagic peptides. *Biochemical Journal*, **286**, 671–75.

Perry, A. C. F., Jones, R., Niiang, L. S. P., Jackson, R. M. & Hall, L. (1992c). Genetic evidence for an androgen-regulated epididymal secretory glutathione peroxidase whose transcript does not contain a selenocysteine codon. *Biochemical Journal*, **285**, 863–70.

Perry, A. C. F., Jones, R. & Hall, L. (1993a). Isolation and characterization of a rat cDNA clone encoding a secreted superoxide dismutase reveals the epididymis to be a major site of its expression. *Biochemical Journal*, **293**, 21–5.

(1993b). Sequence analysis of monkey acrosin–trypsin inhibitor transcripts and their abundant expression in the epididymis. *Biochimica et Biophysica Acta*, **1172**, 159–60.

Perry, A. C. F., Hall, L., Bell, A. E. & Jones, R. (1994). Sequence analysis of a mammalian phospholipid-binding protein from testis and epididymis and its distribution between spermatozoa and extracellular secretions. *Biochemical Journal*, **301**, 235–42.

Perry, A. C. F., Jones, R. & Hall, L. (1995). The monkey ESP 14.6 mRNA, a novel transcript expressed at high levels in the epididymis. *Gene*, **153**, 291–2.

Rankin, T. L., Ong, D. E. & Orgebin-Crist, M.-C. (1992). The 18-kDa mouse epididymal protein (MEP10) binds retinoic acid. *Biology of Reproduction*, **46**, 767–71.

Regalado, F., Esponda, P. & Nieto, A. (1993). Temperature and androgens regulate the biosynthesis of secretory proteins from rabbit cauda epididymidis. *Molecular Reproduction and Development*, **36**, 448–53.

Robaire, B. & Hermio, L. (1988). Efferent ducts, epididymis, and vas deferens: structure, functions and their regulation. In *The physiology of reproduction*, 1st edn, vol. 1, ed. E. Knobil & J. D. O'Neill, pp. 999–1080. New York: Raven Press.

Rowley, M., Teshima, J. F. & Heller, C. C. (1970). Duration of transit of spermatozoa through the human male ductular systems. *Fertility and Sterility*, **21**, 390–6.

Schoysman, R. (1993). Clinical situations challenging the established concept of epididymal physiology in the human. *Acta Europea Fertilitas*, **24**, 55–60.

Schoysman, R. & Bedford, J. M. (1986). The role of the human epididymis in sperm maturation and sperm storage as reflected in the consequences of epididymovasectomy. *Fertility and Sterility*, **46**, 293–99.

Setchell, B. P. (1978). *The mammalian testis*. London: Paul Elek.

Siiteri, J. E., Enstrud, K. M., Moore, A. & Hamilton, D. W. (1995). Identification of osteopontin (OPN) mRNA and protein in the rat testis, and epididymis, and on sperm. *Molecular Reproduction and Development*, **40**, 16–28.

Silber, S. J. (1980). Vasoepididymovasectomy to the head of the epididymis: recovery of normal spermatozoal motility. *Fertility and Sterility*, **34**, 149–53.

(1988). Pregnancy caused by sperm from vasa efferentia. *Fertility and Sterility*, **49**, 373–75.

(1989). Apparent fertility of human spermatozoa from the caput epididymidis. *Journal of Androlgoy*, **10**, 263–9.

Silber, S. J., Ord, T., Balmaceda, J. P., Patrizio, P. & Asch, R. H. (1990). Congenital absence of the vas deferens: the fertilizing capacity of human epididymal sperm. *New England Journal of Medicine*, **32**, 1788–92.

Smith, G. D., Wolf, D. P., Trautman, K. C., da Cruz e Silva, E. F., Greengard, P. & Vijayaraghavan, S. (1996). Primate sperm contain protein phosphatase I, a biochemical mediator of motility. *Biology of Reproduction*, **54**, 719–27.

Snell, G. D. (1933). X-ray sterility in the male house mouse. *Journal of Experimental Zoology*, **65**, 421–41.

Sonneberg-Reithmacher, E., Walter, B., Riethmacher, D., Godecke, S. & Birchmeier, C. (1996). The c-*ros* tyrosine kinase receptor controls regionalization and differentiation of epithelial cells in the epididymis. *Genes and Development*, **10**, 1184–93.

Storey, B. T. (1995). Interactions between gametes leading to fertilization – the sperms eye view. *Reproduction, Fertility and Development*, **7**, 927–42.

Sylvester, S. R., Morales, C., Oko, R. & Griswold, M. D. (1991). Localization of sulphated glycoprotein-2 (clusterin) on spermatozoa and in the reproductive tract of the male rat. *Biology of Reproduction*, **45**, 195–207.

Syntin, P., Dacheux, F., Druant, X., Gatti, J. L., Okamura, N. & Dacheux, J.-L. (1996). Characterization and identification of proteins secreted in the various regions of the adult boar epididymis. *Biology of Reproduction*, **55**, 956–74.

Tesh, J. M. & Glover, T. D. (1969). Ageing of spermatozoa in the male tract and its effect on fertility. *Journal of Andrology*, **16**, 292–98.

Turner, T .T. (1995). On the epididymis and its role in the development of the fertile ejaculate. *Journal of Reproduction and Fertility*, **16**, 292–8.

Turner, T. T., Gleavy, J. L. & Harris, J. M. (1990). Fluid movement in the lumen of the rat epididymis: effect of vasectomy and subsequent vasovasostomy. *Journal of Andrology*, **11**, 422–8.

Usselman, M. C. & Cone, R. A. (1983). Rat sperm are mechanically immobilized in the caudal epididymis by 'immobilin', a high molecular weight glycoprotein. *Biology of Reproduction*, **29**, 1241–53.

Vierula, M. E., Araki, Y., Raukin, T. L., Tulsiani, D. R. P. & Orgebin-Crist, M.-C. (1992). Immunolocalization of a 25-kilodalton protein in mouse testis and epididymis. *Biology of Reproduction*, **47**, 844–56.

Vijayaraghavan, S., Stephans, D. T., Trautman, K., Smith, G. D., Khatra, B., da la Cruz e Silva, E. F. & Greengard, P. (1996). Sperm motility development in the epididymis is associated with decreased glycogen synthase kinase-3 and protein phosphatase I activity. *Biology of Reproduction*, **54**, 709–18.

Waites, G. M. H. & Einer-Jensen, N. (1974). Collection and analysis of rete testis fluid from macaque monkeys. *Journal of Reproduction and Fertility*, **41**, 505–8.

Wang, C., McDonald, V., Leung, A., Superlano, L., Berman, N., Hull, L. & Swerdloff, R. S. (1997). Effect of increased scrotal temperature on sperm production in normal men. *Fertility and Sterility*, **68**, 334–9.

Wasylyk, C., Flores, P., Gutman, A. & Wasylyk, B. (1989). PEA3 is a nuclear target for transcription activation by non-nuclear oncogenes. *EMBO Journal*, **8**, 3371–8.

Winer, M. A. & Wolgemuth, D. J. (1995). The segment-specific pattern of a-raf expression in the mouse epididymis is regulated by testicular factors. *Endocrinology*, **136**, 2561–72.

Wong, P. Y. D., Au, C. L. & Bedford, J. M. (1982). Biology of the scrotum. II. Suppression by abdominal temperature of transepithelial ion and water transport in the cauda epididymidis. *Biology of Reproduction*, **26**, 683–9.

Yeung, C.-H., Cooper, T. G., Bergmann, M. & Schulze, H. (1991). Organization of tubules in the human caput epididymides and the ultrastructure of their epithelia. *American Journal of Anatomy*, **191**, 261–79.

Yeung, C.-H., Cooper, T.-G., Oberpenning, F., Schulze, H. & Nieschlag, E. (1993). Changes in movement characteristics of human spermatozoa along the length of the epididymis. *Biology of Reproduction*, **49**, 274–80.

Yeung, C.-H., Schröter, S., Wagenfeld, A., Kirchhoff, C., Kliesch, S., Poser, D., Weinbauer, G. F., Nieschlag, E. & Cooper, T. G. (1997). Interaction of the human epididymal protein CD52 (HE5) with epididymal spermatozoa from men and cynomolgus monkeys. *Molecular Reproduction and Development*, **48**, 267–75.

Young, W. C. (1929). A study of the function of the epididymis. II. The importance of an ageing process in sperm for the length of the period during which fertilizing capacity is retained by sperm isolated in the epididymis of the guinea-pig. *Journal of Morphology and Physyiology*, **48**, 475–91.

(1931). A study of the function of the epididymis. II. Functional changes undergone by spermatozoa during their passage through the epididymis and vas deferens in the guinea-pig. *Journal of Experimental Biology*, **8**, 151–62.

6 Transport of spermatozoa to the egg and fertilization success

JACKSON BROWN, STEVE PUBLICOVER AND CHRIS BARRATT

The primary aim of this chapter is to highlight selected recent developments encompassing the dynamic transport of spermatozoa to the egg and sperm interaction with the egg vestments, emphasizing potential lines for future research. One area specifically explored, in some detail, is the role of calcium in the acrosome reaction (AR). In this section, comparison with our detailed understanding of the role of Ca^{2+} in the release of neurotramsmitter is used to identify future areas of research that can be explored to further our basic understanding of the AR. In this chapter, little attention is given to fertilization events after sperm–egg fusion, and, for details of this, the interested reader is referred to several recent reviews (Swann & Lai, 1997; Sakkas et al., 1997). Throughout this chapter we concentrate primarily on data from the human.

How does the spermatozoon reach the egg?

Remarkably, we know very little about the transport of spermatozoa to the fallopian tube in the human. In fact, there are only a handful of studies which have investigated this process in vivo. Usually, such studies have attempted to answer the very basic questions of how many spermatozoa are in the uterus and/or fallopian tube. Such studies were completed in the 1970s and early 1980s and, by their very design, failed to take into account many factors that we now know, at least from other animal data, to affect the transport process. For example, time between sperm recovery and ovulation was often not documented accurately. In addition, techniques used to recover sperm were often inadequate thus, results were usually qualitative not quantitative (for a review and details of such studies, see Barratt & Cooke, 1991). As a consequence, we simply do not know how many spermatozoa reach the fallopian tube in the pre-, peri- and post-ovulatory period. In our own studies, which controlled for the time between insemination and recovery of spermatozoa, time of ovulation and efficiency of recovery techniques, low numbers of spermatozoa were consistently recovered from the oviducts of ten women (Williams et al., 1993a). Such studies need to be extended to include more subjects as there was great variability between individuals (median number of spermatozoa 251; range 79–1386). However, we found no evidence of an isthmic reservoir, which was surprising as an isthmic reservoir has been demonstrated in many mammal studies to date (pigs, Hunter, 1984; hamsters, Smith & Yanagimachi, 1990; cows, Wilmut & Hunter, 1984; sheep, Hunter & Nicol, 1983). If an isthmic reservoir exists, it is certainly not as obvious as that in animals. Perhaps the cervix acts as the main sperm reservoir in the human. It is a reflection of our lack of understanding about sperm transport in the human that such basic questions remain unanswered.

Undoubtedly, studying sperm transport *in vivo* provides enormous ethical, technical and logistical problems. Until such problems can be overcome, we will remain relatively ignorant about the numbers, distribution and function of spermatozoa in the human reproductive tract. A thorough understanding of the intricate nature of sperm transport remains a challenging scientific goal. Improvements in our understanding are likely to have practical implications: for example, we will enhance our knowledge of insemination techniques (intra-uterine and intra-tubal) and, with such knowledge probably construct more effective insemination regimens. Considering the enormous number of artificial insemination cycles that are performed each year it is surprising that we still remain ignorant about optimal insemination doses, times of insemination and methods of insemination. For example, the benefits of intra-uterine insemination without ovulation induction remain controversial (Hughes, 1997). If spermatozoa can be recovered from the fallopian tube, and their functional status examined, this will provide a quantum leap in our understanding of sperm function – perhaps we can then improve the efficiency of our *in vitro* fertilization (IVF) techniques just by selecting the good spermatozoa as has been demonstrated in the mouse (see Siddiquey & Cohen, 1982). In animal experiments, detailed knowledge of sperm distribution within the female tract following insemination has been critical in developing effective insemination regimens (Wilmut & Hunter, 1984; Hunter & Nicol, 1983; Stevernick *et al.*, 1997).

In contrast to our comprehensive understanding of the detection and prediction of ovulation, we know little about the optimum width of the insemination window. A recent study by Wilcox and colleagues has shown clearly that this window, at least for natural intercourse, covers a 6 day period, ending on the day of ovulation (Wilcox *et al.*, 1995). This is the first study to identify such a wide window and shows that human spermatozoa can survive, in a fully functional state, in the female tract for at least 6 days. The implications of this to the timing of assisted reproductive techniques, which often deal with compromised gamete quality, has yet to be determined. It is likely, at least when using frozen donor spermatozoa that the window is narrower, but how much narrower remains uncertain. Data from the Centres d'Études et de Conservation des Oeufs et des Spermes Humaines (CECOS) suggest optimal success rates when inseminations are performed within a 2 day window (Lansac *et al.*, 1997), but additional experiments, using more accurate techniques to detect ovulation, are likely to define the length of this window more accurately.

Recently, both in animals and humans, *in vitro* culture systems have been developed to examine the interaction between the oviductal epithelium and spermatozoa. *In vivo*, sperm–epithelium interactions are important to establish and maintain the isthmic reservoir, at least in animals. Although limited sperm–epithelium interaction takes place in the human female tract (see Williams *et al.*, 1993*b*) it remains to be fully categorized. The molecular basis of sperm–epithelium interactions has not been determined, although in hamsters carbohydrate residues are important (Demott *et al.*, 1995). Several *in vitro* oviductal culture systems have been established in the human (see Pacey *et al.*, 1995*a,b*; Morales *et al.*, 1996; Baillie *et al.*, 1997). Human spermatozoa make strong transient interactions with the epithelium *in vitro*. Surprisingly, preliminary studies indicated that neither menstrual cycle nor addition of mid cycle levels of oestrogens had any significant effect on sperm binding (Baillie *et al.*, 1997). Such *in vitro* systems are valuable models that will allow detailed investigation on the nature and importance of sperm–epithelium interactions.

In addition to co-culture systems, *in vitro* systems examining the interactions between spermatozoa and the female reproductive tract have concentrated on the effects of reproductive tract secretions on sperm function. Such studies indicate that cervical mucus can rapidly initiate capacitation, although paradoxically it can maintain spermatozoa in a functional state for several days (see Zinamen *et al.*, 1989). Such a dual role may be important for sperm storage in the cervix, which, to date, has not been clearly demonstrated to occur in the human. The paucity of oviductal fluid has limited the number of *in vitro* studies that could be performed. From the preliminary information available, oviductal fluid may perform a paradoxical function similar to that of human mucus (see De Jonge *et al.*, 1993; Zhu *et al.*, 1994*a,b*; Barratt & Hornby, 1995); however, such experiments were performed on a very limited number of samples and require a larger data base before definitive conclusions can be drawn. Interestingly, in bovines, several oviductal glycoproteins which enhance sperm capacitation have been identified (King & Killian, 1994). Experiments in humans, using homologous glycoproteins isolated from human oviductal fluid combined with tissue culture systems, are likely to provide useful experimental tools for investigating this process. In addition, screening and subsequent expression of glycoproteins from cDNA oviductal libraries will allow the cellular and molecular interactions to be understood in more detail.

The immunological status of spermatozoa, and the response by the human female tract, remains an enigma (for recent reviews, see Barratt & Pockley, 1998; Barratt, 1997; Clark *et al.*, 1996, 1997). Paradoxically, when spermatozoa enter the human female tract they initiate a massive influx of leukocytes (primarily neutrophils), i.e. the leukocytic cell reaction (Pandya

& Cohen, 1985; Thompson *et al.*, 1991, 1992). The stimulus for this reaction and its function is unknown. In bovines, these leukocytes predominately phagocytose non-motile spermatozoa (Mattner, 1969). Whilst it is tempting to suggest that the leukocytes selectively phagocytose defective 'non-fertilizing' human spermatozoa, there is no evidence to support or reject this hypothesis. The primary question is: why does not the female produce anti-sperm antibodies when exposed to spermatozoa? Limited expression of histocompatability antigens, immunosuppressive effects of seminal plasma and cervical mucus may play a role (see Pallanen & Cooper, 1994; Barratt & Pockley, 1998). However, with the development of the 'danger hypothesis' the current immunological paradigm of self and non-self is now being modified (Ridge *et al.*, 1996). In the context of sperm–female reproductive tract interactions it is possible that spermatozoa do not induce an immune response because the danger signal is not presented, i.e. spermatozoa are not dangerous to the female and thus an immune response is not mounted. This is an attractive hypothesis but has yet to be critically examined in the context of sperm–female tract interactions (see Barratt & Pockley, 1998). Many fundamental questions remain to be addressed about the immunological interaction of spermatozoa with the female tract – the time has come to integrate modern immunological thinking into reproductive biology (see Fearon & Locksley, 1996; Fearon, 1997; Medzhitov & Janeway, 1997)

Interactions between spermatozoa and the egg vestements

Penetration of the cumulus

Although the cumulus is the first egg vestment to be penetrated by the spermatozoon we known comparatively little about this process. In the main, studies have focused on the induction of the AR by the cumulus. At present, it is unclear if a complete AR is induced in spermatozoa as they pass through the cumulus. Progesterone, which is probably in relatively high levels in the cumulus, is likely to activate spermatozoa – for example, inducing a calcium influx (Aitken *et al.*, 1996a, see below) – and, as a consequence, when they reach the zona pellucida the spermatozoa may have started to undergo the AR. In fact, progesterone may act to augment the AR, as has been shown in mice (Roldan *et al.*, 1994). It is generally accepted that spermatozoa need to be capacitated to successfully penetrate the cumulus, although the results of such studies are not conclusive. Now that we have more defined tests of sperm function, e.g. tyrosine phosphorylation status as a marker of capacitation (Aitken, 1997), and a clearer concept of what consitutes hyperactivation (Mortimer *et al.*, 1997), further studies that re-examine sperm penetration into and through the cumulus can now be performed. It is anticipated that using such methods clearer answers will be forthcoming in the near future.

Interactions with the zona pellucida

Following the initial work of Paul Wassarman and Jurrien Dean there have been significant advances in our understanding of sperm–zona interactions (Chamberlin & Dean, 1990; Wassarman, 1992). In the mouse, about which most is known, the zona pellucida contains three heterogeneous glycoproteins (ZP1, ZP2 and ZP3). The primary initial interaction of spermatozoa with the zona pellucida is via ZP3, which stimulates induction of the AR (Beebe *et al.*, 1992). Expression of recombinant proteins, both in the hamster and in the mouse, indicate that the O-linked carbohydrate moieties of ZP3 are important for initial gamete recognition (Beebe *et al.*, 1992; Kinloch *et al.*, 1991, 1995). The nature of the carbohydrates moieties is still a matter of some debate, but in the mouse those located on the C-terminal region are crucial (Kinloch *et al.*, 1995). Equivalent studies in pigs, primarily using native zona proteins, also point to the importance of carbohydrate moieties (although in this case both N- and O-linked) in the initial gamete recognition (Koyama *et al.*, 1994; Gupta *et al.*, 1995; for a review, see Benoff, 1997). The main function of the polypeptide backbone of ZP3 is to cross-link the complementary receptors on the sperm plasma membrane for induction of the AR, although a direct role in gamete recognition remains to be examined (Leyton & Saling, 1989). Complementary progress in our understanding of human sperm–zona interaction has been hampered by the paucity of human zona and the technical difficulties in expressing various forms of biologically active recombinant human zona proteins (see Whitmarsh *et al.*, 1996; Chapman & Barratt, 1996, 1997). It is likely that the human system is not greatly different from those of the pig and the mouse. However, specific experiments have yet to be completed. In our studies we have shown, surprisingly, that non-glycosylated recombinant human ZP3 will induce the AR when incubated with capacitated spermatozoa for long periods (Whitmarsh *et al.*, 1996; Chapman *et al.*, 1998). The significance of this remains to be established but the protein may have a more significant role in human than in the other mammals studied. In addition, we need to further extend our experiments to examine the role of ZP2 and ZP1 as practically nothing is known about their function in humans. Clinical studies have clearly demonstrated the importance of the interaction between the zona pellucida and spermatozoa as failure and/or poor binding is associated with fertilization defects (Liu & Baker, 1992, 1994; Oehninger *et al.*, 1992). In addition, failure to undergo the AR in response to native human zona pellucida is a well-defined cause of male infertility (Liu & Baker, 1994, 1996). It is therefore important that we understand the molecular nature of these interactions to aid in the potential treatment of male fertility as well as for the potential development of new contraceptive vaccines.

There is much debate about the nature of the complementary receptors on spermatozoa for the zona proteins. Several well-defined and well-discussed candidates include: P95 zona receptor kinase, Burks *et al.*, 1995; β1–4-galactosyltransferase, Lu & Shur, 1997; and fertilization antigen 1, Zhu & Naz, 1997. In truth, clear unequivocal evidence to identify one candidate is not forthcoming, although, zona receptor kinase is probably the best candidate recognized so far in the human (see Brewis & Moore, 1997). Interesting experiments using knockout mice have added confusion to the field; for example, mice which have had the β1–4-galactosyltransferase gene deleted (Lu & Shur, 1997) are fertile! This highlights the biological redundancy that exists in the fertilization mechanism. In this context, it is interesting that other unexpected candidates may play an important role in sperm–zona binding. For example, mice that have had the calmegin gene deleted produce normal numbers of spermatozoa but they fail to bind to the zona pellucida (Ikawa *et al.*, 1997). Calmegin is a chaperone protein that may play a role in transporting molecules important in binding the zona to the sperm plasma membrane. We await with interest to see whether there is a complementary defect in man. In order to make significant progress in this field it is necessary to use recombinant molecular techniques to produce clearly defined molecules that can be studied (see Chapman & Barratt, 1996, 1997). Quite simply there is not enough native biological material available to obtain an in-depth understanding.

Interaction with the oolema

There is now almost universal acceptance that mammalian spermatozoa need to be acrosome reacted in order to bind and fuse with the oolema. Spermatozoa bind to the oolema via the sperm plasma membrane overlying the apical margin of the equitorial segment. This region is preserved after the AR and is modified just before and/or after the AR to permit binding and fusion, i.e. it acquires fusiogenic competence. There are a plethora of studies that review sperm–oocyte binding (for reviews, see Snell & White, 1996; Allen & Green, 1997; Brewis & Moore, 1997). Primarily, studies have focused on the oocyte integrins and sperm-bound disintegrins. However, the mechanisms of binding and fusion are still poorly understood. For example, there remains considerable controversy over the role of fertilin (formerly known as PH30). Fertilin consists of an α and a β subunit that probably exist as a heterodimer *in vivo* (Waters & White, 1997). Traditionally, the α subunit has been assigned a role in fusion and the β subunit a role in binding (because of the presence of a disintegrin domain). Recent experiments challenge this simplistic view; for example, the bovine fertilin α subunit has a disintegrin-like domain (Waters & White, 1997). Interestingly, the human α subunit may not play a role in gamete interaction as the α fertilin gene is a pseudogene in the human (Jury *et al.*, 1997). Green and colleagues suggest that, using viral fusion as a model, much can be determined about the molecular interactions of the spermatozoa and the oolema (Allen & Green, 1997). In addition, as with studies on the zona pellucida, recombinant protein production will enhance our understanding. In this context both recombinant fertilin α and β have been expressed and their biological activity determined (see Evans *et al.*, 1997*a*,*b*). Using these approaches, rapid progress in this field will be made in the next 3–5 years. However, as a cautionary note, whatever molecules are identified as being involved in binding and/or fusion their location on spermatozoa must be clearly documented, as some molecules thought to be critical in the sperm–oolema fusion (e.g. fertilin) are not located in the equatorial region and thus may not play a critical role in fusion (for discussion, see Brewis & Moore, 1997).

Excitation–secretion coupling: acrosome reaction as a parallel to transmitter release

The AR of mammalian spermatozoa, as with virtually all other forms of stimulus-activated exocytotic secretion, is mediated by an elevation of $[Ca^{2+}]_i$. Induction of the AR by the zona pellucida-derived protein ZP3 involves aggregation of ZP3 receptors (Leyton & Saling, 1989) and, in addition to modulation of $[Ca^{2+}]_i$, is accompanied by various biochemical processes that are known to have significance in intracellular signalling. These include activation of tyrosine kinase (Aitken, 1997), phospholipase Cγ1 (PLC γ1; Tomes *et al.*, 1996) and adenylyl cyclase (Ward & Kopf, 1993). However, the central importance of elevated $[Ca^{2+}]_i$ in activating exocytosis of the acrosome is clear in that: (1) physiological activation of the AR, by solubilized zona pellucida or by progesterone (PR), is effective only in the presence of a normal or near-normal $[Ca^{2+}]_o$; (2) activation of AR, either by ZP3 or by PR is always accompanied by elevation of $[Ca^{2+}]_i$ (Thomas & Meizel, 1989; Bailey & Storey, 1994; Florman, 1994; Tesarik *et al.*, 1996); and (3) artificial elevation of $[Ca^{2+}]_i$ by the use of calcium ionophores such as A23187 is sufficient to induce the AR.

Dependence of ligand-induced AR on $[Ca^{2+}]_o$ is consistent with participation of membrane Ca^{2+} channels in both ZP3- and PR-induced responses. The identity of the channel responsible for the initial PR-induced Ca^{2+} transient has not been elucidated beyond the fact that it is sensitive to La^{3+} (Aitken *et al.*, 1996*b*). However, there is considerable evidence that voltage operated Ca^{2+} channels (VOCCs) are responsible for at least part of the Ca^{2+}-influx induced by ZP3, that activation of this pathway involves depolarization of the membrane and that blockade of VOCCs is sufficient to greatly attenuate the AR (Florman *et al.*, 1992; Zeng *et al.*, 1995). The AR can therefore be considered to be a Ca^{2+}-mediated, voltage-regulated secretory activity with some similarities to secretion by somatic cells, including the release of neurotransmitter (Florman *et al.*, 1995). There are striking differences between the two processes, particularly the kinetics of stimulus–secretion coupling. Transmitter is mobilized and secreted within 1 ms whereas the AR can take up to 10 min between presentation of a stimulus and exocytosis of the acrosomal contents (Roldan & Harrison, 1989; Thomas & Meizel, 1989;

Tesarik *et al.*, 1996). However, in other respects there are clear similarities that are worthy of consideration. The physiology and ultrastructure of excitation–secretion coupling at presynaptic terminals have been the subject of intense research for many years and have been elucidated in considerable detail. The molecular mechanisms underlying the fusion of the plasmalemma and secretory vesicles are now also beginning to be understood. In comparison, understanding of the secretory event known as the AR is poorly understood. Current understanding of the AR can be compared with understanding of synaptic transmitter release 10–20 years ago, when mobilization of Ca^{2+} and the ultrastructural events had been described, but virtually nothing was known of the molecular basis (Ceccarelli & Hurlbut, 1980; Rahamimoff *et al.*, 1980; Fig. 6.1). The synaptic model is therefore potentially of considerable value both in interpreting data concerning control of the AR, and also in the design of experiments to elucidate events underlying exocytosis of the acrosome.

Ca^{2+} and secretion of neurotransmitter

Participation of Ca^{2+} in excitation–secretion coupling at the nerve terminal was first established in the 1960s by Katz & Miledi (Katz & Miledi, 1965, 1967), who also demonstrated that, in the presence of Ca^{2+}, focal presynaptic depolarisation was sufficient to induce transmitter secretion (Katz & Miledi, 1969). VOCCs, known to occur in squid giant axon, were believed to mediate this action of Ca^{2+}. Subsequently, Llinas and colleagues, working

Fig. 6.1. Models of transmitter release and the acrosome reaction. Left panel shows a model for the control of transmitter release, similar to those published 15–20 years ago (e.g. Statham & Duncan, 1976; Rahamimoff *et al.*, 1980). Depolarization by the action potential causes voltage-operated Ca^{2+} channel (VOCC) gating, allowing Ca^{2+} influx and activation of transmitter release via the Ca^{2+} receptor 'X'. Right panel is derived from the model for activation of the AR by ZP3, proposed by Florman *et al.* (1995). Activation involves opening of a nonselective cation channel. Consequent depolarizataion opens Ca^{2+} channels and allows influx of Ca^{2+}, which triggers events resulting in acrosome reaction. The proposed modulation of VOCCs by G-protein-dependent intracellular alkalinization is not included in this simplified version. 'X' indicates the unknown binding site for Ca^{2+}, now suspected to be synaptotagmin (see the text); ZP3, zona pellucida-derived glycoprotein 3; R, ZP3 receptor.

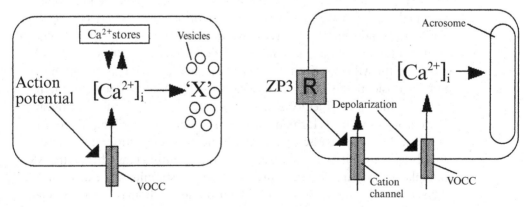

on aequorin-injected squid giant synapse, showed that a $[Ca^{2+}]_i$ transient was a necessary step in stimulus–secretion coupling (Llinas *et al.*, 1972; Llinas & Nicholson, 1974). Taken together, these data led to the model for transmitter release shown in Fig. 6.1, which is not dissimilar to current models for participation of Ca^{2+} in the AR.

Structure of the transmitter release site

Since the establishment of a role for Ca^{2+} in neurotransmitter secretion, most progress has concerned the ultrastructure of release and the molecules underlying Ca^{2+}-activated exocytosis. The use of freeze–fracture electron microscopy has allowed detailed examination of the structural events that occur during transmitter secretion, particularly at neuromuscular synapses (Heuser *et al.*, 1979). One of the most striking findings is that secretion occurs only at specialized sites on the presynaptic membrane, known as active zones (AZs), around which the synaptic vesicles cluster. AZs vary in their arrangement but always include organized clusters or strips of paired, intramembrane proteins of about 10 nm diameter, spaced at intervals of about 50 nm. Fusion of vesicles with the membrane normally occurs within 20–50 nm of the particle rows. Use of fluorescently labelled VOCC ligands has confirmed that at least some of these proteins are VOCCs (Robitaille *et al.*, 1990; Cohen *et al.*, 1991). The standardized spatial arrangement of VOCCs and membrane fusion sites is consistent with the idea of an array of 'secretion proteins', possibly assembled into a functional unit that includes VOCC(s), secretory vesicle recognition site and a Ca^{2+}-sensitive, fusion-activation site. Evidence for such association between VOCCs and components of the exocytotic apparatus already exists (Bennett, 1997; Stanley, 1997). A further feature of AZs is that in resting nerve terminals a proportion of the synaptic vesicles are closely associated with the membrane. These are referred to as 'docked' and are assumed to be immediately releasable. The majority of vesicles are 'clustered' behind the AZ. These clustered vesicles are apparently held in position by interaction with elements of the cytoskeleton (possibly synapsin), which links vesicles to the cytoskeleton and prevents their premature release (Landis *et al.*, 1988). Vesicles are released from the cluster by action of calmodulin kinase II, which when activated by Ca^{2+}-calmodulin, phosphorylates synapsin, causing it to detach from the vesicle membrane (Huttner *et al.*, 1983). Upon detaching from the cytoskeleton, vesicles can diffuse to and dock at the AZ, where they have to undergo a Mg-ATP -dependent priming before being competent to undergo rapid exocytosis (Sudhof, 1995). $[Ca^{2+}]_i$ in the bulk of the cytoplasm (but not at the AZ), therefore regulates the recharging of vesicle docking sites, and so determines the size of the store of immediately releasable secretory vesicles.

The structure of AZs is clearly ideal for producing the extremely rapid secretory response that is a feature of transmitter release. It also means that, during a presynaptic action potential, intracellular buffering of $[Ca^{2+}]$ will have relatively little effect on $[Ca^{2+}]_i$ surrounding the docked vesicles (which presumably includes the Ca^{2+}-sensitive site). For a brief period (1–2 ms; Smith & Augustine, 1988) $[Ca^{2+}]$ may greatly exceed that which is recorded by the techniques used to monitor $[Ca^{2+}]_i$. Calculations suggest that concentrations of well over 20–100 μM may be reached at distances of 20–50 nm from the mouth of a single VOCC (Smith & Augustine, 1988; Stanley, 1997). These estimates are in accord with evidence that the exocytotic machinery has a remarkably low sensitivity to Ca^{2+}, requiring concentrations of 20 μM up to 200 μM (Roberts et al., 1990; Heidelberger et al., 1994) and make clear the importance of the close association between VOCCs and vesicle docking sites. Thus the secretory system has two requirements for Ca^{2+}. Release of clustered vesicles for docking is mediated by calmodulin and shows a Ca^{2+}-sensitivity typical of most Ca^{2+}-mediated cellular responses (activation at 1 μM or lower), whereas exocytosis of vesicles requires much higher concentrations of Ca^{2+} and occurs close to the mouth of the VOCC, in an area referred to as the 'ion domain' (Stanley, 1997). With reference to secretion by spermatozoa and other non-neuronal cells, it is worthy of note that a similar, low affinity for Ca^{2+} is also characteristic of Ca^{2+}-induced exocytosis in endocrine cells, where 'instant', short-duration secretion is not required (Thomas et al., 1993; Heinemann et al., 1994).

Proteins of transmitter release

The second area in which significant progress is being made is in identification of proteins participating in the control of exocytosis by Ca^{2+}. Though, in theory, fusion of phospholipid membranes might be activated directly by the presence of high concentrations of divalent cations (e.g. Duzgunes et al., 1981), the involvement of proteins which form a multimeric, Ca^{2+}-sensitive fusion complex has long been suspected and is now well established (Sudhof, 1995; Troy Littleton & Bellen, 1995).

A number of proteins located either on the vesicle or both the vesicle and plasma membranes (Stanley, 1997) have been implicated in release of transmitter. Some of these proteins, such as synaptotagmin, have been proposed as Ca^{2+}-sensitive sites, conferring Ca^{2+} sensitivity on the process. Others appear to be parts of (or homologues of) a ubiquitous fusion apparatus that is not constitutively Ca^{2+} dependent and may participate in intracellular membrane trafficking (Troy Littleton & Bellen, 1995; O'Connor et al., 1996; Knepper & Inoue, 1997).

Promotion of exocytosis by this protein complex, in both neuronal and non-neuronal cells, appears to include formation of a fusion pore. This pore is a multimeric protein ion channel that spans both vesicle and plasma membranes, initiating the release of vesicle contents and facilitating collapse of the exocytotic vesicle and fusion of the lipid domains (Bruns & Jahn, 1995; Lindau & Almers, 1995; Lollike et al., 1995). Direct monitoring of exocytosis can be carried out either by micro-voltametry to detect release of vesicle contents or by capacitance measurement of the cell membrane when held in the whole-cell patch clamp configuration. Data obtained by both of these techniques suggest that initially a small opening is formed, followed by rapid collapse of the vesicle and explosive release of its contents (Matthews, 1996). It appears that almost all 'exocytoxins' (toxins targeted against exocytosis) interact with the proteins responsible for formation of the fusion complex. These include botulinum toxins, tetanus toxin and alpha-latrotoxin (a component of black widow spider venom), which associates with synaptotagmin and induces massive, Ca^{2+}-independent transmitter release (Adams & Swanson, 1996).

The acrosome reaction

Participation of VOCCs in the acrosome reaction
The grounds for accepting that VOCCs are of importance in the process of stimulus–secretion coupling in spermatozoa are primarily phar-macological, since currents have not been observed directly. Many organic compounds, vertebrate and invertebrate toxins and metal ions that block VOCCs (with varying degrees of efficacy) have been identified. A number of these show sufficient specificity in their actions that they can be used as probes for participation of VOCCs in physiological processes. One group of compounds, the dihydropyridines (DHPs) has proved particularly useful in this respect. The action of DHPs, when used at sufficiently low doses (nor-mally micromolar levels) is considered to be specific to a class of VOCCs referred to as L-channels (Triggle, 1990) and has been used widely, to probe L-channel involvement in many activities of somatic cells. These com-pounds, as well as other, less-specific, organic blockers (phenylalkylamines, benzothiazapines) and divalent metal ions that block VOCCs in excitable cells (Ni^{2+}, Co^{2+}) greatly attenuate the ZP3-induced AR in human and other mammalian spermatozoa (Babcock & Pfeiffer, 1987; Florman *et al.*, 1992; O'Toole *et al.*, 1996). Other than the anomalous finding that Ni^{2+} is a more effective antagonist than Co^{2+}, a characteristic of a different type of VOCC (T-channels) (Florman *et al.*, 1992), these data indicate an involvement of L-type VOCCs in stimulus–secretion coupling in mammalian spermatozoa, at least in response to ZP3. As would be expected with such a Ca^{2+} influx pathway, activation of AR is associated with membrane depolarization (Arnoult *et al.*, 1996*a*) which is presumably necessary for gating of the VOCCs. Furthermore, in both mouse and bovine spermatozoa, membrane hyperpolarization of 15–30 mV occurs during capacitation, such that one of the functions of capacitation could be to release VOCCs from steady-state inactivation (Zeng *et al.*, 1995).

Recently patch-clamping has been applied to mouse spermatogenic cells on the grounds that mature sperm lack a protein synthesis capability and that channel expression in spermatogenic cells is liable to be similar to that in mature spermatozoa (Arnoult *et al.*, 1996*b*; Lievano *et al.*, 1996; Santi *et al.*,

1996). These studies have produced evidence that the VOCC of rodent spermatozoa is different from any previously identified VOCCs of somatic cells. Whole cell clamp of spermatogenic cells revealed the presence of only a single VOCC type, which has the biophysical properties (voltage sensitivity, kinetics) of a T-type VOCC, but shows characteristic, L-channel-like sensitivity to DHPs. Molecular analysis of the expression of VOCC subunits in these cells revealed primarily the α_1E-type channel (Lievano et al., 1996). Initial studies on a rat α_1E clone showed that expression of this subunit in *Xenopus* oocytes produced a low-voltage-activated, T-like current (Soong et al., 1993). Subsequent work on clones from other mammalian species suggests that expression of α_1E is normally responsible for a high voltage activated channel. A much more convincing candidate for the α_1 subunit of the neuronal T-channel (α_1G) has recently been described (Perez-Reyes et al., 1998), though it is conceivable that the α_1E subunit could produce a low-voltage activated, T-like current in spermatozoa. Direct measurement of channel conductance (currently not possible in spermatozoa) may help to resolve the identity of the sperm membrane VOCC.

The sensitivity of this T-like current to various inhibitors resembles the sensitivity of the ZP3–induced AR (including a greater efficacy of Ni^{2+} than Co^{2+}; Arnoult et al., 1996b) and it therefore appears that the T-current that has been characterized in spermatogenic cells is responsible for at least part of the Ca^{2+} influx induced by ZP3. This interpretation, if correct, leads to the intriguing conclusion that activation of the T-current leads to a slowly developing, prolonged elevation of $[Ca^{2+}]_i$. As discussed by Arnoult et al. (1996a), the T-channel is normally responsible for generating rhythmic activity rather than allowing significant influx of Ca^{2+}. Under voltage clamp the channel inactivates within 60–100 ms and does not provide prolonged influx. It therefore appears that if, as indicated by the pharmacological data, the VOCCs of spermatozoa play a necessary role in stimulus–secretion coupling, it must be to provide a signal leading to mobilization of Ca^{2+} from another source (Arnoult et al., 1996a). A peculiarity of the T-current expressed in mouse spermatogenic cells is a slowly decaying, voltage-dependent facilitation of current amplitude, probably due to temporary tyrosine dephosphorylation (Arnoult et al., 1997). The function of this voltage sensitivity (if it is indeed functional) is not known. The only similar modulation of T-currents that has been described so far occurs in stromal cells of rat bone marrow (Publicover et al., 1995).

Ca^{2+} in the acrosome reaction

Responses of $[Ca^{2+}]_i$ of mammalian spermatozoa to agonists or drug treatments that induce the AR have been observed using fluorescent probes, either by spectrofluorimetry or imaging. Studies with ratioing probes have allowed some estimates of $[Ca^{2+}]_i$ during induction of the AR. These mostly lie in the range 0.5–1 μM (e.g. Blackmore, 1993; Zeng *et al.*, 1995; Brewis *et al.*, 1996), though Meizel and colleagues have recorded progesterone-induced responses of 8–10 μM in the anterior head of individual human spermatozoa (Meizel *et al.*, 1997). These values are comparable with those recorded during stimulus–secretion coupling in a range of cell types (including neurons), but do not compare with measurements and model-generated estimates of $[Ca^{2+}]$ at the AZ. However, fluorescent techniques even when using imaging, give an average signal for a volume of cytoplasm significantly larger than that which determines whether membrane fusion occurs. It is therefore still possible that localized, high $[Ca^{2+}]$ 'ion zones' are formed between the acrosome and plasma membranes, similar to those occurring at the AZ.

Participation of such localized areas of high $[Ca^{2+}]_i$ in the AR has recently been proposed (Spungin & Breitbart, 1996, Breitbart & Spungin, 1997). Using a cell-free system (purified plasma and outer acrosomal membranes) derived from bovine spermatozoa, these authors have provided evidence that actin filaments are formed on the plasma and outer acrosomal membranes during capacitation (Spungin *et al.*, 1995). Attachment of a phosphatidylinositol 4,5-bisphosphate-specific phospholipase (PLC) to this actin then occurs. The authors suggest that activation of PLC allows actin dispersion, permitting membrane fusion. Inhibition of such dispersion by phalloidin prevents membrane fusion and inhibits the AR in intact cells (Spungin *et al.*, 1995). Fifty per cent activation of release of actin from extracted plasma membranes occurs at 80 μM Ca^{2+}, a concentration orders of magnitude higher than those reported for spermatozoa undergoing the AR (Spungin & Breitbart, 1996). The authors suggest that the necessary large rise in $[Ca^{2+}]_i$ could be achieved by Ca^{2+} influx, through a protein kinase C (PKC)-regulated, DHP-sensitive VOCC but that initial activation of PLC occurs at a lower $[Ca^{2+}]_i$ resulting from release of stored Ca^{2+} (Spungin & Breitbart, 1996).

If such high concentrations of Ca^{2+} occur then they will almost certainly be achieved by localization of Ca^{2+} channels, either in the plasmalemma or the acrosomal membrane. Little work has been done on localization of VOCCs in spermatozoa. Goodwin *et al.* (1997) report that antibodies directed against the $\alpha 1$ subunit of rabbit skeletal muscle L-channels ($\alpha 1$ S) are detected in the postacrosomal region of human spermatozoa (though on the basis of a parallel reverse transcriptase/PCR study on rat testis, the authors suggest that the expressed channel subunit is cardiac ($\alpha 1$c) L-type). This is clearly not consistent with clustering of VOCCs at the membrane fusion site. The situation is further confused by the fact that the VOCC subunit identified in this study is not the one detected by PCR carried out on mouse spermatogenic cells (Lievano *et al.*, 1996; see above) and is not believed to be responsible for currents of the type detected in spermatogenic cells of rat and mouse (see above).

Other sources of Ca²⁺ for the acrosome reaction

Stimulus–secretion coupling at a nerve terminal relies entirely on influx through VOCCs as a source of Ca^{2+}, though stored Ca^{2+} may be of significance in synaptic modulation. However, there is evidence that release of stored Ca^{2+} may occur during initiation of the AR (Breitbart & Spungin, 1997). Treatment of mouse spermatozoa with solubilized zonae pellucidae or purified ZP3 stimulates tyrosine kinase activity leading to activation of PLCγ. PLCγ 1 localizes to the posterior acrosome and postacrosomal region (Tomes *et al.*, 1996). PLC β (a G-protein-activated form) and associated G-proteins can be localized to the anterior acrosomal region of mouse spermatozoa (Walensky & Snyder, 1995). Activation of one or both of these enzymes by ZP3 should lead to generation of diacylglycerol (and consequent activation of PKC) and inositol 1,4,5-triphosphate (IP_3). IP_3 receptors have been localized to the acrosome cap of rat, hamster, mouse and dog spermatozoa (Walensky & Snyder, 1995). These authors also showed that IP_3 reduced Ca^{2+} loading of digitonin-permeabilized spermatozoa and that this effect was inhibited by heparin, a blocker of the IP_3 receptor. Thapsigargin, a compound that selectively blocks the Ca^{2+}-ATPase of intracellular (non-mitochondrial) membranes, causes elevation of $[Ca^{2+}]_i$ in human spermatozoa (Blackmore, 1993), liberation of stored Ca^{2+} in rat spermatozoa (Walensky & Snyder, 1995) and activates the AR of mouse and human sperm (Meizel & Turner, 1993; Walensky & Snyder, 1995). These data are consistent with an IP_3-Ca^{2+} signalling system in spermatozoa (activated by G-protein and/or tyrosine kinase activation), involving release of Ca^{2+} stored within the acrosome. Evidence has also been presented for the existence of a cAMP-gated Ca^{2+} channel in the acrosomal membrane of bovine spermatozoa (Spungin & Breitbart, 1996). Elevation of [cyclic AMP] during the AR could activate such a channel (Ward & Kopf, 1993).

Future research

Clearly, evidence exists to support the involvement of a variety of mechanisms by which $[Ca^{2+}]_i$ may be elevated during the AR. These include influx through VOCCs mediated by depolarization or by activity of PKC, release of Ca^{2+} from the acrosome induced by IP_3 (through either G-protein or tyrosine kinase pathways) and activation of cyclic AMP-gated channels. These pathways could operate in parallel, to increase the probability of AR and thus fertilization, or could be activated in sequence, to provide various Ca^{2+} signals of different magnitudes and localized to different sites within the spermatozoon. To grasp the significance of these biochemical data it is necessary that efforts are made to understand the control of membrane fusion during the AR. In particular, future work should include elucidation of the structure and organization of the secretory apparatus and the secretory event, as has been, and is being, achieved in the study of transmitter release. Some important questions to be answered include:

1 Are the Ca^{2+} channels that participate in the AR clustered, similarly to other secretory systems?

2 Does membrane fusion occur at predefined sites?

3 Are there specific Ca^{2+}-regulated fusion proteins in the acrosome and/or plasma membrane, possibly producing fusion pores?

The progress that has been made in the elucidation of the processes that underlie secretion of neurotransmitter suggests that it is probable that the structural and regulatory aspects of the AR will be far better understood within the next 5–10 years.

References

Adams, M. E. & Swanson, G. (1996). Neurotoxins. *Trends in Neuroscience,* 19, suppl.

Aitken, R. J. (1997). Molecular mechanisms regulating human sperm function. *Molecular Human Reproduction,* 3, 169–73.

Aitken, R. J., Buckingham, D. W., Harkiss, D. *et al.* (1996a). The extragenomic action of progesterone on human spermatozoa is influenced by redox regulated changes in tyrosine phosphorylation during capacitation. *Molecular and Cellular Endocrinology,* 117, 83–93.

Aitken, R. J., Buckingham, D. W. & Irvine, D. S. (1996b). The extragenomic action of progesterone on human spermatozoa: evidence for a ubiquitous response that is rapidly down-regulated. *Endocrinology,* 137, 3999–4009.

Allen, C. A. & Green, D. P. L. (1997). The mammalian acrosome reaction: gateway to sperm fusion with the oocyte? *BioEssays,* 19, 241–7.

Arnoult, C., Cardullo, R. A., Lemos, J. R. & Florman, H. M. (1996a). Activation of mouse sperm T-type Ca^{2+} channels by adhesion to the egg zona pellucida. *Proceedings of the National Academy of Sciences, USA,* 93, 13004–9.

Arnoult, C., Zeng, Y. & Florman, H. M. (1996b). ZP3–dependent activation of sperm cation channels regulates acrosomal secretion during mammalian fertilization. *Journal of Cell Biology,* 134, 637–45.

Arnoult, C., Lemos, J. R. & Florman, H. M. (1997). Voltage-dependent modulation of T-type calcium channels by protein tyrosine phosphorylation. *EMBO Journal,* 16, 1593–9.

Babcock, D. F. & Pfeiffer, D. R. (1987). Independent elevation of cytosolic Ca^{2+} and pH of mammalian sperm by voltage dependent and pH-sensitive mechanisms. *Journal of Biological Chemistry,* 262, 15041–7.

Bailey, J. L. & Storey, B. T. (1994). Calcium influx into mouse spermatozoa activated by solubilized mouse zona pellucida, monitored with the calcium fluorescent indicator, fluo-3. *Molecular Reproduction and Development,* 39, 297–308.

Baillie, H. S., Pacey, A. A., Warren, M. A. *et al.* (1997). Greater numbers of human spermatozoa associate with endosalpingeal cells derived from the isthmus compared to those from the ampulla. *Human Reproduction,* 12, 1985–92.

Barratt, C. L. R. (1997). Hypothesis to unify an embryonic defence system and HIV infection. *Molecular Human Reproduction,* 3, 81–2.

Barratt, C. L. R. & Cooke, I. D. (1991). Sperm transport in the human female reproductive tract – a dynamic interaction. *International Journal of Andrology*, **14**, 394–411.

Barratt, C. L. R. & Hornby, D. P. (1995). Induction of the acrosome reaction by rhuZP3. In *Human sperm acrosome reaction*, ed. P. Fenichel & J. Parinaud, pp. 105–12. John Libbey Eurotext, Colloque INSERM **236**.

Barratt, C. L. R. & Pockley, G. (1998). Sperm survival in the female reproductive tract: presence of immunosuppression or absence of recognition? *Molecular Human Reproduction*, **4**, 309–16.

Beebe, S. J., Leyton, L., Burks, P., *et al.* (1992). Recombinant mouse ZP3 inhibits sperm binding and induces the acrosome reaction. *Development Biology*, **151**, 48–54.

Bennett, M. K. (1997). Ca^{2+} and the regulation of neurotransmitter secretion. *Current Opinion in Neurobiology*, **7**, 316–22.

Benoff, S. (1997). Carbohydrates and fertilisation. *Molecular Human Reproduction*, **3**, 599–637.

Blackmore, P. F. (1993). Thapsigargin elevates and potentiates the ability of progesterone to increase intracellular free calcium in human sperm: possible role of perinuclear calcium. *Cell Calcium*, **14**, 53–60.

Breitbart, H. & Spungin, B. (1997). The biochemistry of the acrosome reaction. *Molecular Human Reproduction*, **3**, 195–202.

Brewis, I. A. & Moore, H. D. M. (1997). Molecular mechanisms of gamete recognition and fusion at fertilization. *Human Reproduction, National Supplement, Journal of the British Fertility Society*, **2**, 156–65.

Brewis, I. A., Clayton, R., Barratt, C. L. R. *et al.* (1996). Recombinant human zona pellucida glycoprotein 3 induces calcium influx and acrosome reaction in human spermatozoa. *Molecular Human Reproduction*, **2**, 583–9.

Bruns, D. & Jahn, R. (1995). Real-time measurement of transmitter release from single synaptic vesicles. *Nature*, **377**, 62–5.

Burks, D. J., Carballada, R., Moore, H. D. M. *et al.* (1995). Interaction of a tyrosine kinase from human sperm with the zona pellucida at fertilization. *Science*, **269**, 83–6.

Ceccarelli, B. & Hurlbut, W. P. (1980). Vesicle hypothesis of the release of quanta of transmitter. *Physiological Review*, **60**, 396–441.

Chamberlin, M. E. & Dean, J. (1990). Human homolog of the mouse sperm receptor. *Proceedings of the National Academy of Sciences, USA*, **87**, 6014–18.

Chapman, N. R. & Barratt, C. L. R. (1996). The role of carbohydrate in spermatozoa-ZP3 adhesion. *Molecular Human Reproduction*, **2**, 767–74.

(1997). Sperm–zona interaction and recombinant DNA technology. *Molecular Human Reproduction*, **3**, 646–50.

Chapman, N. R., Kessopoulou, E., Andrews, P. D. *et al.* (1998). The polypeptide backbone of recombinant human zona pellucida glycoprotein-3 initiates acrosomal exocytosis in human spermatozoa *in vitro*. *Biochemical Journal*, **330**, 839–45.

Clark, G. F., Oehninger, S., Patankar, M. S. *et al.* (1996). A role for glycoconjugates in human development: the human feto-embryonic defence hypothesis. *Human Reproduction*, **11**, 467–73.

Clark, G. F., Dell, A., Morris, H. R., Patankar, M. S. *et al.* (1997). Viewing AIDS from a glycobiological perspective: potential links to the human fetoembryonic defence system hypothesis. *Molecular Human Reproduction*, **3**, 5–14.

Cohen, M. W., Jones, O. T. & Angelides, K. J. (1991). Distribution of Ca^{2+} channels on frog motor-nerve terminals revealed by fluorescent omega-conotoxin. *Journal of Neuroscience*, **11**, 1032–9.

De Jonge, C. J., Barratt, C. L. R., Radwanska, E. & Cooke, I. D. (1993). The acrosome reaction-inducing effect of human follicular and oviductal fluid. *Journal of Andrology*, **14**, 359–65.

Demott, R. P., Lefebvre, R. & Suarez, S. (1995). Carbohydrates mediate the adherence of hamster sperm to oviductal epithelium. *Biology of Reproduction*, **52**, 1395–403.

Duzgunes, N., Wilschut, J., Fraley, R. & Papahadjopoulos, D. (1981). Studies on the mechanism of membrane fusion: Role of head-group composition in calcium- and magnesium-induced fusion of mixed phospholipid vesicles. *Biochimica et Biophysica Acta*, **642**, 182–95.

Evans, J. P., Kopf, G. S. & Schultz, R. M. (1997*a*). Characterization of the binding of recombinant mouse sperm fertilin α subunit to mouse eggs: evidence for adhesive activity via an egg β1 integrin-mediated interaction. *Developmental Biology*, **187**, 79–93.

Evans, J. P., Schultz, R. M. & Kopf, G. S. (1997*b*). Characterization of the binding of recombinant mouse sperm fertilin α subunit to mouse eggs: evidence for function as a cell adhesion molecule in sperm–egg binding. *Developmental Biology*, **187**, 94–106.

Fearon, D. T. (1997). Seeking wisdom in innate immunity. *Nature*, **388**, 323–4.

Fearon, D. T. & Locksley, R. M. (1996). The instructive role of innate immunity in the acquired immune response. *Science*, **272**, 50–60.

Florman, H. M. (1994). Sequential focal and global elevations of sperm intracellular Ca^{2+} are initiated by zona pellucida during acrosomal exocytosis. *Developmental Biology*, **165**, 152–64.

Florman, H. M., Corron, M. E., Kim, T. D. H. & Babcock, D. F. (1992). Activation of voltage-dependent calcium channels of mammmalian sperm is required for zona pellucida-induced acrosomal exocytosis. *Developmental Biology*, **152**, 304–14.

Florman, H. M., Lernos, J. T., Arnoult, C. *et al.* (1995). Exocytotic ion channels in mammalian sperm. In *Human acrosome reaction*, ed. P. Fenichel & J. Parinaud, pp. 179–89. Colloque INSERM 236.

Goodwin, L. O., Leeds, N. B., Hurley, I. *et al.* (1997). Isolation and characterization of the primary structure of testis-specific L-type calcium channel: implications for contraception. *Molecular Human Reproduction*, **3**, 255–68.

Gupta, S. K., Yurewicz, Y. C., Afzalpurar, A. *et al.* (1995). Localisation of epitopes for monoclonal antibiodies at the N-terminus of the porcine zona pellucida glycoprotein pZPC. *Molecular Reproduction and Development*, **42**, 220–5.

Heidelberger, R., Heinemann, C., Neher, E. & Matthews, G. (1994). Calcium dependence of the rate of exocytosis in a synaptic terminal. *Nature*, **371**, 513–15.

Heinemann, C., Chow, R. H., Neher, E. & Zucker, R. S. (1994). Kinetics of the secretory response in bovine chromaffin cells following flash photolysis of caged Ca^{2+}. *Biophysical Journal*, **67**, 2546–57.

Heuser, J. E., Reese, T. S., Dennis, M. J. *et al.* (1979). Synaptic vesicle exocytosis captured by quick freezing and correlated with quantal transmitter release. *Jorunal of Cell Biology*, **81**, 275–300.

Hughes, E. G. (1997). The effectiveness of ovulation induction and IUI in the treatment of persistent infertility – a metaanalysis. *Human Reproduction*, **12**, 1865–72.

Hunter, R. H. F. (1984). Pre-ovulatory arrest and peri-ovulatory redistribution of competent spermatozoa in the isthmus of the pig oviduct. *Journal of Reproduction and Fertility*, **72**, 203–11.

Hunter, R. H. F. & Nicol, R. (1983). Transport of spermatozoa in the sheep oviduct: preovulatory sequestering of cells in the caudal isthmus. *Journal of Experimental Zoology*, **228**, 121–8.

Huttner, W. B., Schlieber, W., Greengard, P. & De Camilli, P. (1983). Synapsin 1 (protein 1), a nerve terminal specific phosphoprotein. 3. Its association with synaptic vesicles studied in a highly purified synaptic vesicle preparation. *Journal of Cell Biology*, **96**, 1374–88.

Ikawa, M., Wada, I., Kominami, K. *et al.* (1997). The putative chaperone calmegin is required for sperm fertility. *Nature*, **387**, 607–11.

Jury, J. A., Frayne, J. & Hall, L. (1997). The human fertilin alpha gene is non-functional: implications for its proposed role in fertilisation. *Biochemical Journal*, **321**, 577–81.

Katz, B. & Miledi, R. (1965). The effect of calcium on acetylcholine release from motor nerve terminals. *Proceedings of the Royal Society of London, B*, **161**, 496–544.

(1967). The timing of calcium action during neuromuscular transmission. *Journal of Physiology*, **189**, 535.

(1969). Spontaneous and evoked activity of motor nerve terminals in calcium ringer. *Journal of Physiology*, **203**, 689–706.

King, R. S. & Killian, G. J. (1994). Purification of bovine estrus associated protein and localisation of binding on sperm. *Biology of Reproduction*, **51**, 34–42.

Kinloch, R. A., Mortillo, S. A., Stewart, C. L. *et al.* (1991). Embryonal carcinoma cells transfected with ZP3 genes differentially glycosylate similar polypeptides and secrete active mouse sperm receptor. *Journal of Cell Biology*, **115**, 655–64.

Kinloch, R. A., Sakai, Y. & Wassarman, P. M. (1995). Mapping the mouse ZP3 combining sites for sperm by exon swapping and site-directed mutagenesis. *Proceedings of the National Academy of Sciences, USA*, **92**, 263–7.

Knepper, M. A. & Inoue, T. (1997). Regulation of aquaporin-2 water channel trafficking by vasopressin. *Current Opinion in Cell Biology*, **9**, 560–4.

Koyama, K., Hasegawa, A., Inoue, M. *et al.* (1994). Blocking of human sperm zona interaction by monoclonal antibodies to a glycoprotein family (ZP4) of porcine zona pellucida. *Biology of Reproduction*, **45**, 727–35.

Landis, D. M. D., Hall, A. K., Weinstein, L. A. & Reeses, T. S. (1988). The organisation of cytoplasm at the presynaptic active zone of a central nervous-system synapse. *Neuron*, **1**, 201–9.

Lansac, J., Thepot, F., Mayaux, M. J. *et al.* (1997). Pregnancy outcomes after artificial insemination or IVF with frozen donor semen: a collaborative study of the French CECOS Federation. *European Journal of Obstetrics, Gynaecology and Reproductive Biology*, 74, 223–8.

Lenton, E. A. (1993). Ovulation timing. In *Donor insemination*, ed. C. L. R. Barratt & I. D. Cooke, pp. 97–110. Cambridge: Cambridge University Press.

Leyton, L. & Saling, P. (1989). Evidence that aggregation of mouse sperm receptors by ZP3 triggers the acrosome reaction. *Journal of Cell Biology*, 108, 2163–8.

Lievano, A., Santi, C. M., Serrano, C. J., Trevino, C. L., Bellve, A. R., Hernandez-Cruz, A. & Darszon, A. (1996). T-type channels and alpha1E expression in spermatogenic cells, and their possible relevance to the sperm acrosome reaction. *FEBS Letters*, 388, 150–4.

Lindau, M. & Almers, W. (1995). Structure and function of fusion pores in exocytosis and ectoplasmic membrane fusion. *Current Opinion in Cell Biology*, 7, 509–17.

Liu, D. Y. & Baker, H. W. G. (1992). Tests of human sperm function and fertilisation *in vitro*. *Human Reproduction*, 58, 465–83.

(1994). Disordered acrosome reaction of spermatozoa bound to the zona pellucida: a newly discovered sperm defect causing infertility with reduced sperm–zona pellucida penetration and reduced fertilisation *in vitro*. *Human Reproduction*, 9, 1694–700.

(1996). A simple method for assessment of the human acrosome reaction of spermatozoa bound to the zona pellucida: lack of a relationship with ionophore A23187-induced acrosome reaction. *Human Reproduction*, 11, 551–7.

Llinas, R. & Nicholson, C. (1974). Calcium role in depolarization–secretion coupling: an aequorin study in squid giant synapse. *Proceedings of the National Academy of Sciences, USA*, 72, 187–90.

Llinas, R., Blinks, J. R. & Nicholson, C. (1972). Calcium transient in the presynaptic terminal of squid giant synapse: detection with aequorin. *Science*, 176, 1127–9.

Lollike, K., Borregaard, N. & Lindau, M. (1995). The exocytotic fusion pore of small granules has a conductance similar to anion channel. *Journal of Cell Biology*, 129, 99–104.

Lu, Q. X. & Shur, B. D. (1997). Sperm from β 1-4-galactosyltransferase null mice are refractory to ZP3 induced acrosome reactions and penetrate the zona pellucida poorly. *Development*, 124, 4121–31.

Matthews, G. (1996). Synaptic exocytosis and endocytosis: capacitamce measurements. *Current Opinion in Neurobiology*, 6, 358–64.

Mattner, P. E. (1969). Phagocytosis of spermatozoa by leucocytes in bovine cervical mucus *in vitro*. *Journal of Reproduction and Fertility*, 20, 133–4.

Medzhitov, R. & Janeway, C. A. Jr (1997). Innate immunity: impact on the adaptive immune response. *Current Opinion in Immunology*, 9, 4–9.

Meizel, S. & Turner, K. O. (1993). Initiation of the human sperm acrosome reaction by thapsigargin. *Journal of Experimental Zoology*, 267, 350–5.

Meizel, S., Turner, K. O. & Nuccitelli, R. (1997). Progesterone triggers a wave of increased free calcium during the human sperm acrosome reaction. *Developmental Biology*, 182, 67–75.

Morales P., Palma V., Salgado A. M. *et al.* (1996). Sperm interaction with human oviductal cells *in vitro*. *Human Reproduction*, **11**: 1504–9.

Mortimer, S. T., Schoevaert, D., Swan, M. A. & Mortimer, D. (1997). Quantitative observations of the flagellar beat patterns of capacitating human spermatozoa. *Human Reproduction*, **12**, 1006–12.

O'Connor, V., Pellegrini, L., Bommert, K., Dresbach, T., El Far, O., Betz, H., Debello, W., Hunt, J. M., Schweizer, F., Augustine, G. & Charlton, M. P. (1996). Protein–protein interactions in synaptic vesicle exocytosis. *Biochemical Society Transactions*, **24**, 666–70.

Oehninger, S., Toner, J. P., Muasher, S. J. *et al.* (1992). Prediction of fertilization *in vitro* with human gametes: Is there a litmus test? *American Journal of Obstetrics and Gynaecology*, **167**, 1760–7.

O'Toole, C. M. B., Roldan, E. R. S. & Fraser, L. R. (1996). Role for Ca^{2+} channels in the signal transduction pathway leading to acrosomal exocytosis in human spermatozoa. *Molecular Reproduction and Development*, **45**, 204–11.

Pacey, A. A., Hill, C. J., Scudamore, I. W. *et al.* (1995a). The interaction *in vitro* of human spermatozoa with epithelial cells from the human uterine (Fallopian) tube. *Human Reproduction*, **10**, 360–6.

Pacey, A. A., Davies, N., Warren, M. A. *et al.* (1995b). Hyperactivation may assist human spermatozoa to detach from intimate association with the endosalpinx. *Human Reproduction*; **10**, 2603–9.

Pallanen, P. & Cooper, T. G. (1994). Immunology of the testicular excurrent ducts. *Journal of Reproduction and Immunology*, **26**, 167–216.

Pandya, I. J. & Cohen, J. (1985). The leukocytic reaction of the human uterine cervix to spermatozoa. *Fertility and Sterility*, **43**, 417–21.

Perez-Reyes, E., Cribbs, L. L., Dand, A. *et al.* (1998). Molecular characterization of a neuronal low-voltage-activated T-type calcium channel. *Nature*, **391**, 896–900.

Publicover, S. J., Preston, M. R. & El Haj, A. J. (1995). Voltage-dependent potentiation of low-voltage-activated Ca^{2+} channel currents in cultured rat bone marrow cells. *Journal of Physiology*, **489**, 649–61.

Rahamimoff, R., Lev-Tov, A. & Meiri, H. (1980). Primary and secondary regulation of quantal transmitter release: calcium and sodium. *Journal of Experimental Biology*, **89**, 5–18.

Ridge, J. P., Fuchs, E. J. & Matzinger, P. (1996). Neonatal tolerance revisited: turning on newborn T cells with dendritic cells. *Science*, **271**, 1723–6.

Roberts, W. M., Jacobs, R. A. & Hudspeth, A. J. (1990). Colocalization of ion channels involved in frequency selectivity and synaptic transmission at presynaptic active zones of hair cells. *Journal of Neuroscience*, **6**, 221–3.

Robitaille, R., Adler, E. M. & Charlton, M. P. (1990). Strategic location of calcium channels at transmitter release sites of frog neuromuscular synapses. *Neuron*, **5**, 773–9.

Roldan, E. R. S. & Harrison, R. A. P. (1989). Polyphosophoinositide breakdown and subsequent exocytosis in the Ca^{2+}/ionophore-induced acrosome reaction in mammalian spermatozoa. *Biochemical Journal*, **259**, 397–406.

Roldan, E. R. S., Murane, T. & Shi, Q. X. (1994). Exocytosis in spermatozoa in response to progesterone and zona pellucida. *Science*, **266**, 1578–81.

Sakkas, D., Bianchi, P. G., Manicardi, G. *et al.* (1997). Chromatin packaging anomalies and DNA damage in human sperm: their possible implications in the treatment of male factor infertility. In *Genetics of human male fertility*, ed. C. L. R. Barratt, C. De Jonge, D. Mortimer & J. Parinaud, pp. 205–22. Paris: EDK Press.

Santi, C. M., Darszon, A. & Hernandez-Cruz, A. (1996). Dihydropyridine-sensitive T-type Ca^{2+} channel is the main Ca^{2+} current carrier in mouse primary spermatocytes. *American Journal of Physiology*, **40**, C1585–C1593.

Siddiquey, A. K. S. & Cohen, J. (1982). *In-vitro* fertilisation in the mouse and the relevance of different sperm–egg concentrations and volumes. *Journal of Reproduction and Fertility*, **66**, 237–42.

Smith, S. J. & Augustine, G. J. (1988). Calcium ions, active zones and synaptic transmitter release. *Trends in Neuroscience*, **11**, 458–64.

Smith, T. T. & Yanagimachi, R. (1990). The viability of hamster spermatozoa stored in the isthmus of the oviduct: the importance of sperm–epithelium contact for sperm survival. *Biology of Reproduction*, **42**, 450–7.

Snell, W. J. & White, J. M. (1996). The molecules of mammalian fertilisation. *Cell*, **85**, 629–37.

Soong, T. W., Stea, A., Hodson, C. D., Dubel, S. T., Vincent, S. R. & Snutch, T. P. (1993). Structure and functional expression of a member of the low voltage-activated calcium channel family. *Science*, **260**, 1133–6.

Spungin, B. & Breitbart, H. (1996). Calcium mobilisation and influx during sperm exocytosis. *Journal of Cell Science*, **109**, 1947–55.

Spungin, B., Margalit, I. & Breitbart, H. (1995). Sperm exocytosis reconstructed in a cell-free system: evidence for the involvement of phospholipase C and actin filaments in membrane fusion. *Journal of Cell Science*, **108**, 2525–35.

Stanley, E. F. (1997). The calcium channel and the organization of the presynaptic transmitter release face. *Trends in Neuroscience*, **20**, 404–9.

Statham, H. E. & Duncan, C. J. (1976). Dantrolene and the neuromuscular junction: evidence for intracellular calcium stores. *European Journal of Pharmacology*, **39**, 143–50.

Stevernick, D. W. B., Soede, N. M., Bouwman, E. G. & Kemp, B. (1997). Influence of insemination–ovulation interval and sperm cell dose on fertilisation in sows. *Journal of Reproduction and Fertility*, **111**, 165–71.

Sudhof, T. C. (1995). The synaptic vesicle cycle: a cascade of protein–protein interactions. *Nature*, **375**, 645–53.

Swann, K. & Lai, F. A. (1997). A novel signalling mechanism for generation of calcium oscillations at fertilisation in mammals. *Bioessays*, **19**, 371–8.

Tesarik, J., Carreras, A. & Mendoza, C. (1996). Single cell analysis of tyrosine kinase dependent and independent Ca^{2+} fluxes in progesterone induced acrosome reaction. *Molecular Human Reproduction*, **2**, 225–32.

Thomas, P. & Meizel, S. (1989). Phosphatidylinositol-4,5–bisphosphate hydrolysis in human sperm stimulated with follicular fluid or progesterone is dependent on Ca^{2+} influx. *Biochemical Journal*, **264**, 539–46.

Thomas, P., Wong, J. G., Lee, A. K. & Almers, W. (1993). A low affinity Ca^{2+} receptor controls the final steps in peptide secretion from pitiutary melanotrophs. *Neuron*, **11**, 93–104.

Thompson, L. A., Tomlinson, M. J., Barratt, C. L. R. *et al.* (1991). Positive immu-
noselection: a method of isolating leukocytes from leukocytic reacted
human cervical mucus. *American Journal of Reproduction and
Immunology*, **26**, 58–61.

Thompson, L. A., Barratt, C. L. R., Bolton, A. E. & Cooke, I. D. (1992). The leukocytic reaction of the human uterine cervix. *American Journal of
Reproduction and Immunology*, **28**, 85–9.

Tomes, C. N., McMaster, C. R. & Saling, P. M. (1996). Activation of mouse sperm
phosphatidylinositol 4,5-bisphosphate phospholipase C by zona pellucida
is modulated by tyrosine phosphorylation. *Molecular Reproduction and
Development*, **43**, 196–204.

Triggle, D. J. (1990). Calcium, calcium channels and calcium channel antagonists.
Canadian Journal of Physiological Pharmacology, **68**, 1474–81.

Troy Littleton, J. & Bellen, H. J. (1995). Synaptotagmin controls and modulates
synaptic vesicle fusion in a Ca^{2+}-dependent manner. *Trends in
Neuroscience*, **18**, 177–83.

Walensky, L. D. & Snyder, S. H. (1995). Inositol 1,4,5-trisphosphate receptors selectively localized to acrosomes of mammalian sperm. *Journal of Cell Biology*,
130, 857–69.

Ward, C. R. & Kopf, G. S. (1993). Molecular events mediating sperm activation.
Developmental Biology, **158**, 9–34.

Waters, S. I. & White, J. M. (1997). Biochemical and molecular characterization of
bovine fertilin α and β (ADAM 1 and ADAM 2): a candidate sperm-egg
binding/fusion complex. *Biology of Reproduction*, **56**, 1245–54.

Wassarman, P. M. (1992). Mouse gamete adhesion molecules. *Biology of
Reproduction*, **146**, 86–191.

Whitmarsh, A. J., Woolnough, M. J., Moore, H. D. M. *et al.* (1996). Biological
activity of recombinant human ZP3 produced *in vitro*: potential for a
sperm function test. *Molecular Human Reproduction*, **2**, 911–19.

Wilcox, A. J., Weinberg, C. R. & Baird, D. D. (1995). Timing of sexual intercourse
in relation to ovulation – effects on the probability of conception, survival
of the pregnancy, and sex of the baby. *New England Journal of Medicine*,
333, 1517–65.

Williams, M., Hill, C. J., Scudamore, I. *et al.* (1993*a*). Sperm numbers and distribution within the human fallopian tube around ovulation. *Human
Reproduction*, **8**, 2019–26.

Williams, M., Thompson, L. A., Li, T. C. *et al.* (1993*b*). Uterine flushing: a method
to recover spermatozoa and leukocytes. *Human Reproduction*, **8**, 925–8.

Wilmut, I., Hunter, R. H. F. (1984). Sperm transport into the oviducts of heifers
mated early in oestrus. *Reproduction, Nutrition, Développement*, **24**, 461–8.

Zeng, Y., Clark, E. N. & Florman, H. M. (1995). Sperm membrane potential:
hyperpolarization during capacitation regulates zona pellucida-dependent
acrosomal secretion. *Developmental Biology*, **171**, 554–63.

Zinamen, M., Drobnis, P., Morales *et al.* (1989). The physiology of sperm recovered from the human uterine cervix: acrosomal status and response to
inducers of the acrosome reaction. *Biology of Reproduction*, **41**, 790–7.

Zhu, X. & Naz, R. (1997). Fertilization antigen 1: cDNA cloning, testis specific, and immunocontraceptive effects. *Proceedings of the National Academy of Sciences, USA,* **94**, 4704–9.

Zhu J., Barratt, C. L. R., Lippes, J., Pacey, A. A., Lenton, E. A. & Cooke, I. D. (1994*a*). Human oviductal fluid prolongs sperm survival. *Fertility and Sterility,* **61**, 360–6.

Zhu, J. J., Barratt, C. L. R., Lippes, J., *et al.* (1994*b*). The sequential effect of human cervical mucus, oviductal and follicular fluid on sperm function. *Fertility and Sterility,* **61**, 1129–35.

7 Changes in human male reproductive health

STEWART IRVINE

Introduction

During the past two decades, a number of reports have appeared which have raised serious concerns about the development of reproductive problems in animals and man (Colborn *et al.*, 1996; Cadbury, 1997). There have been reports of alligators with abnormal male genital development (Guillette *et al.*, 1994) and of reproductive changes in fish and birds (Giesy *et al.*, 1994; Sumpter & Jobling, 1995). At the same time, there have been controversial reports of changes in human semen quality (Carlsen *et al.*, 1992; Auger *et al.*, 1995; Irvine *et al.*, 1996), alongside reports of an increasing incidence of congenital malformations of the male genital tract, such as cryptorchidism and hypospadias (Kallen *et al.*, 1986; Ansell *et al.*, 1992), and of an increasing incidence of testicular cancer (Adami *et al.*, 1994; Hoff Wanderas *et al.*, 1995). However, there is controversy over whether or not these reported changes in male reproductive health are genuine (Setchell, 1997), and if so, what the causes and implications are, in particular the implications for clinicians caring for couples with infertility.

Testicular cancer

Although many of the changes seen in male reproductive health are controversial, there seems little argument that testicular cancer is increasing in frequency, with unexplained increases in the age-standardized incidence observed in Europe (Adami *et al.*, 1994; Bergstrom *et al.*, 1996; Hernes *et al.*, 1996) and the USA (Devesa *et al.*, 1995; Zheng *et al.*, 1996). In the west of Scotland, for example, the number of testicular germ cell tumours registered has more than doubled between 1960 and 1990 (Hatton *et al.*, 1995), while a recent study from Norway reported that the age-standardized incidence for testicular cancer increased from 2.7 per 100 000 in 1955 to 8.5 per 100 000 in 1992. (Hoff Wanderas *et al.*, 1995). A similar study reported a 61% increase in testicular cancer in southern Norway from 1986–7 to 1991–2 (Hernes, *et al.*, 1996). In parts of the USA, the overall age-adjusted incidence rate of testicular cancer has increased 3.5-fold during the past 60 years (Zheng *et al.*, 1996).

There is substantial geographical variation in both the incidence of testicular cancer and in the observed rate of increase (Adami *et al.*, 1994). This geographical variation may be linked with that seen in semen quality – testicular cancer is four times more common in Denmark, where studies have revealed rather low sperm counts (Jensen *et al.*, 1996), than in Finland where semen quality is better (Vierula *et al.*, 1996).

Interestingly, the observed increases, both in Europe and theUSA would appear to be a birth cohort effect (Bergstrom *et al.*, 1996; Zheng *et al.*, 1996). Bergstrom and colleagues (1996) evaluated data from Denmark, Norway, Sweden, the former German Democratic Republic, Finland and Poland, including data on over 30 000 cases of testicular cancer from 1945 to 1989 in men aged 20–84. They found considerable regional variation in both the incidence of testicular cancer and in the observed rate of increase, ranging from a 2.3% increase annually in Sweden to 5.2% annually in the former East Germany. Of note, in all six countries, birth cohort was a stronger determinant for testicular cancer risk than calendar time, such that men born in 1965 had a risk of testicular cancer that was 3.9 times (95% CI 2.7–5.6; Sweden) to 11.4 times (95% CI 8.3–15.5; former East Germany) higher than for men born in 1905. Similarly, Zheng *et al.*, (1996), working in the USA, concluded that the increase in testicular cancer seen in men born after 1910 was explained mainly by a strong birth cohort effect.

The aetiology of testicular cancer is ill understood, and space does not permit a detailed discussion of this complex topic here. However, it is clear that men with a history of cryptorchidism have a significantly increased risk, estimated to be about 3.6-fold (95% confidence intervals (CI) 1.8–6.9) in one study (Møller *et al.*, 1996) and 5.2-fold (95% CI 2.1–13.0) in another (Prener *et al.*, 1996). The risk of testicular cancer has also been found to be elevated in association with other congenital malformations of the genital tract including inguinal hernia, hypospadias and hydrocoele (Prener *et al.*, 1996). It has been suggested that paternal (but not maternal) occupation before conception may alter the subsequent testicular cancer risk of offspring (Knight & Marrett, 1997), as may the parental use of agricultural fertilizers (Kristensen *et al.*, 1996) or childhood residence in areas with a high nitrate concentration in ground water (Møller, 1997). Whilst fathers of testicular cancer sufferers have been found to have a slight increase in their own risk of the disease (about 2-fold, 95% CI 1.01–3.43), a much more significant risk attaches to the brothers of men with testicular cancer, who have been estimated to have a 12-fold increase in their own risk (95% CI 3.3–31.5) (Westergaard *et al.*, 1996). These latter observations support the possible involvement of a genetic component in the aetiology of testicular cancer, but also leave room for the possible role of factors acting during intrauterine or early neonatal life, and which might be shared by brothers. The notion that exposure during development to environmental factors is perhaps supported by the observation that milk consumption in adolescence was increased in cases of adult testicular cancer. In a case control study in the UK, Davies *et al.* (1996) found that, while cryptorchidism was a major risk factor for testicular cancer (7.19, 95% CI 2.36–21.9), each extra quarter pint of milk consumed increased the risk by 1.39 (95% CI 1.19–1.63).

Cryptorchidism and congenital malformations of the male genital tract

The incidence of congenital malformation of the male genital tract may also be changing, with increases observed in the prevalence of cryptorchidism and hypospadias (Editorial, *Lancet*, 1985). Cryptorchidism, for example, has increased by as much as 65–77% over recent decades in the UK (Ansell *et al.*, 1992). In contrast, data from the USA have tended to suggest that rates of cryptorchidism have not changed (Berkowitz *et al.*, 1993), although one recent large study from the USA reported that rates of hypospadias have doubled between the 1970s and 1980s (Paulozzi *et al.*, 1997). Here, too, regional differences have been observed, although the data are perhaps less robust than is the case with testicular cancer. In one multicentre study of 8122 boys from seven malformation surveillance systems around the world, Kallen *et al.* (1986), concluded that, even when differences in ascertainment were taken into account, true geographical differences exist in the prevalence of hypospadias at birth. Intriguingly, this study also concluded that there seemed to be an inverse correlation between the fertility of a population (estimated from mean parity in control women) and the prevalence of isolated hypospadias at birth.

In looking at risk factors for cryptorchidism, Berkowitz *et al.*, (1995) and Berkowitz & Lapinski (1996) suggested that maternal obesity, low birth weight, preterm delivery, the presence of other congenital malformations, ethnic group and a family history of the condition may be relevant. Others have found strong associations between cryptorchidism and low social class (Møller & Skakkebaek, 1996).

Changing semen quality: historical evidence in normal men

The suggestion that semen quality may be changing is not new. In 1974, Nelson & Bunge (1974) reported data on 386 men presenting for vasectomy in Iowa, USA. The mean sperm concentration of this group was 48×10^6/ml, only 7% having sperm concentrations above 100×10^6/ml. In speculating about secular trends in semen quality, they compared their data with values previously published in studies of semen quality in fertile men. These studies had reported average values for sperm concentration of 120×10^6/ml ($n = 200$) (Hotchkiss, 1938), 145×10^6/ml ($n = 49$) (Farris, 1949) and 100.7×10^6/ml ($n = 100$) (Falk & Kaufman, 1950). In 1951, MacLeod & Gold had published their landmark study of semen quality in 1000 male partners in infertile relationships, together with a similar number of men of proven fertility. In this group they found an average sperm concentration of 107×10^6/ml, with 5% having sperm concentrations below 20×10^6/ml, and 44% having greater than 100×10^6/ml. Nelson & Bunge (1974) thus interpreted their data as suggesting that the earlier studies were broadly consistent with each other, implying that sperm concentration had fallen. They speculated that their data 'would tend to incriminate an environmental factor to which the entire population has been exposed' (Nelson & Bunge, 1974).

This study was followed by several reports of semen quality in fertile men which found intermediate values for average sperm concentration of 70×10^6 to 81×10^6/ml (Rehan *et al.*, 1975; Sobrero & Rehan, 1975; Smith & Steinberger, 1977). These data were reviewed by MacLeod & Wang (1979), who drew together much of the available information on semen quality in fertile and infertile men and relied heavily on their extensive data on semen quality in the male partners of infertile marriages. They concluded that there was no evidence of a general fall in semen quality, although a number of further papers suggested that there may in fact be a downward trend. Leto & Frensilli (1981), for example, reported a decline in semen quality amongst potential semen donors, 77% of volunteer donors having acceptable semen quality (by AATB (American Association of Tissue Banks) standards) in 1973, compared to only 37%, by the same standards, in 1980. In addition, they observed a significant overall decline in the donors' sperm concentration over the same time. In 1980, James (1980) reported the first (admittedly non-systematic) review of published data on semen quality in men of proven fertility and in unselected normal men. Using the simple technique of unweighted rank correlation (recognizing its shortcomings), he noted significant negative correlations, between year of publication and average sperm concentration, amongst 17 papers containing data on 7639 fertile men and amongst 12 papers containing data on 354 unselected men.

Changing semen quality: historical data on infertile men

Whilst MacLeod & Wang (1979) had not seen any change in the semen quality of the male partners of infertile couples presenting in New York, two European studies reached different conclusions. In Denmark, Bostofte *et al.* (1983) compared 1077 men presenting for assessment of infertility in 1952 with 1000 similar men presenting 20 years later in 1972. They observed a significant fall in sperm concentration, a decrease in qualitative motility and an increase in the proportion of spermatozoa with abnormal morphology. Unfortunately, the two populations were not directly comparable, the men examined in 1972 being younger and of slightly higher social class. Notwithstanding this, the median sperm concentration appeared to fall from 73.4×10^6/ml in 1952 to 54.5×10^6/ml 20 years later, whilst no change was noted in ejaculate volume. Similar findings were reported in a Swedish study, the median sperm concentration amongst 185 men being investigated for infertility in 1960–1 being 109×10^6/ml, falling to 65×10^6/ml in 1980–1 (Osser *et al.*, 1984).

Although controversial in their way, these early publications failed to raise major public health concerns, perhaps because the data came from selected groups of men, unrepresentative of the general population, including men attending infertility clinics (Bostofte *et al.*, 1983; Osser *et al.*, 1984; Menkveld *et al.*, 1986), semen donors (Leto & Frensilli, 1981) or candidates for vasectomy (Nelson & Bunge, 1974). Perhaps also because the matter was debated in 'the peaceful obscurity of the specialist journals' (Farrow, 1994).

Changing semen quality: meta-analysis

In 1992, Carlsen *et al.* reawakened concern over the possibility of secular trends in semen quality, publishing a meta-analysis of data on semen quality in normal men. The authors undertook a systematic review of available data in normal men, published since 1930. Standard techniques applicable to meta-analysis were used to identify relevant papers, and care was taken to exclude data on infertile couples, men selected on the basis of their semen quality and data generated using non-classical approaches to semen analysis. Data were obtained on 14 947 men, published in 61 papers between 1938 and 1990. Unfortunately most of the data published related to mean values for sperm concentration, with only 19/61 studies reporting the more appropriate median value. Using weighted linear regression, the authors observed a decline in average ejaculate volume from 3.40 ml in 1940 to 2.75 ml in 1990. A similar analysis for sperm concentration suggested an apparent decline from 113×10^6/ml in 1940 to 66×10^6/ml in 1990, along with a decline in the proportion of men with a sperm concentration above 100×10^6/ml. A similar significant decline in mean sperm concentration was seen when the 39 papers reporting data on men of proven fertility were analysed separately. There was no change in the average age of the men studied, and no apparent influence of age on the observed secular trend in semen quality. Given that a high proportion of the reported studies emanated from the USA (28 studies, including data on 8329 men), this subgroup was analysed separately and a similar trend observed. In discussing the implications of this review, the authors considered the possibilities that racial, geographical or other aspects of the populations studied could be important, together with the obvious difficulties of methodological and selection bias inherent in meta-analysis.

Predictably, the central message of this meta-analysis, that sperm counts had declined by about 50% over the past 50 years, attracted enormous attention and generated much controversy (Brake & Krause, 1992; Bromwich *et al.*, 1994; Farrow 1994; Olsen *et al.*, 1995). Several workers published reanalyses and reinterpretations of the data presented. Bromwich and colleagues (1994) noted that sperm concentration data tend not to be normally distributed and that mean sperm concentration is thus not an ideal measure of central tendency. They went on to speculate that much of the apparent change in semen quality could be accounted for by a change in the 'accepted' definition of the lower limits of 'normal' semen from around 60×10^6/ml in the 1920s (Macomber & Sanders, 1929) to 20×10^6/ml, which is the figure commonly accepted today (World Health Organization, 1992). This change might have led to the exclusion of men with sperm concentrations of between 20×10^6 and 60×10^6/ml in the earlier studies. However, it has been pointed out that at least some of the earlier papers did include men with semen quality in this range (Keiding et al., 1994).

Others presented different statistical approaches to the data, suggesting that alternative models including the quadratic, spline fit and stairstep provided a better fit than the linear regression used by Carlsen et al., (1992) and might lead to a different interpretation. For example, the use of linear or quadratic models tends to suggest that any change in semen quality is gradual and may be continuing, whereas the stairstep model tends to suggest that 'something happened' that is not continuing. A sudden apparent fall in semen quality may be due to substantial changes in analytical methodology, subject selection criteria and study selection criteria, or to the widespread introduction of a global environmental factor. Yet as Keiding & Skakkebaek (1996) pointed out, all of the statistical models agree on one qualitative message – a decline in semen quality over time.

It is very clear that the numerous epidemiological pitfalls of work in this area mean that 'answering even simple questions is difficult' (Farrow, 1994). However, the concern of the Danish group, and of others, was not based only upon the results of this meta-analysis, but also on data from other medical disciplines and from wildlife research that pointed to the development of other male reproductive problems. Given the potential seriousness of the problem, it is surely legitimate that all the available data be mustered and presented, even if imperfect, if only to help define questions and priorities for future study.

Changing semen quality: contemporary data in favour

Most of the papers that appeared immediately following the meta-analysis of Carlsen et al. (1992) provided alternative interpretations of the data; new data have since emerged. These data have been able to address some of the inherent problems in a meta-analysis that used data collected in different countries, at different times, on different populations and with different methods of semen analysis. Unfortunately, the available data still fail to reach a conclusion as to whether or not there is any secular trend in semen quality.

Auger et al. (1995) published data on semen quality in fertile Parisian men. They examined data on 1750 men in a single geographical area, with consistent methods of subject recruitment and laboratory technique, during a 20 year period. All their study subjects were men of proven fertility, those presenting for vasectomy and the siblings of infertile men being specifically excluded. They observed a fall in all of the classical measures of semen quality over time. Because of the size of their data set, and the length of the data collection period, these workers were able to examine the independent effects of age at donation, and year of birth, taking into account any effect of the duration of abstinence. Sperm concentration was found to be affected by age with each year of advancing age being associated with a 3.3% fall in sperm concentration. Of particular importance is the fact that men born later were found to have poorer semen quality, each later year of birth being associated with a 2.6% fall in sperm concentration. Similar although less dramatic falls were noted in the other parameters of semen quality. An accompanying editorial by Sherins (1995) unfortunately misinterpreted this study as being concerned with men selected as sperm donors, rather than potential donors, and thus raised concerns about selection bias that were not well founded.

A number of other groups have published data suggesting a secular trend in semen quality amongst normal men. In a study of 577 unselected candidate semen donors in Scotland, born between 1951 and 1973, Irvine et al. (1996) noted that the median sperm concentration fell from 98×10^6/ml amongst donors born before 1959 to 78×10^6/ml amongst donors born after 1970, whilst the median total sperm number/ejaculate fell from 301×10^6 to 214×10^6. In a similar study of 416 consecutive candidate semen donors in Belgium, Van Waeleghem et al. (1996) observed declines in sperm concentration, motility and morphology. They observed a fall in sperm concentration from a mean of 71×10^6/ml to 58.6×10^6/ml, when donors assessed between 1977 and 1980 were compared with those assessed between 1990 and 1995. Corresponding figures for grade a motility, were 52.7 vs. 31.7% and for normal morphology 39.2 vs. 26.6%.

Changing semen quality: contemporary data against

In contrast, a number of reports have failed to find any evidence of a secular trend in semen quality. In Finland, Vierula et al. (1996) studied 238 normal men and 5481 men from infertile couples. They found a mean sperm concentration of 133.9×10^6/ml, a median of 90×10^6/ml, with the comparable figures for total sperm number/ejaculate being 396.6×10^6 and 309×10^6, respectively, amongst the normal men. Interestingly, these figures are significantly higher than other recent European data, being comparable to the data published in the USA in the 1950s (MacLeod & Gold, 1951). Unfortunately, no analysis of secular trends was presented in the group of normal men. In a similar way, a study of 302 volunteer semen donors in Toulouse, France, between 1977 and 1992 found no evidence of changes in semen quality with time (Bujan et al., 1996). Handelsman (1997b) examined the semen quality of 509 volunteer semen donors with a mean age of 33, presenting to one Australian unit between 1980 and 1995, and observed a median sperm concentration of 69×10^6/ml, but found no evidence of any effect of year of observation or year of birth on sperm concentration, total sperm number or ejaculate volume. In the same report, they included data on 180 men contributing semen samples in the course of clinical studies, and found that men who volunteered for studies conducted in 1987–9 had higher sperm counts (103×10^6 to 142×10^6/ml) than men volunteering for similar studies in 1990–4 (63×10^6 to 84×10^6/ml). They concluded that significant biases are introduced by subject self-selection in this area, and advocated caution in generalizing from such data to the population when the sample cannot be shown to be representative of that population. This leaves open the question of whether a representative sample can ever be obtained?

Two significant papers from the USA have provided evidence of unchanging semen quality in the populations studied. Fisch *et al.* (1996) conducted a retrospective review of data on 1283 men electing to store spermatozoa with a commercial semen banking service, prior to vasectomy, between 1970 and 1974. This study involved data collection in three locations within the USA: Minnesota in the north ($n = 600$), New York in the east ($n = 400$) and Los Angeles in the west ($n = 221$). Unfortunately, the data were complicated by the fact that some subjects were represented by data from one semen sample, whilst others were represented by the arithmetic mean of several samples. In addition, different techniques for semen analysis were used in the different locations, at different times. Overall, this group of workers found a small but significant increase in sperm concentration with time, equivalent to about 0.65% per year. Sperm concentration rose from 77×10^6/ml in 1970 to 89×10^6/ml in 1994, and there were no significant changes in ejaculate volume or sperm motility. Of interest, there was no apparent effect of age on sperm concentration, although they did observe a (positive) effect of abstinence on sperm count and ejaculate volume. The duration of abstinence did not appear to change during the period of data collection, and, notably, was not affected by age. What was particularly interesting, however, were the very marked regional variations in semen quality apparent between the three geographical locations contributing subjects to the study. For example, sperm concentrations were highest in New York (mean $= 131.5 \times 10^6$/ml), intermediate in Minnesota (100.8×10^6/ml), and lowest in California (72.7×10^6/ml). Regrettably, interpretation of these striking regional differences is complicated by the fact that there were differences between the centres in respect of the mean age of subjects, in their reported duration of abstinence and in the techniques of semen analysis.

In a study published at the same time, Paulsen *et al.* (1996) presented data on multiple semen samples from 510 normal men participating in research studies in Seattle, north-western USA, between 1972 and 1993. These men were highly selected on the basis of normal blood chemistry, endocrine profiles and physical examination. Between 4 and 30 samples per subject were analysed and, in contrast to all previous studies discussed above, sperm concentrations were determined by Coulter counter. The (geometric) mean sperm concentration in 1972 was 46.5×10^6/ml, and regression analysis showed a weak increase with time, which was statistically significant, but regarded by the authors as clinically insignificant.

In addition to the Finnish data mentioned above (Vierula et al., 1996), two substantial reports have addressed the question of semen quality in the male partners of infertile couples. De Mouzon et al. (1996) have published what is (at the time of writing) the largest retrospective review of semen quality data. On the basis of the French national in vitro fertilization (IVF) register, they reviewed the results of 19848 semen analyses from 7714 men undergoing IVF for tubal disease, and having a normal semen analysis prior to IVF. They found a significant decrease in semen quality with later year of birth, the average sperm concentration in men born before 1939 being 92.5×10^6/ml, falling to 77.1×10^6/ml for men born after 1965. In a smaller study, Berling & Wölner-Hanssen (1997) reported on semen quality in 718 semen samples submitted by infertile men from 1985 to 1995 in one Swedish centre and found no relationships with age or date of birth, although ejaculate volume seemed to decrease and normal morphology, motility and sperm penetration of hyaluronic acid polymer increased during the study period.

Changing semen quality?

Most recently, a very careful reanalysis of the historical data (Carlsen et al., 1992) on semen quality in normal men has been published (Swan et al., 1997). These workers used multiple linear regression models, controlling for abstinence time, age, the proportion of the sample with proven fertility, specimen collection method, study goal and geographical location to examine regional differences and the interaction between region and year of publication. Using a linear model, they found that sperm concentrations and the rate of decline in sperm concentration differed significantly across regions. They concluded that there was evidence of a decline in sperm concentrations in the USA of -1.5×10^6/ml per year (95% CI -1.9 to -1.1), and in Europe of -3.13×10^6/ml per year (95% CI -4.96 to -1.30), but not in non-Western countries. Results were similar when other (non-linear) models were used, and these workers concluded that their results were unlikely to be due to either confounding or selection bias (Swan et al., 1997).

Thus, the available literature on secular changes in semen quality is, at best, inconclusive. To a greater or lesser extent, all of the available data suffer from the problems of being retrospective, collected in different countries, at different times, using different methods of subject selection and recruitment and different laboratory methodology. The retrospective nature of the data means that control of important confounding variables is often imperfect, weakening the conclusions reached. More evidence is clearly needed, yet one is tempted to wonder whether the inherent difficulties in laboratory methodology, subject selection and the large number of potential confounding variables involved mean that it may never be possible to resolve the issue of secular trends in human semen quality with certainty.

Regional variations: a possible clue?

Whilst the position with regard to secular changes in semen quality remains unresolved, an important observation to emerge from this work is the striking regional differences that are apparent: for example, the above-mentioned study by Fisch *et al.* (1996), in which sperm concentrations were highest in New York (mean = 131.5×10^6/ml), intermediate in Minnesota (100.8×10^6/ml), and lowest in California (72.7×10^6/ml). The Seattle data, with a geometric mean of 46.5×10^6/ml, is not directly comparable (Paulsen, *et al.*, 1996). Within Europe, similar patterns can be observed. Semen quality in normal Finnish men would appear to be high, with a mean sperm concentration of 133.9×10^6/ml being reported (Vierula *et al.*, 1996), whilst in Paris and Edinburgh lower mean values of 98.8×10^6/ml and 104.5×10^6/ml have been reported (Auger *et al.*, 1995; Irvine *et al.*, 1996). In contrast, semen quality in normal men in Belgium has been reported at 66.8×10^6/ml, and in Denmark at 69.2×10^6/ml (Jensen *et al.*, 1996; Van Waeleghem *et al.*, 1996). Whether or not there are also regional differences in the occurrence or otherwise of secular changes in semen quality is unknown (Bujan *et al.*, 1996), but it is clear that geography is an important confounding variable which requires to be taken into account when examining such data (Fisch & Goluboff, 1996; Lipshultz, 1996). An example of how local this effect might be was provided by one study that found evidence of deteriorating semen quality in a group of patients resident within the area of one water supply company, but no change in the semen of similar patients living nearby (Ginsberg *et al.*, 1994). Data from the Centres d'Étude et de Conservation des Oeufs et des Spermes Humaines (CECOS) (see CECOS *et al.*, 1997) has provided strong support for the existence of regional differences within France, and the recent meta-analysis by Swan *et al.* (1997) noted that intraregional differences were at least as large as the mean decline in sperm concentration.

It is possible that these regional differences, which might be due to ethnic, environmental or lifestyle factors, could provide a valuable tool in addressing the hypothetical causes of changes in semen quality (Irvine, 1996). Why, for example is the quality of semen in Finland and Denmark so apparently different? The 'Finnish exception' has already provided the first evidence that these differences in semen quality may be reflected in real changes in the biological fertility of the population. Using time taken to achieve a pregnancy in fertile couples as a measure of fertility (Joffe *et al.*, 1995), Joffe (1996) examined antenatal population and cross-sectional studies in Finland and the UK. In both comparisons, fertility was significantly greater in Finland than the UK. The author therefore concluded that 'the previously reported difference in sperm counts between Finland and elsewhere in north-west Europe (including Britain) is probably not artefactual'. This suggests that the reported worldwide decline in semen quality is also real.

The cause of changes in male reproductive health?

The cause of any observed changes in male reproductive health remains unknown. It is clear that lifestyle factors such as occupation (Thonneau *et al.*, 1997), smoking (Vine *et al.*, 1994), dress habits (Tiemessen *et al.*, 1996) and even time spent commuting (Thonneau *et al.*, 1996, 1997) may be relevant. However, the hypothesis that has attracted most attention concerns exposure to environmental xenooestrogens during development (Sharpe & Skakkebaeck, 1993). This is now a large and complex field, reviewed recently by the Danish EPA (Danish Environmental Protection Agency, 1995).

Sertoli cells play an important role in regulating the environment within the seminiferous tubules, each Sertoli cell supporting the development of a limited number of germ cells (Orth *et al.*, 1988). Any perturbation in the development of the reproductive system that leads to a reduction in Sertoli cell number will reduce the individual's ultimate capacity for sperm production in adult life. In most mammals, Sertoli cell replication occurs during fetal and postnatal life, Sertoli cell number becoming fixed at some stage of development. In the rat, Sertoli cell multiplication commences around 19–20 days of gestation and ceases around 15 days of postnatal life (Orth, 1982). In some primates there is a rapid and substantial proliferation of Sertoli cells at the onset of puberty (Marshall & Plant, 1996). In man, the total number of Sertoli cells increases significantly between late fetal and prepubertal life, with a further increase during puberty (Cortes *et al.*, 1987). Hence any 'window' for adverse effects on Sertoli cell multiplication may be longer in humans than in other species.

The idea that exposure to 'oestrogens' may affect male reproductive development is founded on the observation that follicle-stimulating hormone (FSH) is involved in determining Sertoli cell number (Orth, 1984) and that oestrogens produced by Sertoli cells may keep FSH levels in check by negative feedback whilst Sertoli cell number is being determined. Hence, short-term exposure of neonatal rats to oestradiol results in a suppression of FSH levels and in consequence reductions in testicular weight and spermatogenesis in adult life, whilst exposure of rodents *in utero* to the synthetic oestrogen diethylstilboestrol (DES) results not only in reductions in testis size and spermatogenesis in adult life, but also in an increased incidence of cryptorchidism and hypospadias (Sharpe, 1993). In a similar way, the male offspring of women exposed to diethylstilboestrol during pregnancy have an increased incidence of cryptorchidism and hypospadias at birth, and of abnormal spermatogenesis in adult life (Stillman, 1982). It is not, however, clear whether they are any less fertile as a result (Wilcox *et al.*, 1995). The effect on testicular descent, and perhaps also on increase in testis cancer risk, would presumably be mediated through interference with the secretion of müllerian inhibiting substance (MIS) (Kuroda *et al.*, 1990; Hirobe *et al.*, 1992). Testicular cancer may also be a congenital condition that becomes manifest at or after puberty (Skakkebaek *et al.*, 1987).

Thus, our understanding of the development of the male reproductive system leads to the conclusion that exposure to exogenous oestrogens may perturb it in such a way as to give rise to the changes which appear to be emerging in human health. This raises two important questions: are we exposed to more exogenous oestrogens than hitherto, and can exposure to exogenous oestrogens cause these changes in animal models?

There is certainly concern over the growing number of chemicals that may be viewed as 'endocrine disrupters'. The Danish EPA has recently released a report raising concern over environmental chemicals with oestrogenic effects (Danish Environmental Protection Agency, 1995), whilst recent commentaries in the *Lancet* (Ginsburg, 1996) and *British Medical Journal* (de Kretser, 1996) have highlighted the need for further research in this complex area. It is clear that there are chemicals in the environment which are 'oestrogenic', and which can perturb sexual development in exposed animals (White *et al.*, 1994; Jobling *et al.*, 1995; Jobling *et al.*, 1996). In mammals, it has been shown that exposure of pregnant mice to ethinyloestradiol increases the frequency of gonadal dysgenesis, cryptorchidism and testicular cancer, in association with impaired Leydig cell development and reduced Sertoli cell numbers (Yasuda *et al.*, 1985a; Walker *et al.*, 1990) Gestational exposure of rats to xenooestrogens has been shown to result in reduced testicular size and sperm production (Sharpe *et al.*, 1995) and we now know that exposure of pregnant sheep to xenooestrogens supresses fetal FSH. In an attempt to estimate the familial and genetic contributions to variation in human testicular function, Handelsman (1997a) has studied 11 pairs of monozygotic and 6 pairs of dizygotic twins, and observed that sperm concentration, testicular size and sex hormone binding globulin (SHBG) all had a strong familial effect, but was unable to confirm any genetic component.

Conclusions

Although the 'environmental oestrogen' hypothesis has attracted much attention, and there exist some biological data to confirm its plausibility, evidence that it is causally related to changes in human male reproductive health remains circumstantial. The evidence for secular changes in semen quality and other changes in male reproductive health is inconclusive, with the exception of testicular cancer, although evidence for regional differences in male reproductive health would appear to be stronger. In both cases, association does not imply causality, and several other possible explanations require to be considered. As far as semen quality is concerned, sperm count is a poor index of fertility, and there are as yet, no data on secular changes or regional differences in sperm function, although there may be some evidence of regional differences in fertility.

Whilst the available evidence is inconclusive and circumstantial, its weight is considerable and at the very least it should raise concerns that deserve to be addressed by properly designed, coordinated and funded research. Delay may compromise the fertility and reproductive health of future generations (de Kretser, 1996; Irvine, 1996).

References

Adami, H. O., Bergstrom, R., Mohner, M., Zatonski, W., Storm, H., Ekbom, A., Tretli, S., Teppo, L., Ziegler, H., Rahu, M., Gurevicius, R. & Stengrevics, A. (1994). Testicular cancer in nine northern European countries. *International Journal of Cancer*, **59**, 33–8.

Ansell, P. E., Bennet, V., Bull, D., Jackson, M. B., Pike, L. A., Pike, M. C., Chilvers, C. E.D., Dudley, N. E., Gough, M. H., Griffiths, D. M., Redman, C., Wilkinson, A. R., Macfarlane, A. & Coupland, C. A. C. (1992). Cryptorchidism: a prospective study of 7500 consecutive male births, 1984–8. *Archives of Disease in Childhood*, **67**, 892–9.

Auger, J., Kunstmann, J. M., Czyglik, F. & Jouannet, P. (1995). Decline in semen quality among fertile men in Paris during the past 20 years. *New England Journal of Medicine*, **332**, 281–5.

Bergstrom, R., Adami, H. O., Mohner, M., Zatonski, W., Storm, H., Ekbom, A., Tretli, S., Teppo, L., Akre, O. & Hakulinen, T. (1996). Increase in testicular cancer incidence in six European countries: a birth cohort phenomenon. *Journal of the National Cancer Institute*, **88**, 727–33.

Berkowitz, G. S. & Lapinski, R. H. (1996). Risk factors for cryptorchidism: a nested case-control study. *Paediatric and Perinatal Epidemiology*, **10**, 39–51.

Berkowitz, G. S., Lapinski, R. H., Dolgin, S. E., Gazella, J. G., Bodian, C. A. & Holzman, I. R. (1993). Prevalence and natural history of cryptorchidism. *Pediatrics*, **92**, 44–9.

Berkowtiz, G. S., Lapinski, R. H., Godbold, J. H., Dolgin, S. E. & Holzman, I. R. (1995). Maternal and neonatal risk factors for cryptorchidism. *Epidemiology*, **6**, 127–31.

Berling, S. & Wölner-Hanssen, P. (1997). No evidence of deteriorating semen quality among men in infertile relationships during the last decade: a study of males from southern Sweden. *Human Reproduction*, **12**, 1002–5.

Bostofte, E., Serup, J. & Rebbe. H. (1983). Has the fertility of Danish men declined through the years in terms of semen quality? A comparison of semen qualities between 1952 and 1972. *International Journal of Fertility*, **28**, 91–5.

Brake, A. & Krause, W. (1992). Decreasing quality of semen (letter). *British Medical Journal*, **305**, 1498.

Bromwich, P., Cohen, J., Stewart, I. & Walker, A. (1994). Decline in sperm counts: an artefact of changed reference range of 'normal'? *British Medical Journal,* **309,** 19–22.

Bujan, L., Mansat, A., Pontonnier, F. & Mieusset, R. (1996). Time series analysis of sperm concentration in fertile men in Toulouse, France, between 1977 and 1992. *British Medical Journal,* **312,** 471–2.

Cadbury, D. (1997). *The feminization of nature: our future at risk.* London: Hamish Hamilton Ltd.

Carlsen, E., Giwercman, A., Keiding, N. & Skakkebaek, N. E. (1992). Evidence for decreasing quality of semen during past 50 years. *British Medical Journal,* **305,** 609–13.

CECOS, Féderation Française de, Auger, J. & Jouannet, P. (1997). Evidence for regional differences of semen quality among fertile french men. *Human Reproduction,* **12,** 740–5.

Colborn, T., Dumanoski, D. & Myers, J. P. (1996). *Our stolen future.* London: Penguin Group.

Cortes, D., Muller, J. & Skakkebaek, N. E. (1987). Proliferation of Sertoli cells during development of the human testis assessed by stereological methods. *International Journal of Andrology,* **10,** 589–96.

Danish Environmental Protection Agency (1995). *Male reproductive health and environmental chemicals with oestrogenic effects.* Copenhagen: Ministry of Environment and Energy.

Davies, T. W., Palmer, C. R., Ruja, E. & Lipscombe, J. M. (1996). Adolescent milk, dairy product and fruit consumption and testicular cancer. *British Journal of Cancer,* **74,** 657–60.

de Kretser, D. M. (1996). Declining sperm counts. Environmental chemicals may be to blame. *British Medical Journal,* **312,** 457–8.

De Mouzon, J., Thonneau, P., Spira, A. & Multigner, L. (1996). Semen quality has declined among men born in France since 1950. *British Medical Journal,* **313,** 43.

Devesa, S. S., Blot, W. J., Stone, B. J., Miller, B. A., Tarone, R. E. & Fraumeni, J. F. Jr (1995). Recent cancer trends in the United States. *Journal of the National Cancer Institute,* **87,** 175–82.

Editorial (1985). An increasing incidence of cryptorchidism and hypospadias. *Lancet* i, 1311.

Falk, H. C. & Kaufman, S. A. (1950). What constitutes a normal semen? *Fertility and Sterility,* **1,** 489–503.

Farris, E. J. (1949). The number of motile spermatozoa as an index of fertility in man: a study of 406 semen specimens. *Journal of Urology,* **61,** 1099–104.

Farrow, S. (1994). Falling sperm quality: fact or fiction? *British Medical Journal,* **309,** 1–2.

Fisch, H. & Goluboff, E. T. (1996). Geographic variations in sperm counts: a potential cause of bias in studies of semen quality. *Fertility and Sterility,* **65,** 1044–6.

Fisch, H., Goluboff, E. T., Olson, J. H., Feldshuh, J., Broder, S. J. & Barad, D. H. (1996). Semen analyses in 1283 men from the United States over a 25-year period: no decline in quality: *Fertility and Sterility,* **65,** 1009–14.

Giesy, J. P., Ludwig, J. P. & Tillit, D. E. (1994). Deformities in birds of the Great Lakes region. *Environmental Science and Technology*, **28**, 128–35.

Ginsburg, J. (1996). Tackling environmental endocrine disrupters. *Lancet*, **347**, 1501–2.

Ginsburg, J., Okolo, S., Prelevic, G. & Hardiman, P. (1994). Residence in the London area and sperm density (letter). *Lancet*, **343**, 230.

Guillette, L. J., Jr, Gross, T. S., Masson, G. R., Matter, J. M., Percival, H. F. & Woodward, A. R. (1994). Developmental abnormalities of the gonad and abnormal sex hormone concentrations in juvenile alligators from contaminated and control lakes in Florida. *Environmental Health Perspectives*, **102**, 680–8.

Handelsman, D. J. (1997a). Estimating familial and genetic contributions to variability in human testicular function: a pilot twin study. *International Journal of Andrology*, **20**, 215–21.

Handelsman, D. J. (1997b). Sperm output of healthy men in Australia: magnitude of bias due to self-selected volunteers. *Human Reproduction*, **12**, 2701–5.

Hatton, M. Q. F., Paul, J., Harding, M., MacFarlane, G., Robertson, A. G. & Kaye, S. B. (1995). Changes in the incidence and mortality of testicular cancer in Scotland with particular reference to the outcome of older patients treated for non-seminomatous germ cell tumours. *European Journal of Cancer, Part A: General Topics*, **31**, 1487–91.

Hernes, E. H., Harstad, K. & Fossa, S. D. (1996). Changing incidence and delay of testicular cancer in southern Norway (1981–1992). *European Urology*, **30**, 349–57.

Hirobe, S., He, W. W., Lee, M. M. & Donahoe, P. K. (1992). Müllerian inhibiting substance messenger ribonucleic acid expression in granulosa and Sertoli cells coincides with their mitotic activity. *Endocrinology*, **131**, 854–62.

Hoff Wanderas, E., Tretli, S. & Fossa, S. D. (1995). Trends in incidence of testicular cancer in Norway, 1955–1992. *European Journal of Cancer, Part A: General Topics*, **31**, 2044–8.

Hotchkiss, R. S. (1938). Semen analysis of two hundred fertile men. *American Journal of Medical Science*, **196**, 362.

Irvine, S. (1996). Is the human testis still an organ at risk? *British Medical Journal*, **312**, 1557–8.

Irvine, D. S., Cawood, E. H. H., Richardson, D. W., MacDonald, E. & Aitken, R. J. (1996). Evidence of deteriorating semen quality in the UK: birth cohort study in 577 men in Scotland over 11 years. *British Medical Journal*, **312**, 476–1.

James, W. H. (1980). Secular trend in reported sperm counts. *Andrologia*, **12**, 381–8.

Jensen, T. K., Giwercnam, A., Carlsen, E., Scheike, T. & Skakkebaek, N. E. (1996). Semen quality among members of organic food associations in Zealand, Denmark. *Lancet*, **347**, 1844.

Jobling, S., Reynolds, T., White, R., Parker, M. G. & Sumpter, J. P. (1995). A variety of environmentally persistent chemicals, including some phthalate plasticizers, are weakly estrogenic. *Environmental Health Perspectives*, **103**, 582–7.

Jobling, S., Sheahan, D., Osborne, J. A. Matthiessen, P. & Sumpter, J. P. (1996). Inhibition of testicular growth in rainbow trout (*Oncorhynchus mykiss*) exposed to estrogenic alkylphenolic chemicals. *Environmental Toxicology and Chemistry*, **15**, 194–202.

Joffe, M. (1996). Decreased fertility in Britain compared with Finland. *Lancet*, **347**, 1519–22.

Joffe, M., Villard, L., Li, Z., Plowman, R. & Vessey, M. (1995). A time to pregnancy questionnaire designed for long term recall: validity in Oxford, England. *Journal of Epidemiology and Community Health*, **49**, 314–19.

Kallen, B., Bertollini, R., Castilla, E., Czeizel, A., Knudsen, L. B., Martinez-Frias, M. L., Mastroiacovo, P. & Mutchinick, O. (1986). A joint international study on the epidemiology of hypospadias. *Acta Paediatrica Scandinavica, Suppl.*, **324**, 1–52.

Keiding, N. & Skakkebaek, N. E. (1996). Sperm decline – real or artefact? *Fertility and Sterility*, **65**, 450–1.

Keiding, N., Giwercman, A., Carlsen, E. & Skakkebaek, N. E. (1994). Commentary: importance of empirical evidence. *British Medical Journal*, **309**, 22.

Knight, J. A. & Marrett, L. D. (1997). Parental occupational exposure and the risk of testicular cancer in Ontario. *Journal of Occupational and Environmental Medicine*, **39**, 333–8.

Kristensen, P., Andersen, A., Irgens, L. M., Bye, A. S. & Vagstad, N. (1996). Testicular cancer and parental use of fertilizers in agriculture. *Cancer Epidemiology, Biomarkers and Prevention*, **5**, 3–9.

Kuroda, T., Lee, M. M., Haqq, C. M., Powell, D. M., Manganaro, T. F. & Donahoe, P. K. (1990). Müllerian inhibiting substance ontogeny and its modulation by follicle-stimulating hormone in rat testes. *Endocrinology*, **127**, 1825–32.

Leto, S. & Frensilli, F. J. (1981). Changing parameters of donor semen. *Fertility and Sterility*, **36**, 766–70.

Lipshultz, L. I. (1996). 'The debate continues' – The continuing debate over the possible decline in semen quality. *Fertility and Sterility*, **65**, 909–11.

MacLeod, J. & Gold, R. Z. (1951). The male factor in fertility and infertility. II. Spermatozoon counts in 1000 men of known fertility and in 1000 cases of infertile marriage. *Journal of Urology*, **66**, 436–49.

MacLeod, J. & Wang, Y. (1979). Male fertility potential in terms of semen quality: a review of the past, a study of the present. *Fertility and Sterility*, **31**, 103–16.

Macomber, D. & Sanders, M. B. (1929). The spermatozoa count. Its value in the diagnosis, prognosis and treatment of sterility. *New England Journal of Medicine*, **200**, 981–4.

Marshall, G. R. & Plant, T. M. (1996). Puberty occurring either spontaneously or induced precociously in rhesus monkey (*Macaca mulatta*) is associated with a marked proliferation of Sertoli cells. *Biology of Reproduction*, **54**, 1192–9.

Menkveld, R., Van Zyl, J. A., Kotze, T. J. W. & Joubert, G. (1986). Possible changes in male fertility over a 15-year period. *Archives of Andrology*, **17**, 143–4.

Møller, H. (1997). Work in agriculture, childhood residence, nitrate exposure, and testicular cancer risk: a case-control study in Denmark. *Cancer Epidemiology, Biomarkers and Prevention*, **6**, 141–4.

Møller, H. & Skakkebaek, N. E. (1996). Risks of testicular cancer and cryptorchidism in relation to socio-economic status and related factors: case-control studies in Denmark. *International Journal of Cancer*, **66**, 287–93.

Møller, H., Prener, A. & Skakkebaek, N. E. (1996). Testicular cancer, cryptorchidism, inguinal hernia, testicular atrophy, and genital malformations: case-control studies in Denmark. *Cancer Causes and Control*, **7**, 264–74.

Nelson, C. M. K. & Bunge, R. G. (1974). Semen analysis: evidence for changing parameters of male fertility potential. *Fertility and Sterility*, **25**, 503–7.

Olsen, G. W., Bodner, K. M., Ramlow, J. M., Ross, C. E. & Lipshultz, L. I. (1995). Have sperm counts been reduced 50 percent in 50 years? A statistical model revisited. *Fertility and Sterility*, **63**, 887–93.

Orth, J. M. (1982). Proliferation of Sertoli cells in fetal and postnatal rats: a quantitative autoradiographic study. *Anatomical Record*, **203**, 485–92.

(1984). The role of follicle-stimulating hormone in controlling Sertoli cell proliferation in testes of fetal rats. *Endocrinology*, **115**, 1248–55.

Orth, J. M., Gunsalus, G. L. & Lamperti, A. A. (1988). Evidence from Sertoli cell-depleted rats indicates that spermatid number in adults depends on numbers of Sertoli cells produced during perinatal development. *Endocrinology*, **122**, 787–94.

Osser, S., Liedholm, P. & Ranstam, J. (1984). Depressed semen quality: a study over two decades. *Archives of Andrology*, **12**, 113–16.

Paulozzi, L. J., Erickson, J. D. & Jackson, R. J. (1997). Hypospadia trends in two US surveillance systems. *Pediatrics*, **100**, 831–4.

Paulsen, C. A., Berman, N. G. & Wang, C. (1996). Data from men in greater Seattle area reveals no downward trend in semen quality: further evidence that deterioration of semen quality is not geographically uniform. *Fertility and Sterility*, **65**, 1015–20.

Prener, A., Engholm, G. & Jensen, O. M. (1996). Genital anomalies and risk for testicular cancer in Danish men. *Epidemiology*, **7**, 14–19.

Rehan, N. E., Sobrero, A. J. & Fertig, J. W. (1975). The semen of fertile men: statistical analysis of 1300 men. *Fertility and Sterility*, **26**, 492–502.

Setchell, B. P. (1997). Sperm counts in semen of farm animals, 1932–1995. *International Journal of Andrology*, **20**, 209–14.

Sharpe, R. M. (1993). Declining sperm counts in men – is there an endocrine cause? *Journal of Endocrinology*, **136**, 357–60.

Sharpe, R. M. & Skakkebaeck, N. E. (1993). Are oestrogens involved in falling sperm counts and disorders of the male reproductive tract. *Lancet*, **341**, 1392–5.

Sharpe, R. M., Fisher, J. S., Millar, M. M., Jobling, S. & Sumpter, J. P. (1995). Gestational exposure of rats to xenoestrogens results in reduced testicular size and sperm production. *Environmental Health Perspectives*, **103**, 2–9.

Sherins, R. J. (1995). Are semen quality and male fertility changing? *New England Journal of Medicine*, **332**, 327–8.

Skakkebaek, N. E., Berthelsen, J. G., Giwercman, A. & Muller, J. (1987). Carcinoma-in-situ of the testis: possible origin from gonocytes and precursor of all types of germ cell tumours except spermatocytoma. *International Journal of Andrology*, **10**, 19–28.

Smith, K. D. & Steinberger, E. (1977). What is oligospermia? In *The testis in normal and infertile men*, ed P. Troen & H. R. Nankin, pp. 489–503. New York: Raven Press.

Sobrero, A. J. & Rehan, N.- E. (1975). The semen of fertile men. II. Semen characteristics of 100 fertile men. *Fertility and Sterility*, **26**, 1048–56.

Stillman, R. J. (1982). *In utero* exposure to diethylstilbestrol: adverse effects on the reproductive tract and reproductive performance in male and female offspring. *American Journal of Obstetrics and Gynecology*, **142**, 905–21.

Sumpter, J. P. & Jobling, S. (1995). Vitellogenesis as a biomarker for estrogenic contamination of the aquatic environment. *Environmental Health Perspectives*, **103**, 173–8.

Swan, S. H., Elkin, E. P. & Fenster, L. (1997). Have sperm densities declined? A reanalysis of global trend data. *Environmental Health Perspectives*, **05**, 1228–32.

Thonneau, P., Ducot, B., Bujan, L., Mieusset, R. & Spira. A. (1996). Heat exposure as a hazard to male fertility. *Lancet*, **347**, 204–5.

(1997). Effect of male occupational heat exposure on time to pregnancy. *International Journal of Andrology*, **20**, 274–8.

Tiemessen, C. H. J., Evers, J. L. H. & Bots, R. S. G. M. (1996). Tight-fitting underwear and sperm quality. *Lancet*, **347**, 1844–5.

Van Waeleghem, K., De Clercq, N., Vermeulen, L., Schoonjans, F. & Comhaire, F. (1996). Deterioration of sperm quality in young healthy Belgian men. *Human Reproduction*, **11**, 325–9.

Vierula, M., Niemi, M., Keiski, A., Saaranen, M., Saarikoski, S. & Suominen, J. (1996). High and unchanged sperm counts of Finnish men. *International Journal of Andrology*, **19**, 11–17.

Vine, M. F., Margolin, B. H. & Morrison, H. I. (1994). Cigarette smoking and sperm density: a meta-analysis. *Fertility and Sterility*, **61**, 35–43.

Walker, A. H., Bernstein. L., Warren, D. W., Warner, N. E., Zheng, X. & Henderson, B. E. (1990). The effect of *in utero* ethinyl oestradiol exposure on the risk of cryptorchid testis and testicular teratoma in mice. *British Journal of Cancer*, **62**, 599–602.

Westergaard, T., Olsen, J. H., Frisch, M., Kroman, N., Nielsen, J. W. & Melbye, M. (1996). Cancer risk in fathers and brothers of testicular cancer patients in Denmark. A population-based study. *International Journal of Cancer*, **66**, 627–31.

White, R., Jobling, S., Hoare, S. A., Sumpter, J. P. & Parker, M. G. (1994). Environmentally persistent aklylphenolic compounds are estrogenic. *Endocrinology*, **135**, 175–82.

Wilcox, A. J., Baird, D. D., Weinberg, C. R., Hornsby, P. P. & Herbst, A. L. (1995). Fertility in men exposed prenatally to diethyl stilbestrol. *New England Journal of Medicine*, **332**, 1411–16.

World Health Organization (1992). *WHO laboratory manual for the examination of human semen and sperm–cervical mucus interaction*. Cambridge: Cambridge University Press.

Yasuda, Y., Kihara, T. & Tanimura. T. (1985*a*). Effects of ethinyl estradiol on the differentiation of mouse fetal testis. *Teratology*, **32**, 131–18.

Yasuda, Y., Kihara, T., Tanimura, T. & Nishimura, H. (1985*b*). Gonadal dysgenesis induced by prenatal exposure to ethinyl estradiol in mice. *Teratology*, **32**, 219–27.

Zheng, T., Holford, T. R., Ma, Z., Ward, B. A., Flannery, J. & Boyle, P. (1996). Continuing increase in incidence of germ-cell testis cancer in young adults: experience from Connecticut, USA, 1935–1992. *International Journal of Cancer*, **65**, 723–9.

Part 2 **Implications of the new technologies**

8   ICSI: the revolution and the portents

HERMAN TOURNAYE

Introduction

For years, both the understanding and the treatment of male infertility have been disappointing. A specific treatment could be offered only in rare selected cases in which the pathological background was recognized and for which a treatment was available. In an attempt to optimize semen characteristics, the majority of patients suffering from male infertility have therefore been given gonadotrophins, anti-oestrogens, androgens or even antibiotics, without any pathophysiological rationale. Since controlled trials have not been able to demonstrate any significant benefit from such aspecific treatments (O'Donovan *et al.*, 1993), techniques of assisted reproduction, i.e. intra-uterine insemination and *in vitro* fertilization and embryo transfer (IVF-ET), became more popular in the 1980s.

Results after IVF-ET in patients with male infertility, however, continued to be limited because *in vitro* fertilization relies on several conditions, among them an adequate number of selected functional spermatozoa and normal gamete interaction. The latter is deficient in many cases involving sperm disorders. In the 1990s, the use of micromanipulation led to hopes of greater success, but the initial techniques of assisted fertilization, i.e. partial zona dissection (PZD) or subzonal insemination (SUZI) failed to increase the success rates in cases with severe male infertility. The most dramatic improvement was achieved only by the introduction of the technique of intracytoplasmic sperm injection (ICSI) (Palermo *et al.*, 1992, Van Steirteghem *et al.*, 1993*a*,*b*).

Because ICSI needs only one spermatozoon in order to fertilize an oocyte, most subfertile and infertile men, i.e. men with either no spermatozoa in their ejaculate (azoospermia) or very few spermatozoa in their ejaculate (extreme oligozoospermia) can now father a child. By means of ICSI, fertilization and pregnancies can be obtained with spermatozoa recovered either from the ejaculate, or from the epididymis, or from the seminiferous tubules, irrespective of whether spermatogenesis is normal or deficient and irrespective of whether the underlying pathophysiology is understood or not. Today, ICSI is the most powerful tool available to the reproductive andrologist for treating severe male infertility and five years after its introduction the technique has by now become a routine treatment in most IVF centres.

The ICSI revolution

In 1993, two years after the first pregnancy obtained after ICSI, only 35 centres participated in the ESHRE (European Society for Human Reproduction) collaborative study on ICSI (Tarlatzis, 1996), involving a total of 3157 ICSI cycles. By 1995 the number of ICSI cycles recorded was already 37 098, 1519 of which were performed with epididymal sperm and 1005 with testicular sperm. These cycles represent only the tip of the iceberg, since not all centres report their cycles to the ESHRE collaborative study.

The reasons why ICSI is becoming one of the most widely used assisted-reproductive techniques are clear: once beyond the learning curve, ICSI presents itself as a very robust technique. In the 1991–5 update of the ESHRE collaborative study, a fertilization rate of 62% per succesfully injected metaphase-II oocytes, was reported where ejaculated sperm was used. In 88% of these cycles, embryos were transferred and an overall pregnancy rate (with the aid of human chorionic gonadotrophin (hCG) assessment) of 28% was realized. When epididymal spermatozoa were used, 57% of the oocytes were fertilized, the embryo transfer rate was 89% and the overall pregnancy rate was 32%. The fertilization rate with testicular spermatozoa was 49% and, in 89% of the cycles, embryos were transferred. The overall pregnancy rate was 28%. The high transfer rate is typical of ICSI and, together with the favourable pregnancy rates, reflects its power.

Because of the highly predictive results and low failure rates, ICSI is currently being practised more and more to treat moderate male subfertility too. A few randomized controlled trials have compared fertilization after conventional IVF and after ICSI, both having been used for the treatment of moderate male subfertility (Aboulgar *et al.*, 1995; Calderon *et al.*, 1995; Fishel *et al.*, 1995; Hamberger *et al.*, 1995). All these studies used a similar design: sibling oocytes were randomly allocated to either IVF or ICSI. Meta-analysis (Table 8.1) shows that after IVF an average of 26% of the oocytes were fertilized compared to an average of 58% after ICSI. The odds of fertilization were four times higher after ICSI than after IVF (95% CI 3.4 to 5.0). The relative risk of complete fertilization failure was 0.16 (95% CI 0.08 to 0.32), which means in other words that the risk of fertilization failure was six times lower after ICSI than after IVF. One complete fertilization failure after conventional IVF for moderate male-factor infertility may be prevented by performing about three ICSI treatments (number needed to treat 3.2 with a 95% CI of 2.5 to 4.2). Since current functional tests for assessing IVF after conventional methods of insemination have a low negative predictive value, i.e. inaccurate prediction of IVF failure, the use of ICSI to treat long-standing male infertility will probably gain in importance in the years to come.

Table 8.1. Meta-analysis of randomized controlled trials (RCTs) comparing fertilization on sibling oocytes after ICSI and IVF in couples suffering from moderate male subfertility

	ICSI		IVF			
Reference	No. of oocytes injected	No. of oocytes fertilized	No. of oocytes inseminated	No. of oocytes fertilized	OR	95% CI
Fishel *et al.*, 1995	86	50	84	31	2.4	1.3–4.4
Hamberger *et al.*, 1995	382	242	342	116	3.3	2.5–4.6
Aboulgar *et al.*, 1995	361	217	199	36	6.8	4.5–10.4
Calderon *et al.*, 1995[a]	210	104	174	34	4.0	2.5–6.4
Calderon *et al.*, 1995[b]	52	27	27	2	13.5	2.9–63.0
				Common OR	4.2	2.8–6.4

OR, odds ratio.
[a] Couples with male subfertility.
[b] Couples with failed fertilization after conventional IVF.

It remains to be seen whether ICSI will replace standard IVF for the treatment of long-standing non-male infertility. Studies comparing both techniques in a controlled set-up found only a marginal benefit for unexplained infertility (Aboulgar *et al.*, 1996*a*) and no benefit for tubal infertility (Aboulgar *et al.*, 1996*b*).

The ICSI failures

Although ISCI is a highly predictable technique in terms of achieving fertilization and embryo transfer, fertilization failures occur. Fertilization failure after ICSI is due mainly to defective oocyte activation (Sousa & Tesarik, 1994; Flaherty *et al.*, 1995). A review of the fertilization failures occurring after ICSI showed that no fertilization ensued in only 3% of the cycles (76/2732 cycles) (Liu *et al.*, 1995*a*). In 49% of these failed cycles, fertilization failure was related to a sperm factor, i.e. the absence of motile spermatozoa for injection, or for the injection of morphologically abnormal spermatozoa, such as those without acrosomes.

Injection of immotile spermatozoa makes fertilization after ICSI unpredictable and it decreases the fertilization rate (Nagy *et al.*, 1995*a*). In 12 out of 901 ICSI cycles (11 couples) retrospectively analysed (1.3%), no motile spermatozoa had been available for ICSI in the ejaculate and the injection of immotile spermatozoa led to a significant drop in the 2-pronuclei (2-PN) fertilization rate (10.9%) and transfer rate (42%). Moreover, no pregnancies ensued in this small series. Although most patients occasionally had no motile spermatozoa in their ejaculates, some patients had ultrastructural sperm defects whilst others had only non-viable spermatozoa.

The use of the hypo-osmotic swelling test may be very useful where patients are diagnosed as having 100% immotile sperm, in order to select non-senescent spermatozoa (Casper *et al.*, 1996), although this test will be of no value at all where all spermatozoa have short or stump tails. If only dead spermatozoa are present in repeated ejaculates (necrozoospermia), viable spermatozoa may be recovered from a testicular biopsy and give rise to normal 2-PN fertilization rates (Tournaye *et al.*, 1996*a*).

In patients with axonemal defects or functional sperm tail defects, results after ICSI are generally poor and unpredictable. This may be due to associated ultrastructural deficiencies interfering with the microtubule assembly after ICSI, e.g. centrosome abnormalities (Hewitson *et al.*, 1996). One day such ICSI failures may be cured by centrosome transplantation or by the insertion of human centrosomes from transgenic animals.

Patients with globozoospermia are often sterile because their spermatozoa lack an acrosome, so hindering normal gamete interaction. ICSI may overcome this deficient gamete interaction and restore fertility (Hamberger *et al.*, 1995; Liu *et al.*, 1995*b*), but, again, ICSI may not be successful in all patients with globozoospermia.

In some patients oocyte activation may be deficient leading to ICSI failure (Battaglia *et al.*, 1997). In the future, co-injection of recombinant oscillin may overcome fertilization failure in these patients (see p. 161 n1).

The ICSI assault on infertility surgery in the male

Microsurgery has long been one of the few successful specific treatments available to cure infertility caused by obstruction of the excretory ducts. However, in patients with congenital bilateral absence of the vas deferens (CBAVD), surgical creation of a sperm reservoir led to pregnancy rates lower than 5%. IVF using spermatozoa retrieved by microsurgical epididymal sperm aspiration (MESA) yielded only comparable success rates (Silber *et al.*, 1994). It was only after the introduction of ICSI that epididymal sperm began to be used more efficiently and acceptable pregnancy rates were obtained (Tournaye *et al.*, 1994). While in patients with CBAVD, MESA-ICSI is the only efficient treatment, MESA-ICSI can also be performed in patients where microsurgery, i.e. vasoepididymostomy or vasovasostomy, has failed. MESA-ICSI may be a valuable alternative to vasoepididymostomy, whose results now tend to be limited since most obstructions are now caused by *chlamydia trachomatis*, which induces multifocal obstructions. Since the surgical skills needed to perform MESA are less demanding than those needed to perform vasoepididymostomy, MESA-ICSI may become a substitute for reconstructive microsurgery. On the other hand, there is no doubt that vasovasostomy must be preferred over MESAA-ICSI because the benefits of this microsurgical reversal procedure outweigh the costs (Pavlovich & Schlegel, 1997).

The introduction of percutaneous epididymal sperm aspiration (PESA)

Table 8.2. Results of 469 ICSI with testicular spermatozoa from patients with azoospermia

	Aplasia	Arrest	Hypoplasia	Normal
No. of ICSI procedures[a]	81	49	29	310
No. of mature oocytes injected	1039	524	338	3632
2-PN fertilization rate	53%	45%	61%	66%
Cleavage rate	73%	76%	78%	71%
No. of pregnancies (+hCG)[b]	16 (19.8%)	9 (18.4%)	11 (37.9%)	104 (33.5%)
No. of fetal hearts[c]	21 (9.1%)	7 (6.7%)	11 (15.9%)	103 (11.8%)

hCG, human chorionic gonadotrophin; 2-PN, 2 pronuclei.
[a] Cycles with positive sperm recovery.
[b] Pregnancy rate/ICSI within parentheses.
[c] Implantation rate defined as positive heartbeat/embryo transferred.
Adapted from Tournaye *et al.*, 1998 (in press).

(Tsirogotis *et al.*, 1996) and testicular-sperm recovery procedures (Schoysman *et al.*, 1993) have put male microsurgery under even higher pressure.

Epididymal spermatozoa obtained after percutaneous aspiration gives rise to comparable success rates after ICSI to those for microsurgically retrieved epididymal spermatozoa. The use of both frozen–thawed epididymal spermatozoa (Devroey *et al.*, 1995*a*) and testicular spermatozoa (Romero *et al.*, 1996) have proved successful in conjunction with ICSI. On the other hand, percutaneous fine-needle aspiration of testicular spermatozoa gives results after ICSI similar to those where spermatozoa obtained by open biopsy are used. More especially, the high fertilization and pregnancy rates after ICSI, using testicular sperm obtained with simple minimally invasive procedures in patients with normal spermatogenesis may render not only vasoepididymostomy but also MESA and PESA obsolete in the near future. We should not forget however, that microsurgery has the potential to cure obstructive azoospermia while the ICSI approach can only circumvent it.

Azoospermic patients with primary testicular failure may benefit most from techniques of testicular sperm recovery and ICSI (Devroey *et al.*, 1995*b*; Tournaye *et al.*, 1995). Table 8.2 shows the results of sperm recovery in azoospermic patients and testicular sperm extraction (TESE)-ICSI according to testicular histopathology. Fertilization and implantation rates after ICSI, using testicular spermatozoa from men with testicular failure, are generally lower than when spermatozoa from men with normal spermatogenesis are used.

A special category of testicular failure is Klinefelter's syndrome. We have been able to recover testicular spermatozoa in 8 out of 15 azoospermic men with a non-mosaic 47,XXY karyotype in their peripheral blood lymphocytes. In five patients, these spermatozoa were used for ICSI. Three couples achieved a pregnancy, two of which led to the birth of a healthy child

(Tournaye *et al.*, 1996*b*). All embryos were analysed by preimplantation genetic diagnosis (PGD) using fluorescence *in situ* hybridization (FISH) in order to check for sex chromosome normality prior to transfer.

Although spermatozoa may be successfully recovered by multiple excisional testicular biopsies in about half of the patients with testicular failure (Tournaye *et al.*, 1996*c*), some of these patients may experience adverse effects such as testicular haematoma and postsurgical testicular fibrosis. Unfortunately there are no good indicators available for predicting a successful recovery in these patients (Tournaye *et al.*, 1997).

ICSI: the ultimate rape of the oocyte?

Since its introduction, ICSI has given rise to an intense debate because its clinical introduction was not preceded by any suitable research model in animals, mainly because of the technical deficiencies of existing models. The ICSI technique has generated substantial concern, as by the mechanical piercing of the oocyte most of the naturally occurring steps thought to be essential for fertilization are bypassed. This raises questions relating not only to possible damage to the oocyte's contents or ultrastructure, but also to the natural selection process of the spermatozoon.

The introduction of a micropipette and the dislocation of the cytoplasm during injection of the spermatozoon may damage the meiotic spindle present in the metaphase-II oocyte. As yet, however, no significant increase in aneuploidy has been observed in ICSI offspring except for the sex chromosomes (see below) (Bonduelle *et al.*, 1996). When the injection pipette is correctly positioned, the risk of meiotic spindle damage is probably low or non-existent. Furthermore, aneuploidic embryos may not develop further or may not implant after being transferred. Another possible hazard may result from the injection of polyvinylpyrrolidone to slow down sperm movement. To date it is unclear what happens once this compound is injected into the oocyte, but no evidence of a possible toxic effect is currently available.

The selection of the spermatozoon to be injected is made on subjective assessments of motility and shape. This selection may not be adequate to prevent injection of a defective spermatozoon. The chromosomal aberration rate has been found to be higher in human spermatozoa with gross head abnormalities (Lee *et al.*, 1996) and in human spermatozoa from men with unexplained infertility (Moosani *et al.*, 1995). Although many studies found no correlation between overall sperm morphology and the short-term outcome of ICSI, none of these studies assessed the morphology of the individual spermatozoon that was finally injected. In future, the risks associated with the injection of a spermatozoon with abnormal head shape may be anticipated by the development of dedicated real-time computer-assisted sperm morphology analysers, so improving the selection of a spermatozoon with normal size and head shape before injection.

Subfertile men with normal karyotypes produce significantly more disomic spermatozoa (Moosani *et al.*, 1995; Bernardini *et al.*, 1997). This increased disomy rate in subfertile men explains the increase in sex chromosome aneuploidy in ICSI offspring. Whilst in one small series of ICSI pregnancies a high incidence of sex chromosome aneuploidy (4/15) was reported (In't Veldt *et al.*, 1995), all other reports show only a moderate increase (0.8%) in sex chromosome aneuploidy (Govaerts *et al.*, 1995; Bonduelle *et al.*, 1996; Palermo *et al.*, 1996). Assuming no bias when comparing ICSI offspring with newborn children in the general population, the relative risk of sex chromosome aneuploidy after ICSI is 6.3 (95% CI 2.5–15.9). The high incidence reported in one study may be explained by the small sample size of the study or even by technical deficiencies of the ICSI procedure itself. Current methods of sperm selection for ICSI are in themselves, clearly unable to prevent the injection of a disomic spermatozoon, leading to an increased risk of sex chromosome aneuploidy. Since at present this is the only serious adverse outcome demonstrated in offspring after ICSI treatment, more reliable methods should be developed in order to prevent sex chromosome aneuploidy arising in the offspring. In future, disomic sperm may be excluded from the sperm preparations used for ICSI by improved flow cytometric separation techniques which are currently used to separate X- and Y-bearing sperm.

In any case, the general concerns described above and relating to possible damage to the oocytes do not translate into an increased risk of pregnancy wastage (Wisanto *et al.*, 1996) or of congenital birth defects in ICSI offspring (Bonduelle *et al.*, 1996). The combined reported data on major congenital malformations after ICSI (Govaerts *et al.*, 1995; Bonduelle *et al.*, 1996; Palermo *et al.*, 1996) show a malformation rate of 2.6% (32/1226). Compared to the 2.1% (159/7633) rate of major congenital malformations reported in the 1991 collaborative world survey on conventional IVF, the odds ratio for a major congenital malformation after ICSI is 1.3 (95% CI 0.8–1.8). Compared to the general population, the proportional difference between one of the highest major congenital malformation rates reported in a general population survey (2.1%; Leppig *et al.*, 1987) and the above ICSI figure is 0.5% (95% CI −0.5 to 1.5). Although any comparison may be biased and, although the 95% confidence intervals are still wide, all recent evaluations of ICSI offspring have so far failed to show any significant risk of an increase in major congenital malformations (see p.161 n2). But all ICSI series include only small numbers of patients and possible risks may appear only at a later age or in subsequent generations (see p.161 n3).

The brave new world of ICSI

The ingredients for successful ICSI are simple: a metaphase-II oocyte, a functional paternal genome, a functional centrosome and an oocyte-activating factor. For most cases to be treated, these prerequisites can be translated into a mature oocyte and a motile spermatozoon. Whether this spermatozoon is obtained from a man with anti-sperm antibodies, from the testis of a man with incomplete maturation arrest or from a cancer patient in remission who has received chemotherapy is not *in se* important for the short-term outcome of ICSI. If no motile spermatozoon is available, ICSI may be attempted with whatever 'material' is available. Pregnancies have been reported after ICSI with devitalized spermatozoa (Hoshi *et al.*, 1994). ICSI can lead to fertilization in oocytes that have failed to fertilize after conventional *in vitro* insemination procedures and in many IVF clinics, this form of 'rescue-ICSI' has become a routine procedure. Pregnancies have been reported (Tucker *et al.*, 1995), although up to 50% of embryos from reinseminated oocytes have been found to have chromosomal abnormalities (Nagy *et al.*, 1995*b*).

ICSI with elongated spermatids or round spermatids from testicular biopsies or from ejaculates is becoming a standard technique in many IVF programmes (Fishel *et al.*, 1996). Yet the use of these immature haploid germ cells causes much concern. These haploid germ cells have to be distinguished from diploid germ cells by their morphological appearance, which is far from simple. The low success rates after ICSI with spermatids may be due to this failure to select an appropriate haploid germ cell. Round spermatids may be found in up to 70% of the ejaculates of men with azoospermia due to testicular failure (Tesarik *et al.*, 1995). When observed, however, most of these spermatids may have a degenerative aspect and the intactness of their DNA-strand can, therefore, be questioned. There are also questions relating to the immaturity of these germ cells, since during spermatogenesis and epididymal maturation, major nuclear protein changes still have to take place and, in man, genomic imprinting may not be completed by the second meiotic division. In France, the use of spermatids for human reproduction has given rise to an immense debate, since no evidence on safety as regards ICSI offspring was available at the time of its introduction. It was stated that 'For the first time since the Nuremberg code was drafted, we have embarked on human experiments aimed at creating humans without any great urgency for such experiments' and, especially, the use of spermatids for ICSI has been called 'the biggest ethical problem since the development of medically assisted procreation' (Butler, 1995). Nevertheless, viable pregnancies have in the meantime been reported in humans even after ICSI with secondary spermatocytes (Sofikitis *et al.*, 1997), although only a little preliminary research has been published for the mouse. These and other ICSI extravaganza are reported in the literature as major achievements. Maybe they are. The only problem is, that at this moment, we do not know.

ICSI has also had an impact on the clinical approach to the infertile male (Jequier & Cummins, 1997; Tournaye, 1997). Male infertility may become a trivial problem with the advent of a simple approach bypassing any detailed

diagnostic work. Any effort to examine the infertile male patient or to elucidate the cause of the problem may have become futile in the eyes of many.
This 'just look for a spermatozoon and carry out ICSI' approach emanates
from the frustration associated with the fact that the pathophysiology of
most forms of long-standing male infertility are poorly understood and
have no proper cure. However, careful work-up of any infertile male provides the only guarantee to being able to offer a cure whenever it may be possible.

And there is more. The men that may benefit from ICSI treatment are a
distinct subpopulation of subfertile or infertile men who may have a hereditary basis for their fertility problem. ICSI therefore needs more andrological
work-up, not less (Cummins & Jequier, 1994; De Jonge & Pierce, 1995;
Patrizio & Kopf, 1997). Before the introduction of ICSI, the major question
asked was whether a man was able to reproduce. Now the question to be
asked is whether the same man can have a normal child without passing on
genetic or epigenetic disorders.

Many candidates for ICSI may have autosomal karyotype abnormalities
and the incidence of these is inversely related to the number of spermatozoa
in the ejaculate. In patients with moderate oligozoospermia (10×10^6 to
20×10^6 spermatozoa/ml) the aneuploidy rate is about 3% whilst in patients
with extreme oligozoospermia (up to 5×10^6 spermatozoa/ml), this figure is
about 7% (Yoshida *et al.*, 1996). A number of patients undergoing ICSI have
Y chromosome microdeletions associated with their fertility problem and
many patients undergoing ICSI with epididymal sperm, because of congenital bilateral absence of the vas deferens, have mutations in the cystic fibrosis
transmembrane conductance regulator (CFTR) gene.

At present the inheritance pattern of mutations possibly linked to infertility is unknown but it cannot be excluded that ICSI may eventually perpet-
uate male infertility. As well as a complete clinical and genetic work-up, all
candidates for ICSI should be thoroughly counselled and informed that the
use of ICSI may propagate hereditary male infertility.

References

Aboulgar, M. A., Mansour, R. T., Serour, G. I. & Amin, Y. M. (1995). The role of
intracytoplasmic sperm injection (ICSI) in the treatment of patients with
borderline semen. *Human Reproduction*, **11**, 2829–30.

Aboulgar, M. A., Mansour, R. T., Serour, G. I., Sattar, M. A. & Amin, Y. A. (1996*a*).
Intracytoplasmic sperm injection and conventional *in vitro* fertilization for
sibling oocytes in cases of unexplained infertility and borderline semen.
Journal of Assisted Reproduction and Genetics, **13**, 3842–46.

Aboulgar, M. A., Mansour, R. T., Serour, G. I., Amin, Y. A. & Kamal, A. (1996*b*).
Prospective controlled randomized study of *in vitro* fertilization versus
intracytoplasmic sperm injection in the treatment of tubal factor infertility
with normal semen parameters. *Fertility and Sterility*, **66**, 753–6.

Battaglia, D., Koehler, J., Klein, N. & Tucker, M. (1997). Failure of oocyte activation after intracytoplasmic sperm injection using round-headed sperm. *Fertility and Sterility*, **68**, 118–22.

Bernardini, L., Martini, E., Geraedts, J., Hopman, A., Lanteri, S., Conte, N. & Capitanio, G. (1997). Comparison of gonadosomal aneuploidy in spermatozoa of normal fertile men and those with severe male factor detected by *in situ* hybridisation. *Molecular Human Reproduction*, **3**, 431–8.

Bonduelle, M., Wilikens, A., Buysse, A., Van Assche, E., Wisanto, A. Devroey, P., Van Steirteghem, A. C. & Liebaers, I. (1996). Prospective follow-up study of 877 children born after intracytoplasmic sperm injection (ICSI) with ejaculated, epididymal and testicular spermatozoa and after replacement of cryopreserved embryos obtained after ICSI. *Human Reproduction*, **11**, Suppl. 4, 131–55.

Butler, D. (1995). Spermatid injection fertilizes ethics debate. *Nature*, **377**, 277.

Calderon, G., Belil, I., Aran, B., Veiga, A., Gil, Y., Boada, M., Martinez, F., Parera, N., Coroleu, B., Penella, J. & Barri, P. N. (1995). Intracytoplasmic sperm injection (ICSI) versus conventional *in vitro* fertilization, first results. *Human Reproduction*, **10**, 2835–9.

Casper, R. F., Meriano, J. S., Jarvi, K. A., Cowan, L & Lucato, M. L. (1996). The hypo-osmotic swelling test for selection of viable sperm for intracytoplasmic sperm injection in men with complete asthenozoospermia. *Fertility and Sterility*, **65**, 972–6.

Cummins, J. M. & Jequier, A. M. (1994). Treating male infertility needs more clinical andrology, not less. *Human Reproduction*, **9**, 1214–19.

De Jonge, C. J. & Pierce, J. (1995). Intracytoplasmic sperm injection – what kind of reproduction is being assisted? *Human Reproduction*, **10**, 2518–20.

Devroey, P., Liu, J., Nagy, Z., Tournaye, H., Joris, H., Verheyen, G. & Van Steirteghem, A. (1995*a*). Ongoing pregnancies and birth after intracytoplasmic sperm injection with frozen-thawed epididymal spermatozoa. *Human Reproduction*, **10**, 903–6.

Devroey, P., Liu, J., Nagy, P., Goossens, A., Tournaye, H., Camus, M., Van Steirteghem, A. & Silber, S. (1995*b*). Pregnancies after testicular sperm extraction (TESE) and intracytoplasmic sperm injection (ICSI) in non-obstructive azoospermia. *Human Reproduction*, **10**, 1457–60.

Fishel, S., Lisi, F., Rinaldi, L., Lisi, R., Timson, J., Green, S., Hall, J., Fleming, S., Hunter, A., Dowell, K. & Thornton, S. (1995). Intracytoplasmic sperm injection (ICSI) versus high insemination concentration (HIC) for human conception *in vitro*. *Reproduction, Fertility and Development*, **7**, 169–75.

Fishel, S., Aslam, I. & Tesarik, J. (1996). Spermatid conception, a stage too early, or a time too soon? *Human Reproduction*, **11**, 1371–6.

Flaherty, S. P., Payne, D., Swann, N. J. & Matthews, C. D. (1995). Aetiology of failed and abnormal fertilization after intracytoplasmic sperm injection. *Human Reproduction*, **10**, 2623–9.

Govaerts, I., Englert, Y., Vamos, E. & Rodesch, F. (1995). Sex chromosome abnormalities after intracytoplasmic sperm injection (letter). *Lancet*, **346**, 1095–6.

Hamberger, L., Sjögren, A., Lundin, K., Söderlund, B., Nilsson, L., Bergh, C., Wennerholm, U. B., Wikland, M., Svalander, P., Jakobson, A. H. &

Forsberg, A. S. (1995). Microfertilisation techniques – the Swedish experience. *Reproduction, Fertility and Development*, 7, 263–8.

Hewitson, L. C., Simerly, C. R., Tengowski, M. W., Sutovsky, P., Navara, C. S., Haavisto, A. J. & Schatten, G. (1996). Microtubule and chromatin configurations during rhesus intracytoplasmic sperm injection: successes and failures. *Biology of Reproduction*, 55, 271–80.

Hoshi, K., Yanagida, K., Yazawa, H., Katayose, H. & Sato, A. (1994). Pregnancy and delivery after intracytoplasmic sperm injection of an immobilised, killed spermatozoon into an oocyte. *Journal of Assisted Reproduction and Genetics*, 11, 325–6.

In't Veldt, P., Brandenburgh, H., Verhoff, A., Dhont, M. & Los, F. (1995). Sex chromosomal abnormalities and intracytoplasmic sperm injection (letter). *Lancet*, 346, 773.

Jequier, A. M. & Cummins, J. M. (1997). Attitudes to clinical andrology, a time for a change. *Human Reproduction*, 12, 875–6.

Lee, J. D., Kamiguchi, Y. & Yanagimachi, R. (1996). Analysis of chromosome consitution of human spermatozoa with normal and abberant head morphologies after injection into mouse oocytes. *Human Reproduction*, 11, 1942–6.

Leppig, K. A., Werler, M. M., Cann, C. I., Cook, C. A. & Holmes, R. B. (1987). Predictive value of minor anomalies, association with major anomalies. *Journal of Pediatrics*, 110, 531–7.

Liu, J., Nagy, Z. P., Joris, H., Tournaye, H., Camus, M., Devroey, P. & Van Steirteghem, A. C. (1995a). Analysis of 76 total-fertilization-failure cycles out of 2732 intracytoplasmic sperm injection cycles. *Human Reproduction*, 10, 2630–6.

Liu, J., Van Steirteghem, A. C., Nagy, Z., Joris, H., Tournaye, H. & Devroey, P. (1995b). Successful fertilisation and establishment of pregnancies in patients with round-headed spermatozoa. *Human Reproduction*, 10, 626–9.

Moosani, N., Pattinson, H. A., Carter, M. D., Cox, D. M., Rademaker, A. W. & Martin, R. H. (1995). Chromosomal analysis of sperm from men with idiopathic infertility using sperm karyotyping and fluorescence *in situ* hybridisation. *Fertility and Sterility*, 64, 811–17.

Nagy, Z. P., Liu, J., Joris, H., Verheyen, G., Tournaye, H., Camus, M., Derde, M.-P., Devroey, P. & Van Steirteghem, A. C. (1995a). The result of intracytoplasmic sperm injection is not related to any of the three basic sperm parameters. *Human Reproduction*, 10, 1123–9.

Nagy, Z., Staessen, C., Liu, J., Joris, H., Devroey, P. & Van Steirteghem, A. (1995b). Prospective, auto-controlled study on reinsemination of failed-fertilized oocytes by intracytoplasmic single sperm injection. *Fertility and Sterility*, 64, 1130–5.

O'Donovan, P. A., Vandekerckhove, P., Lilford, R. J. & Hughes, E. (1993). Treatment of male infertility, is it effective? Review and meta-analysis of published randomized controlled trials. *Human Reproduction*, 8, 1209–22.

Palermo, G. P., Joris, H., Devroey, P. & Van Steirteghem, A. C. (1992). Pregnancies after intracytoplasmic injection of single spermatozoon into an oocyte. *Lancet*, 1, 826–35.

Palermo, G., Colombero, L., Schattman, G., Davis, O. & Rosenwaks, Z. (1996).

Evolution of pregnancies and initial follow-up of newborns delivered after intracytoplasmic sperm injection. *Journal of the American Medical Association*, **276**, 1893–7.

Patrizio, P. & Kopf, G. S. (1997). Molecular biology in the modern work-up of the infertile male: the time to recognize the need for andrologists. *Human Reproduction*, **12**, 879–83.

Pavlovich, C. P. & Schlegel, P. (1997). Fertility options after vasectomy, a cost-effectiveness analysis. *Fertility and Sterility*, **66**, 133–41.

Romero, J., Remohi, J., Minguez, Y., Rubio, C., Pellicer, A. & Gil-Salom, M. (1996). Fertilisation after intracytoplasmic sperm injection with cryopreserved testicular spermatozoa. *Fertility and Sterility*, **65**, 877–9.

Schoysman, R., Van der Zwalmen, P., Nijs, M., Segal, L., Segal-Bertin, C., Geerts, L., Van Roosdaal, E. & Schoysman, D. (1993). Pregnancy after fertilisation with human testicular spermatozoa (letter). *Lancet*, **342**, 1237.

Silber, S., Nagy, P., Liu, J., Godoy, H., Devroey, P. & Van Steirteghem. A. (1994). Conventional IVF versus intracytoplasmic sperm injection for patients requiring microsurgical sperm aspiration. *Human Reproduction*, **9**, 1705–9.

Sofikitis, N. V., Mantzavinos, T., Loutradis, D., Antypas, S., Miyagawa, I. & Tarlatzis, V. (1997). Treatment of male infertility caused by spermatogenic arrest at the primary spermatocyte stage with ooplasmic injection of round spermatids or secondary spermatocytes isolated from foci of early haploid male gametes. *Human Reproduction, Abstract book* 1, 13th Annual Meeting European Society of Human Reproduction, Edinburgh, June 1997, Abstract O-167.

Sousa, M. & Tesarik, J. (1994). Ultrastructural analysis of fertilization failure after intracytoplasmic sperm injection. *Human Reproduction*, **9**, 2374–80.

Tarlatzis, B. (1996). Report on the activities of the ESHRE Task force on intracyto-plasmic sperm injection. *Human Reproduction*, **11**, Suppl. 4, 160–86.

Tesarik, J., Mendoza, C. & Testart, J. (1995). Viable embryos from injection of round spermatids into oocytes. *New England Journal of Medicine*, **333**, 525–7.

Tournaye, H. (1997). Declining clinical andrology, fact or fiction? *Human Reproduction*, **12**, 876–9.

Tournaye, H., Devroey, P., Liu, J., Nagy, Z., Lissens, W. & Van Steirteghem, A. (1994). Microsurgical epididymal sperm aspiration and intracytoplasmic sperm injection, a new effective approach to infertility as a result of con-genital bilateral absence of vas deferens. *Fertility and Sterility*, **61**, 1445–50.

Tournaye, H., Camus, M. & Goossens, A., Liu, J., Nagy, P., Silber, S., Van Steirteghem, A. C. & Devroey, P. (1995). Recent concepts in the manage-ment of infertility because of non-obstructive azoospermia. *Human Reproduction*, **10**, Suppl. 1, 115–19.

Tournaye, H., Liu, J., Nagy, Z., Verheyen, G., Van Steirteghem, A. C. & Devroey, P. (1996a). The use of testicular sperm for intracytoplasmic sperm injection in patients with necrozoospermia. *Fertility and Sterility*, **66**, 331–4.

Tournaye, H., Staessen, C., Liebaers, I., Van Assche, E., Devroey, P., Bonduelle, M. & Van Steirteghem, A. (1996b). Testicular sperm recovery in 47,XXY Klinefelter patients. *Human Reproduction*, **11**, 1644–9.

Tournaye, H., Liu, J., Nagy, Z., Camus, M., Goossens, A., Silber, S., Van Steirteghem, A. C. & Devroey, P. (1996c). Correlation between testicular histology and outcome after intracytoplasmic sperm injection using testicular sperm. *Human Reproduction*, 11, 127–32.

Tournaye, H., Verheyen, G., Nagy, P., Goossens, A., Ubaldi, F., Silber, S., Van Steirteghem, A. & Devroey, P. (1997). Are there any predictive factors for successful testicular sperm recovery? *Human Reproduction*, 12, 80–6.

Tsirogotis, M., Pelekanos, M., Beski, S., Gregorakis, S., Foster, C. & Craft, I. (1996). Cumulative experience of percutaneous epididymal sperm aspiration (PESA) with intracytoplasmic sperm injection. *Journal of Assisted Reproduction and Genetics*, 13, 315–19.

Tucker, M. J., Morton, P. C., Wright, G., Ingargiola, P. E., Jones, A. E. & Sweitzer, C. L. (1995). Factors affecting success with intracytoplasmic sperm injection. *Reproduction, Fertility and Development*, 7, 229–36.

Van Steirteghem, A. C., Liu, J., Joris, H., Nagy, Z., Janssenswillen, C., Tournaye, H., Derde, M. P., Van Assche, E. & Devroey, P. (1993a). Higher success rate by intracytoplasmic sperm injection than subzonal insemination. Report of a second series of 300 consecutive treatment cycles. *Human Reproduction*, 8, 1055–60.

Van Steirteghem, A. C., Nagy, Z., Joris, H., Liu, J., Staessen, C., Smitz, J., Wisanto, A. & Devroey, P. (1993b). High fertilisation and implantation rates after intracytoplasmic sperm injection. *Human Reproduction*, 8, 1061–6.

Yoshida, A., Miura, K. & Shirai, M. (1996). Chromosome abnormalities and male infertility. *Assisted Reproduction Reviews*, 6, 93–9.

Wisanto, A., Bonduelle, M., Camus, M., Tournaye, H., Magnus, M., Liebaers, I. *et al.* (1996). Obstetric outcome of 904 pregnancies after ICSI. *Human Reproduction*, 11, Suppl. 4, 121–30.

Notes added in proof:
(1) (See p.152) Recently a pregnancy has been reported using a calcium ionophore as oocyte activator (A. Rybouchkin *et al.* (1997), *Fertility and Sterility*, 68, 1144–7).
(2) (See p.155) Further research is, however, necessary since, according to data re-analysis using other criteria, the major birth defect rate was found to be higher in ICSI children (J. J. Kurinczuk & C. Bower (1997), *British Medical Journal*, 315, 1260–6; M. Bonduelle *et al.* (1997), *British Medical Journal*, 315, 1265–6).
(3) (See p.155) Recently there has been an inconclusive debate on whether ICSI may induce a delay in development of the offspring (J. R. Bowen *et al.* (1998), *Lancet*, 2, 1529–34; M. Bonduelle *et al.* (1998), *Lancet*, 2, 1535).

9 The genetic basis of male infertility

PASQUALE PATRIZIO AND DIANA BROOMFIELD

Background information

It is estimated that about 30–40% of couples seeking fertility treatments are diagnosed with male factor infertility. The identification and classification of male infertility still relies on the results of the semen analysis, obtained on at least two separate occasions, and reported according to standard reference values set out by the World Health Organization (1992). Infertile males can be affected by azoospermia, oligozoospermia, asthenozoospermia, teratozoospermia or by any combination of any of these. Once a man is diagnosed as infertile or subfertile, he is usually referred to a reproductive specialist (andrologist or urologist) for evaluation. Today, even the most comprehensive work-up (which includes a detailed history and physical examination, hormonal and immunological assays, ultrasound or Doppler studies and genetic testing) may fail to detect the aetiology responsible for the reproductive disorder in about 60% of the cases. Lately, however, advances in molecular biology and molecular genetics are improving our understanding of many forms of male infertility previously classified as idiopathic. These discoveries are important for many reasons. First, with the use of assisted-reproductive technologies, *in vitro* fertilization (IVF) and intracytoplasmic sperm injection (ICSI), it is possible to offer reproductive hope to men once considered to be irreversibly sterile; however, in these instances, if genetic anomalies (mendelian and chromosomal disorders) are the cause of their infertility, then there is an increased risk of transmitting the genetic defects to future generations. Secondly, it is becoming clearer that abnormalities, both qualitative and quantitative, in semen analysis might be the 'presenting symptom or phenotype' of a variety of pathologies that can also affect non-reproductive organs. An example of the latter is congenital absence of the vas deferens (CAVD). Men with this condition are infertile because spermatozoa, normally produced by the testis, are 'trapped' within the epididymis because they lack the vas deferens. Prior to 1992 the aetiology of CAVD was unknown. Today it is known that CAVD is a variant or mild form of cystic fibrosis and thus every couple undergoing assisted-reproductive technology is screened for mutations in the cystic fibrosis transmembrane regulator gene in order to prevent cystic fibrosis in the offspring (Patrizio *et al.*, 1993). The same can be said of immotile cilia syndrome and some of its variants such as Kartagener's syndrome (Kastury *et al.*, 1997), which phenotypically can present with immotile spermatozoa alone and/or in combination with chronic sinusitis, bronchiectasis and situs inversus. Another variant recently suggested is sperm fibrous sheath dysplasia (Chemes, 1997). Another example is the rare spinobulbar muscular atrophy or Kennedy syndrome, an X-linked condition characterized by late onset, at about age 30, of progressive neurone degeneration and muscular weakness. Here, male infertility with associated testicular atrophy and gynaecomastia is secondary to a defect in the androgen receptor (AR) (Trifiro *et al.*, 1994), and indicates a mild form of androgen insensitivity. The molecular disorder is a significant elongation of the glutamine polymeric region encoded within exon 1 of the *AR* gene. In normal individuals this region has between 17 and 32 glutamine residues, whilst in men with spinal and bulbar muscular atrophy there are between 40 and 52 glutamine residues (Brown, 1995).

There are different approaches to classifing male infertility on a genetic basis. In some textbooks the different forms are divided into pretesticular, testicular and post-testicular forms. Other authors have used the concept of whether virilization is present or not. In this chapter we propose the following scheme of classification:

1 Male infertility with *a single gene defect.*
2 Male infertility with a chromosomal defect (*either numerical or structural*).

According to this classification, a gene or a chromosomal numerical or structural disorder can impair hormonal production or stimulation of spermatogenesis (pretesticular event), or can impact upon the control of the spermatogenic process itself a (testicular event), or can affect sperm transport (a post-testicular event). Only those genetic conditions with the potential for clinical relevance are discussed in detail below.

Male infertility with a gene disorder

Male infertility with a single gene defect, also called mendelian disorders, are due to mutant alleles or a pair of mutant alleles at a single locus. The inheritance of these defects can be dominant or recessive.

In Table 9.1 the most commonly known conditions of male infertility associated with a gene disorder are listed. The last two, Usher's syndrome and AKAP-82 defect are the most recent additions and are mentioned briefly in the last section of this chapter. The list is by no means complete. The rate of genetic discoveries is proceeding at such a pace that it is difficult to keep constantly abreast. The conditions listed below, however, are those with which clinicians dealing with male infertility, and, moreover, those offering reproductive services including ICSI, should be familiar.

Table 9.1. Gene abnormalities in male infertility

Condition/syndrome	Frequency	Phenotype	Inheritance/genotype
Kallmann's	1 in 30 000	Anosmia, delayed puberty, small testes, cleft palate	X-linked recessive *KAL* locus Xp22.3
Immotile cilia	1 in 30 000	Chronic sinusitis, bronchiectasis, immotile spermatozoa, situs inversus	Autosomal recessive chromosome 1p35.1
Cystic fibrosis	1 in 2500	Respiratory infections, pancreatic insufficiency, elevated sweat Cl$^-$, wollfian duct maldevelopment	Autosomal recessive *CFTR* gene Chromosome 7q31.2
CAVD	N/A	Isolated abnormalities in wollfian duct	*CFTR* gene
Androgen insensitivity	1 in 60 000	Different degree of testicular feminization, ? oligo/azoospermia	X-linked recessive androgen receptor Chromosome Xq11–12
Bardet–Biedl	Rare	Obesity, mental retardation, hypogonadism, retinitis pigmentosa	Autosomal recessive Chromosome 16q2.1
Myotonic dystrophy	1 in 8000	Muscle wasting, cataract, testicular atrophy	Autosomal dominant variable penetrance Chromosome 19q13.3
Polycystic kidney disease	1 in 800	Multiple cysts in liver, kidneys, epididymis, seminal vesicles	Autosomal dominant, *PKD*1 chromosome 16p13.3 *PKD*2 chromosome 4q
Usher's	1 in 30 000	Hearing loss, retinitis pigmentosa, sperm axonemal dysfunction	Autosomal recessive *USH*1A–E, type IB more frequent myosin VIIA gene, Chromosome. 11q13.5
? AKAP-82	Unknown	Disturbance of sperm motility	Chromosome Xp11.12

CAVD, congenital absence of the vas deferens; N/A, not applicable; AKAP, A kinase anchoring protein.

Kallmann's syndrome

This disorder is characterized by hypogonadotrophic hypogonadism, anosmia and male infertility. Other abnormalities less frequently observed are unilateral renal aplasia and mirror movement of the extremities and pes cavus (Meschede & Horst, 1997). It is X-linked recessive in most cases, although a second type, autosomal dominant or recessive, has been reported in some families. The gene for the X-linked form is on the Xp22.3 (*KAL* locus) and it is believed that its product encodes for a protein responsible for the neuronal migration from the olfactory placode to the diencephalon. The main endocrinological defect is a lack of hypothalamic secretion of gonadotrophin-releasing hormone (GnRH). These individuals thus have very low or undetectable levels of follicle-stimulating hormone (FSH), luteinizing hormone (LH) and their testosterone is also low. The main mutations detected in the *KAL* locus have been named KALIG-1, KAL-X; however, Kallmann's syndrome can also result from point mutations (Hardelin *et al.*, 1993). These patients have been successfully treated with a combination of FSH or human menopausal gonadotrophin (HMG) and human chorionic gonadotrophin (hCG) up to the point that fertility can be restored.

Immotile cilia syndrome

This syndrome is genetically heterogeneous and perhaps many different clinical entities may belong to this condition. The most frequently cited is Kartagener's syndrome, whose constant features are middle ear infections, sinusitis, bronchiectasis, situs inversus and sperm immotility. The absence or shortening of the inner dynein arms of the axoneme or defective radial spokes are the basis for sperm immotility and ciliary epithelial dysfunction. Recently, immotile strains of the flagellate algae *Chlamydomonas* have been found to have a defect in a gene called *p28* which encodes the inner dynein arms. The human homologue of this gene has been cloned on the short arm of chromosome 1 region p35.1 (Kastury *et al.*, 1997). It is very likely that soon males with different degrees of asthenozoospermia will be assessed for anomaly on 1p35.1. It must be remembered, however, that more than 100 polypeptides have been identified in the constitution of the cilium so there is ample room for genetic heterogeneity!

Cystic fibrosis and congenital absence of the vas deferens

Cystic fibrosis (CF) is an autosomal recessive disease with an incidence of 1:2500 livebirths. The genetic locus has been mapped to the long arm of chromosome 7 (region q31.2), has 27 exons. This is the cystic fibrosis transmembrane conductance regulator gene (*CFTR*). More than 700 mutations have been reported, some of which are defined as severe alleles and some as mild alleles (for a review, see Patrizio & Zielenski, 1996). Classical symptoms of CF are chronic broncopulmonary infections, pancreatic insufficiency, elevated sweat chloride, failure to thrive, and in males, infertility due to congenital absence of the vas deferens (CAVD) (Patrizio *et al.*, 1993). Cystic fibrosis gene mutations have also been found in infertile men with isolated CAVD and no other symptoms suggestive of CF. Extensive testing of men with isolated CAVD revealed that 55% of them carry two mutations, 25% one mutation and in 20% no mutations could be identified. The typical CAVD phenotype combines a severe CFTR allele (i.e. DF 508; W1282X, G542X, etc.) on one chromosome with a mild CFTR allele (R117H, 5T-variant tract, R347H, etc.) on the other. The demonstration of a causative role of the *CFTR* gene in most cases of CAVD illustrates the process of genetic consolidation of diseases previously classified as separate clinical entities. Men with CAVD can father children via the use of epididymal sperm aspiration and ICSI and this has created a new diagnostic dilemma. Since the majority of them carry *CFTR* mutations, it is extremely important to screen their partners and to offer genetic counselling to assess the risk of CF or CAVD in the offspring, before any assisted-reproductive treatment is performed. A recent report (Van Der Ven *et al.*, 1996) demonstrated a high incidence of *CFTR* mutations in men with oligozoospermia compared to control patients. If these data are confirmed, then *CFTR* testing and counselling may be implemented even for males with less severe forms of infertility.

Androgen insensitivity

Among the disorders with androgen insensitivity, the most severe form is complete androgen resistance, formerly called testicular feminization. For the purposes of this chapter, however, the forms of major interest are the infertile male syndrome (IMS) and the spinal and bulbar muscular atrophy (SBMA) (Brown, 1995). Both conditions represent dysfunction of the androgen receptor to the action of circulating androgens. Patients with IMS have been reported to have defective spermatogenesis, oligo or azoospermia and gynaecomastia. While preliminary reports seemed to indicate a high prevalence of AR defects in infertile males, this has not been confirmed in later studies (Meschede & Horst, 1997). The disorder in the AR is inherited as X-linked recessive (Xq11,12) and many mutations ranging from deletions to non-sense mutations, splice variants and point mutations have been described. The other form, SBMA, has age of onset at about 30 years, with cramps and muscular atrophy, and male infertility due to testicular atrophy. The molecular mechanism is the expansion of the trinucleotide repeat sequence (CAG) located in exon 1 of the AR, which causes an abnormal polyglutamine stretch in the receptor protein.

Myotonic dystrophy

Myotonic dystrophy has an incidence of 1:8000 and is transmitted as an autosomal dominant trait with variable penetrance. The gene involved encodes for a member of the serine/threonine protein kinase family and is located on the long arm of chromosome 19 (region q13.3). In myotonic dystrophy there is an expansion (more than 35 repeat motif) of the CTG sequence. Mutant alleles have between 50 and thousands of CTG repeats. Male infertility is observed in about 30% of the subjects, whilst some degree of testicular atrophy occurs in at least 80% of males suffering from this disorder, since the seminiferous tubules are more involved than the Leydig cells. Clinically, the testes of subjects with myotonic dystrophy may appear normal or softer, while in patients with Klinefelter's karyotype the testes are smaller and hard. In affected families, the age of onset of the disease may be anticipated from generation to generation because the triplet repeat motif may become even larger with each reproductive success. During spermatogenesis (male meiosis), expanded alleles may also revert to normal size and this may cause some confusion in genetic counselling.

Table 9.2. Most common numerical and structural abnormalities

Condition/syndrome	Frequency	Phenotype	Genotype
Kleinfelter's	1 in 1000	Tall; small, firm testes; gynaecomastia	47,XXY or mosaic 47,XXY/46,XY
47,XYY	1 in 1000	Tall, either normal fertility or oligozoospermia	47,XYY
Noonan's	1 in 2000	Short stature, webbed neck, cryptorchidism, testicular atrophy	Autosomal dominant mosaicism 46,XY/XO and Chromosome 12q22ter
Prader–Willi's	1 in 16000–25000	Hypotonia, small hands and feet, hypogonadism, obesity	Uniparental disomy Chromosome 15q11.13 (both copies maternal), del. paternal 15q11.13

Male infertility with chromosomal aberrations

Chromosomal anomalies can be numerical or structural and are usually *de novo* events resulting from mutations in the parental germ cell line (Table 9.2). Examples of numerical disorders are polyploidy (when the number of chromosome is a multiple of 23) or aneuploidy when there is gain or loss of one or more chromosomes. Structural anomalies are usually a consequence of breakage that occurs during meiosis. In the simplest case, a single break may result in loss of material (deletion), gain (duplication), or rearrangments (inversions). Rearrangements are further defined as balanced, when all the genetic information is preserved, and as unbalanced when there is loss or gain of genetic information. Translocations in contrast, consist of the exchange of chromosomal segments between non-homologous chromosomes, i.e. chromosomes that have very similar nucleotide sequences and pair with each other during meiosis. Balanced translocations occur in 1 in 500 individuals and the majority do not have any associated clinical problems, except decreased fertility and the risk of abnormalities in the offspring, as a result of malsegregation of the translocation. When a gamete with the unbalanced products of a translocation combines with a normal gamete, the resulting zygote will be partially trisomic for one region of the genome and partially monosomic for another. In some cases, this leads to very early miscarriage, whilst in other cases embryo developmental arrest may occur. In conditions of male factor infertility, particularly when the total sperm count is less than 3 million, a statistically significant rate of arrested embryo developmental arrest has been noted between genomic activation (8-cell stage) and implantation (blastocysts), compared to the rate of development of embryos where a male factor is not involved (Menezo & Janny, 1997). This observation highlights the possibility that genetic anomalies in spermatozoa of borderline or low quality can be responsible for poor embryonic developmental competence. Also, these data stress the concept that spermatozoa participate actively in the steps of embryo development following syngamy. The presence in the karyotype of a constitutional chromosomal anomaly or the presence of chromosome instability can interfere with spermatogenesis. A review of the literature has shown that about 15% of azoospermic males and about 5% of oligozoospermic males have an abnormal karyotype (Van Assche *et al.*,1996). In the azoospermic group, the most common chromosomal abnormality is Klinefelter's syndrome or 47,XXY; in the group of oligozoospermic men, the most frequent cytogenetic anomalies are autosomal robertsonian and reciprocal translocations.

Klinefelter's syndrome

This was the first human sex chromosome abnormality to be reported, and is an example of a germ cell aneuploidy disorder. There are two karyotypes involved:
    1   Classical karyotype XXY (85%).
    2   Mosaic karyotype 47,XXY/46 XY (15%)
The incidence of Klinefelter's syndrome is about 1 in 1000 live births, 1 in 300 spontaneous abortions, 1–2 in 100 any infertile males, and 7 to 13 in 100 azoospermic male populations (Mak & Jarvi, 1996).

The clinical manifestations of patients with Klinefelter's are relatively unremarkable. wolffian (mesonephric) duct differentiation is within normal limits, as are the external genitalia. The prepubertal phenotype is entirely normal, except for the patient being tall with thin, long legs. However, after puberty the manifestations include: the presence of small, firm, atrophic testes (testicular length <2 cm, volume ≤12 cm^3), with impaired secondary sexual characteristics; educational disorders especially dyslexia; normal intelligence, or some mild retardation, poor psychosocial adjustment; gynaecomastia in 50% (secondary to greater amounts of estradiol than testosterone); high LH, high FSH, high E2; low testosterone; thyroid abnormalities; restrictive pulmonary diseases; and the fact that most patients are infertile (Rimoin *et al.*, 1996).

The seminiferous tubules undergo sclerosis and hyalinization and, as a result, only Sertoli cells, which are practically devoid of germ cells, predominate. The severity varies; some tubules may contain abundant Sertoli cells whilst others are completely hyalinized. The complete range of spermatogenesis, with the production of mature spermatozoa, is occasionally seen, especially when there is a mosaic karyotype. Recently, with help from assisted-reproductive technologies these men have been able to father children (Palermo *et al.*, 1998).

In general, the greater the number of X chromosomes the greater is the severity of the syndrome, e.g. greater dysmorphism. Those patients with the mosaic pattern karyotype do not have such severe deformity as those with the classic form. The most common mosaic karyotype is 46,XY/47,XXY.

There are several variants of Klinefelter's syndrome other than 47,XXY; these include 48,XXXY, 48,XXYY, and 49,XXXXY. Thus, patients with Klinefelter's syndrome have at least one Barr body (one of the two X chromosomes is inactivated).

Combined cytogenetic and molecular investigations of the parental origin and meiotic stage of the non-disjunctional error responsible for the syndrome showed that about half of the cases resulted from error in the first stage of paternal meiosis (meiosis-I), a third from errors in maternal meiosis-I (which increases with maternal age), and the remainder from errors in meiosis-II or from a postzygotic meiotic error leading to mosaicism.

Testicular biopsy reveals sclerosis and hyalinization of the seminiferous tubules, absence of spermatogenesis and Leydig cell hyperplasia. Therefore, any male with testicular failure, i.e. high FSH, LH and low testosterone, should be evaluated for Klinefelter's syndrome or other chromosomal disorders before undergoing testicular biopsy alone or in conjunction with testicular sperm extraction (TESE) and ICSI.

47,XYY syndrome

The incidence is 1–4 in 1000 of all live male births (Mak & Jarvi, 1996). These men are phenotypically normal, and they are usually tall (over 2 metres). The origin of this disorder is paternal non-dysjunction at meiosis II, resulting in a YY (diploid rather than haploid 'Y') germ cell. There are less common variants of this disorder, i.e. XXYY and XXXYY, which may result from paternal non-disjunction in meiosis I or meiosis II. These men are at increased risk of antisocial behaviour. Semen analysis typically reveals severe oligozoospermia or azoospermia, and testicular biopsy specimens demonstrate spermatogenic arrest ranging from maturation arrest to complete geminal arrest. Nevertheless, fertility has been documented (Mak & Jarvi, 1996). Greater germ cell damage correlates with higher FSH and LH levels and normal testosterone levels. The risk of producing an abnormal offspring from this condition is minimal, since the extra Y chromosome is lost early from the germ line and thus, it is not passed on to the next generation.

Noonan's syndrome

This syndrome is the male counterpart of Turner's syndrome (XO). It is no surprise that they share similar characteristics, i.e. short stature, webbed neck, lymphedema, low set ears, cubitus valgus and cardiovascular disorders and pulmonary stenosis. The incidence is 1 in 1000–2500 individuals. It is probably inherited as an autosomal dominant disorder. Chromosomal analysis usually reveals 46,XO/XY mosaicism. Most males typically demonstrate cryptorchidism and testicular atrophy, so, Noonan's syndrome is associated with compromised testicular function and elevated gonadotrophins, i.e. FSH and LH. Elsawi *et al.* (1994) conducted a study of genital tract function in 11 adult men with Noonan's syndrome. The study revealed that the mean testicular volume was 21 ml, and that the stretched flaccid penile length was 11.4 cm. They also found that the LH and testosterone levels were within normal limits, but the FSH levels were significantly elevated in those patients with maldescent, and 80% of the men had azoospermia or oligozoospermia. The presence of bilateral maldescent was directly correlated with severe impairment of fertility. Noonan's syndrome has also been associated with other varieties of phenotype, namely lymphatic dysplasia, malignant hyperthermia, perceptual-motor disabilities and endocrinopathies (Mendez & Opitz, 1985).

Prader–Willi's syndrome

The incidence of this disorder is 1 in 16 000–1 in 25 000 and the basic defect is hypothalamic deficiency of GnRH (Mak & Jarvi, 1996). In the majority of cases studied (75%), the deletion of region 15q11. 13 occurred on the chromosome inherited from the patient's father, while in the remaining cases (25%), no deletion was identified but both chromosome 15s were inherited from their mother. Inheritance of two copies of one chromosome from only one of the parents is called uniparental disomy (UPD). Basically, UPD can cause disease by two mechanisms:

1 By having two copies of a recessive gene disorder expressed. Here is a concrete possibility of creating a recessive disease (e.g. cystic fibrosis where only one parent is the carrier).
2 Through the uniparental inheritance of a region of the genome containing an imprinted gene, i.e. genes differentially expressed, depending on whether they are inherited from the male or female parent.

Y-chromosome deletions

About 15% of men with azoospermia and about 10% of men with severe oligozoospermia (total sperm count in the ejaculate not exceeding 5 million) have recently been found to harbour deletions in the azoospermia factor (AZF) locus on the long arm of the Y chromosome (region q11.23) (Reijo et al., 1995, 1996). If we assume that 1 in 1000 men is azoospermic and some 15% of them will be Yq microdeleted, then the frequency of this disorder is estimated to be 1 in 8000–10 000 births. A variety of gene sequences has been identified on the long arm of the Y chromosome as containing possible candidates for the azoospermia gene. However, so far, none has been proved unequivocally to be responsible for azo- or oligozoospermia when deleted (Patrizio, 1997).

Multiple copies (7 tandem repeats of 72 base-pairs each) of a gene called DAZ (deleted in azoospermia) with 16 exons over 42 kilobase-pairs of genomic DNA have been found to be clustered in the AZF region. A DAZ sequence seems to be a strong candidate for AZF since it is the gene sequence most frequently deleted (about 70% of the time) in men with azo- or oligozoospermia. The *DAZ* sequence has also been identified on autosomal chromosome 3 (locus p24) and named *DAZH* (DAZ homologue) (Saxena *et al.*, 1996). Sequence analysis indicated that *DAZ* sequences on the Y chromosome arose during primate evolution by transposition of the autosomal gene to the Y chromosome, followed by amplification and pruning of exons within the transposed gene and by amplification of the modified gene. According to this hypothesis, *DAZH* is the founding member of the *DAZ* family. For both *DAZ* and *DAZH* the precise function is still unclear; *DAZ* has testis-specific expression whilst according to one source author (Saxena *et al.*, 1996), *DAZH* is expressed also in ovarian tissue. However, since *DAZ* is expressed in spermatogonia (Menke *et al.*, 1997) and in ejaculated Y-bearing spermatozoa from men with severe oligozoospermia (Patrizio, 1997), the current hypothesis is that *DAZ* is a gene encoding for an RNA-binding protein of 366 amino acid residues involved in the regulation of meiosis. A *DAZ* sequence, named Boulé, has also been found in *Drosophila* and, when this sequence is disrupted, spermatogenesis in the fly is arrested (Eberhart *et al.*, 1996).

The clinical importance in recognizing microdeletions on the Y chromosome as being responsible for the phenotype azoospermia or oligozoospermia cannot be overemphasized. Today, via ICSI, men with an extremely low sperm count, or even men with spermatozoa harvested directly from testicular biopsies, can successfully father children. In these instances, it is strongly recommended that genetic testing for Y microdeletion is offered to the couple. Non-mosaic Yq-microdeleted individuals will quite predictably produce Y-bearing sperm with the same deletions detected in their peripheral DNA, and thus will have a concrete risk of transmitting male infertility to their sons.

46,XX males

Instead of the one cross-over that usually occurs in the pseudoautosomal region, there is a cross-over between the strictly Y and X chromosome-specific regions proximal to the pseudoautosomal region (Chandley, 1996). Of the four sex chromosomes (gametes) resulting from this meiotic event, two are normal, one is an abnormal X chromosome which has acquired the *SRY* gene (and will thus result in an XX male), and the fourth gamete will have an abnormal Y (without the *SRY* gene). This gamete will give rise to male XY without the *SRY*: thus a phenotypic female with gonadal dysgenesis. Interestingly, there are males with a karyotype of XX who have not acquired the *SRY* gene. Nevertheless, they are still phenotypic males, as is also seen with true XX hermaphrodites. The origin of their testicular tissue is unknown. However, three explanatory hypotheses have been proposed. First, that these males are actually mosaics of cell line with and without a Y chromosome. Secondly, that there is an autosomal gene (of unknown origin) responsible for the testis-determining gene (the result of a mutation). Thirdly that a mutation or an altered level of expression of an X chromosome gene (perhaps related to *SRY* or *TDF*) may result in testicular determination (Chandley, 1996).

The presence or absence of *SRY* usually dictates normality of the male phenotype (in the absence of 45,X cell line). However, this cannot explain all the cases of XX males and XY females (Swyer's syndrome). Interestingly, there are *SRY*-negative 46,XX males and one recent report indicating that complete male development can occur in the absence of the *SRY* gene, with a 46,XX karyotype. Hsu (1994) suggested that these 46,XX subjects without the *SRY* gene may be secondary to an autosomal dominant or X-linked dominant inheritance, whereas the 46,XX males or 46,XX true hermaphrodites who are *SRY* positive may be explained by differential or a non-random inactivation of the *SRY*-bearing X chromosome. It is also possible that, as previously discussed, there may be more than one sex-determining gene, perhaps even on autosomal chromosomes. Alternatively there may be recessive mutations that allow the expression of the male phenotype (McElreavey *et al.*, 1993).

Down's syndrome

Down's syndrome, or trisomy 21, is the most common chromosomal disorder. It is the single most common genetic cause of mental retardation. Its frequency is a function of maternal age at the time of conception. As maternal age increases, the incidence of Down's syndrome increases, secondary to the increased incidence of maternal non-disjunction during meiosis I. For example, at a maternal age of 20, the incidence is 1 in 1667, at 25 years old it is 1 in 1250, at 30 years old it is 1 in 952, at age 35, 1 in 385, at age 40, 1 in 106 and at age 49 1 in 11. Prenatal investigations are usually recommended at maternal age greater than or equal to 35 years. Paternal age is not usually considered to be of significant consequence, unless greater than 60 years.

Down's syndrome is usually diagnosed at birth or shortly thereafter. Phenotypically, these patients have characteristic dysmorphic features, hypotonia, short neck, mental retardation, brachycephaly, flat nasal bridge, low-set ears, eyes with Brushfield spots around the margin of the iris, mouth usually open with protruding tongue, single transverse palmar crease ('simian crease') and clinodactyly. The syndrome is also associated with congenital heart disease, duodenal and tracheoesophageal atresia, and a 15-fold increase in the risk of leukemia. Many if not all of the males have impaired spermatogenesis.

Female patients with trisomy 21 can in some cases become pregnant and bear children, whilst males are almost exclusively sterile. The testicular histology shows spermatogenetic arrest, a reduced number of germ cells and hyalinized tubules. It is unclear how trisomy can ultimately affect testicular histology, although the prevailing hypothesis is that there may be a reduced proliferation of the primordial germ cells during their migration to the gonadal ridge, perhaps associated with an accelerated rate of apoptosis.

Group of rare structural aberrations

Robertsonian and reciprocal translocations

The incidence of robertsonian translocations is about ten times higher in infertile males.

The most common one is 13;14 translocation seen in oligozoospermic males. The testicular biopsy ranges from severe impairment to near normality. Meiotic studies of sterile carriers have shown an increase in the rate of XY bivalent and robertsonian trivalent association during the pachytene stage. The incidence of reciprocal translocations is five times higher in infertile males compared with normal individuals.

Inversions

Paracentric and pericentric inversions are eight times higher in fertile males. The mechanism by which pericentric inversions may affect male infertility is through extensive disturbances of synapses across the inverted region. These occur most frequently on chromosome 1.

Conclusions and future directions

Today, males with extreme oligozoospermia and obstructive or non-obstructive azoospermia can father biological children thanks to the use of assisted-reproductive technologies such as ICSI. This remarkable clinical success, however, is open to criticism because many of the infertile males are being treated without any understanding of the reason for their infertility (Patrizio & Kopf, 1997). Although the small body of literature available implies that these approaches are safe (the 'normal' incidence of major chromosomal anomalies is 2.6%, similar to that of IVF pregnancies), it is apparent that there is an increased risk of sex chromosomal anomalies among the offspring from ICSI. This is especially true when the gametes used are from fathers with an extreme reduction in their sperm output (Tournaye & Van Steirteghem, 1997). Further, these children have not yet reached puberty so their own fertility status cannot be assessed. Aside from fertility problems, manipulations of defective gametes may also cause random mutations or epigenetic abnormalities that cannot yet be objectively detected in the children by any method currently available. Population geneticists use the ability of an individual to reproduce as a marker of his or her genetic fitness. Genetic fitness is, in turn, dependent upon the genetic load of mutations that is proper for each individual. In this context, the inability to reproduce may be seen as a lack of genetic fitness and a selective natural mechanism to control the genetic balance of the gene pool in a whole population. Mapping and sequencing the entire human genome is bringing new technologies and discoveries that underline the role of genetic disorders in the causation of many forms of male infertility. Much remains to be learned. Current ongoing genetic projects are attempting to unravel defects in the competence of male germ cells to undergo proper meiotic recombination and to form spermatids which mature and differentiate to effect fertilization. It is becoming increasingly clear that the regulation of gene expression in germ cells follows defined rules, and mutations in genes affecting meiosis and thus spermiogenesis may cause meiotic arrest and premature germ cell death by apoptosis. The entire process of meiosis and germ cell progression in spermatogenesis, at least as demonstrated in mouse models (Sassoni-Corsi, 1997), appears to be under the control of specific molecules acting as meiotic checkpoints. By the use of targeted gene disruption technology, the function of these molecules can be inferred. For example, altering protamine synthesis in transgenic mice, via modification of the 3' untranslated region of the Prm1 gene, results in the premature nuclear condensation of germ cells and this in turn affects spermatid differentiation (Lee et al., 1995). Moreover, knock-out of the gene encoding retinoic acid receptors ($RAR-\alpha$) in mice, results in high postnatal mortality and sterility in the male survivors, with severe degeneration of the germinal epithelium (Sassone-Corsi, 1997).

Another area of active molecular genetic research is related to sperm motility. Two new potential gene abnormalities associated with sperm motility will be discussed: Usher's syndrome and AKAP-82.

Usher's syndrome

Some individuals with degeneration of the sperm axoneme have been described as having Usher's syndrome (Hunter et al., 1986). Usher's syndrome is the most frequent cause of hereditary deaf–blindness (Levy et al., 1997), and this dual sensorineural deficiency is transmitted as autosomal recessive, affecting 1 child in 30000. Three clinical forms have been described. Usher type I is the most severe and frequent form. Five Usher loci have been mapped so far and they are called USH1A, B, C, D, E. In USH1B, the gene encoding for a type of myosin, called myosin VIIA, is altered. This gene maps to chromosomal region 11q13.5. In the search for USH genes, some histopathological studies have revealed abnormal microtubular organization of the axoneme of the photoreceptor, nasal ciliary cells and sperm tails. In the latter, this translates into poor motility.

AKAP-82

The major phosphoprotein comprising the fibrous sheath of the mouse sperm tail has been identified as a member of the A kinase anchoring protein family of polypeptides (AKAP-82), that anchor the type II regulatory subunit (RII) of the protein kinase A (PK-A) of the fibrous sheath (Carrera *et al.*, 1994). Furthermore, the observation that AKAPs can also anchor the RI subunit of PKA, calcineurin, and protein kinase C suggests that movement of the sperm tail may rely on a sophisticated signal transduction system that acts in discrete regions of the flagellum to bring about coordinated and integrated movement of the axoneme. Defects in such a signalling system may be responsible for some of the immotile or dysfunctional motility sperm phenotypes seen in infertile males with asthenozoospermia. From the work of Carrera *et al.* (1996) it also appears that the AKAP-82 human homologue in the fibrous sheath becomes tyrosine phosphorylated during capacitation. Potentially, it would then link events comprising fertilization competence with those of motility (i.e. hyperactivation). The human homologue of the mouse AKAP-82 exists also in the human sperm fibrous sheath. It is of great interest that the mouse *AKAP* gene is located on the X chromosome (Moss *et al.*, 1997), since this is the first example of an X-linked gene in which both transcription and translation are restricted to haploid male germ cells.

Abnormalities of mitochondrial DNA (mtDNA) may underlie some forms of male infertility (Cummins, 1997). Preliminary data seem to demonstrate increased defective mitochondrial genome in germ cells exposed to testicular ischaemia or other oxidative stress. In particular, a deletion known as 4977 mtDNA has been reported at increased frequency in semen samples from patients with oligozoospermia and teratozoospermia. This mutation and others have also been confirmed recently in testicular biopsy samples (St John *et al.*, 1997). If these preliminary observations hold true, mtDNA mutations should be considered as the next big breakthrough in researching genetic causes of male infertility.

Finally, recent advances in imaging techniques, including laser scanning confocal microscopy, specific antibodies against spermatozoa and egg cytoskeletal proteins, are providing evidence of some novel forms of male infertility occurring after sperm entry into the ooplasm (Simerly *et al.*, 1995). Since the events controlling sperm decondensation, aster formation, oocyte activation and the beginning of mitosis are all controlled by molecular mechanisms, it is likely that anomalies in the genetic control of these molecules may unravel new genetic forms of male infertility.

In summary, before performing ICSI treatment every male with idiopathic infertility should be karyotyped and perhaps fluorescence in-situ-hybridization (FISH) studies on spermatozoa should be carried out, since, as stated earlier in this chapter, both azoospermic and oligozoospermic males have an increased risk of carrying aneuploidy chromosomes. Because of

Table 9.3. Algorithm for the genetic evaluation of the infertile male undergoing ICSI

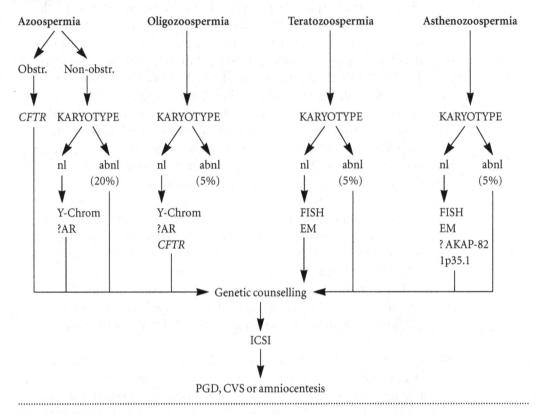

EM, electron microscopy
CFTR, cystic fibrosis transmembrane conductance regulator gene
AR, androgen receptor
AKAP, A kinase anchoring protein gene
PGD, preimplantation genetic diagnosis
CVS, chorionic villi sampling
FISH, fluorescent in situ hybridization
?, still considered as research trials. Obstr., obstructive; Non-obstr., non-obstructive; nl, normal; abnl, abnormal.

mosaicism, we do not know the frequency of chromosomal abnormalities observed in peripheral DNA and, therefore, their occurrence in spermatozoa. By the same token, we do not know when such abnormalities are present on spermatozoa and absent in peripheral DNA. Unfortunately, at present, FISH cannot be used to select the 'best fit sperm' for ICSI. Thus, patients undergoing ICSI with known or unknown genetic defects should ideally be offered preimplantation genetic diagnosis, chorionic villi sampling or amniocentesis as well.

The algorithm in Table 9.3 summarizes the potential genetic evaluation of the infertile male prior to ICSI.

References

Brown, T. R. (1995). Human androgen insensitivity syndrome. *Journal of Andrology*, **16**, 299–303.

Carrera, A., Gerton, G. L. & Moss, S. B. (1994). The major fibrous sheath polypeptide of mouse sperm: structural and functional similarities to the A-kinase anchoring proteins. *Developmental. Biology*, **165**, 272–84.

Carrera, A., Moos, J., Gerton, G. L., Ping, N. P., Tesarik, J., Kopf, G. S. & Moss, S. B. (1996). Regulation of protein tyrosine phosphorylation in human sperm by a calcium /calmodulin dependent mechanism: identification of A kinase anchor protein as a major substrate for tyrosine phosphorylation. *Developmental Biology*, **180**, 284–96.

Chandley, A. C. (1996). Infertility. In *Emery and Rimoin's principles and practice of medical genetics*, 3rd edn, ed. D. L. Rimoin, J. M. Connor & R. E. Pyeritz, pp. 667–75. New York: Churchill Livingstone.

Chemes, H. E. (1997). Dysplasia of the fibrous sheath and dynein deficiency, a cytoskeletal abnormality of human spermatozoa. *Journal of Andrology Suppl.*, [Abstr.4], p. 25

Cummins, J. M. (1997). Mitochondrial DNA: implications for the genetics of human male fertility. In *Genetics of human male fertility*, ed. C. Barratt, C. De Jonge, D. Mortimer & J. Parinaud, pp. 287–307. EDK, Paris.

Eberhart, C. G., Maines, J. Z. & Wasserman, S. A. (1996). Meiotic cell cycle requirement for a fly homologue of human deleted in azoospermia. *Nature*, **381**, 783–5.

Elsawi, M. M., Pryor, J. P., Klufio, G., Barnes, C. & Patton, M.A. (1994). Genital tract function in men with Noonan syndrome. *Journal of Medical Genetics*, **31**, 468–70.

Hardelin, J.-P., Levilliers, J., Blanchard, S., Carel, J. C., Leutenegger, M., Pinard-Bertelletto, J. P., Bouloux, P. & Petit, C. (1993). Heterogeneity in the mutations responsible for X chromosome-linked Kallmann syndrome. *Human Molecular Genetics*, **2**, 373–7.

Hsu, L. Y. F. (1994). Phenotype/karyotype correlations of Y chromosome aneuploidy with emphasis on structural aberrations in postnatally diagnosed cases. *American Journal of Medical Genetics*, **53**, 108–12.

Hunter, D. G., Fishman, G. A., Mehta, R.S. & Kretzer, F. L. (1986). Abnormal sperm and photoreceptor axonemes in Usher's syndrome. *Archives of Ophthalmology*, **104**, 385–9.

Kastury, K., Taylor, W. E.,Arver, S., Gerber, S., Larget-Piet, D., Chenal, V., Liu, X. Z., Newton, V., Steel, K. P. *et al.* (1997). cDNA cloning, chromosomal mapping and tissue distribution of the human axonemal dynein light chain gene: a candidate gene for the immotile cilia syndrome. *Journal of Andrology, Suppl.*,[Abstr.1], p. 25

Lee, K., Haugen, H. S.,Clegg, C. H. & Braun, R. E. (1995). Premature translation of protamine 1 mRNA causes precocious nuclear condensation and arrests spermatid differentiation in mice. *Proceedings of the National Academy of Sciences, USA*, **92**,12451–5.

Levy, G., Levi-Acobas, F., Blanchard, S., Alagappan, R., Brown, L. G., Rosenberg, M., Rozen, S., Jaffre, T., Straus, D. *et al.* (1997). Myosin VIIA gene: heterogeneity of the mutations responsible for Usher syndrome type IB. *Human Molecular Genetics*, **6**, 111–16.

Mak, V., Jarvi, K. A. (1996). The genetics of male infertility. *Journal of Urology*, **156**. 1245–57.

McElreavey, K., Vilian, E., Abbas, N. Herskowitz, I. & Fellous, M. (1993). A regulatory cascade hypothesis for mammalian sex determination: SRY represses a negative regulator of male development. *Proceedings of the National Academy of Sciences, USA*, **90**, 3368–72.

Mendez, H. M. M. & Opitz, J. M. (1985). Noonan syndrome: a review. *American Journal of Medical Genetics*, **21**, 493–506.

Menezo, Y. J. R. & Janny, L. (1997). Influence of paternal factors in early embryogenesis. In *Genetics of human male fertility*, ed. C. Barratt, C. De Jonge, D. Mortimer & J. Parinaud, pp. 246–57. Paris: EDK.

Menke, D. B., Mutter, G. L. & Page, D. C. (1997). Expression of DAZ, an azoospermia factor candidate, in human spermatogonia. *American Journal of Human Genetics*, **60**, 237–41.

Meschede, D. & Horst, J. (1997). The molecular genetics of male infertility. *Molecular Human Reproduction*, **3**, 419–30.

Moss, S. B., Vanscoy, H. & Gerton, G. L. (1997). Mapping of a haploid transcribed and translated sperm specific gene to the mouse X chromosome. *Mammalian Genome*, **8**, 37–8.

Palermo, G. D., Schlegel, P. N., Sills, E. S., Veecl, L. I., Zaninovic, N., Menendez, S. & Rosenwaks, Z. (1998). Births after intracytoplasmic injection of sperm obtained by testicular extraction from men with non-mosaic Klinefelter syndrome. *New England Journal of Medicine*, **338**, 588–90.

Patrizio, P. (1997). Mapping of the Y chromosome and clinical consequences. In *Genetics of human male fertility*, ed. C. Barratt, C. De Jonge, D. Mortimer, & J. Parinaud, pp. 25–42, Paris: EDK.

Patrizio, P. & Kopf, G. S. (1997). Molecular biology in the modern work-up of the infertile male: time to recognize the need for andrologists. *Human Reproduction*, **12**, 879–83.

Patrizio, P. & Zielenski, J. (1996). Congenital absence of the vas deferens: a mild form of cystic fibrosis. *Molecular Medicine Today*, **2**, 24–31.

Patrizio, P., Asch, R. H., Handelin, B. & Silber, S. J. (1993). Aetiology of congenital absence of the vas deferens: genetic study of three generations. *Human Reproduction*, **8**, 215–20.

Reijo, R., Lee, T.-Y., Salo, P., Alagappan, R., Skaletsky, H., Reeve, M. P., Reijo, R., Rozen, S., Dinulos, M. B. *et al*. (1995). Diverse spermatogenic defects in humans caused by Y chromosome deletions encompassing a novel RNA-binding protein gene. *Nature Genetics*, **10**, 383–93.

Reijo, R., Alagappan, R. K., Patrizio, P. & Page, D. C. (1996). Severe oligozoospermia resulting from deletions of azoospermia factor gene on Y chromosome. *Lancet*, **347**, 1290–3.

Rimoin, D. L., Connor, J. M. & Pyeritz, R. E. (1996). *Emery and Rimoin's principles and practice of medical genetics*, 3rd edn, ed. C. Barratt, C. De Jonge, D. Mortimer & J. Parinand, New York: Churchill Livingstone.

Sassone-Corsi, P. (1997). Transcriptional checkpoints determining the fate of male germ cells. *Cell*, **88**, 163–6.

Saxena, R., Brown, L. G., Hawkins, T.,Ord, T., Rawlins, R., Jones, J., Navara, C., Gerrity, M. & Rinehart, J. (1996). The *DAZ* gene cluster on the Y chromosome arose from an autosomal gene that was transposed, repeatedly amplified and pruned. *Nature Genetics*, **14**, 292–9.

Simerly, C., Wu, G., Zoran, S. *et al.* (1995). The paternal inheritance of the centrosome, the cell's microtubule organizing center in humans and its implications for infertility. *Nature Medicine*, **1**, 47–53.

St John, J. C., Cooke, I. D. & Barratt, C. L. R. (1997). The use of long PCR to detect multiple deletions in the mitochondrial DNA of human testicular tissue from azoospermic and severe oligozoospermic patients. In *Genetics of human male fertility*, ed. C. Barratt, C. De Jonge, D. Mortimer & J. Parinaud, 333–47. Paris: EDK.

Tournaye, H. & Van Steirteghem, A. (1997). ICSI concerns do not outweigh its benefit. *Journal of NIH Research*, **9**, 35–40.

Trifiro, M.A., Kazemi-Esfarjani, P. & Pinsky, L. (1994). X-linked muscular athrophy and the androgen receptor. *Trends Endocrinology and Metabolism*, **5**, 416–21.

Van Assche, E., Bonduelle, M., Tournaye, H., Joris, H., Verhayen, F., Devroey, P., Van Steirteghem, A. & Liebaers, I. (1996). Cytogenetics of infertile men. *Human Reproduction*, 11 Suppl. 4, 1–24.

Van Der Ven, K., Messer, L., Van Der Ven, H., Jeyendran, R. S. & Ober, C. (1996): Cystic fibrosis mutation screening in healthy men with reduced sperm quality. *Human Reproduction*, **11**, 513–17.

World Health Organization (1992). *Laboratory manual for the examination of human semen and sperm–cervical mucus interaction*, 3rd edn. Cambridge: Cambridge University Press.

10 The treatment of azoospermia with surgery and ICSI

SHERMAN SILBER

ICSI for oligoasthenospermia

Before 1992, male infertility had been considered in most cases to be untreatable. Then came a surprisingly neat solution: ICSI, i.e the injection of a single spermatozoon into a single egg. Since the publication of the first papers on ICSI for oligozoospermia in 1992 and 1993, an intense flurry of scientific effort has been dedicated to extending its application to virtually every type of male infertility (Palermo *et al.*, 1992; Van Steirteghem *et al.*, 1993; Silber, 1995; Silber *et al.*, 1995*a*). First it was confirmed that the most severe cases of oligoasthenoteratospermia enjoyed the same success rates as mild cases of male factor infertility and that these pregnancy rates were no different from those of couples where men with normal spermatozoa were undertaking conventional IVF (Nagy *et al.*, 1995*a*). Next, it was discovered that it does not really matter how the spermatozoon is pretreated prior to ICSI, and that any method for aspirating the spermatozoon into an injection pipette and transferring it into the oocyte is adequate (Liu *et al.*, 1994*a*). In fact, no sperm defect precluded success with the ICSI technique. Any fertilization failure was always related either to poor egg quality or to sperm non-viability (Liu *et al.*, 1995). It appeared that there was no negative effect on the pregnancy rate with ICSI even with the most severe morphological sperm defects, the most severe reduction in motility, or with the tiniest number of spermatozoa in the ejaculate ('pseudoazoospermia') (see Tables 10.1 and 10.2). Only absolute immotility of ejaculated or epididymal spermatozoa lowered the fertilization rate, and this was found to be due not to the immotility of spermatozoa but rather to their non-viability. Completely non-motile spermatozoa, if viable, were capable of normal fertilization and pregnancy rates (see Fig. 10.1), however few of them there might be in an ejaculate.

Sperm retrieval and ICSI for obstructive azoospermia

Long-term studies of vasoepididymostomy using the single-tubule microsurgical technique has been remarkably successful for obstructive

181

Table 10.1. Result of ICSI with ejaculated sperm not related to sperm quality

	No. of cycles	2PN (%)	Transfer (%)	Clinical pregnancies (%)
Sperm Count (Total)				
'0'	57	58	86	25
up to 1×10^6	97	64	96	26
>1 to 5×10^6	128	70	96	22
>5×10^6	684	71	93	30
Motility				
0^a	12	10	42	0
0	54	60	87	13
>0 to 5%	19	68	100	32
>5 to 50%	479	70	88	31
>50%	337	74	95	26
Morphology				
0	48	68	88	31
>1 to 3	125	70	96	33
>4 to 13	307	71	94	26
>14	203	75	95	29

2PN, 2 pronuclei.

[a] Nagy et al., 1995a.

Table 10.2. Fertilization failure, October 1992 to December 1994

No. of cycles	2PN (%)	Clinical pregnancies
2732	71%	964 (36%)

Failed fertilization in 29 (1%) cycles (28 couples)

of 26 couples with failed fertilization, who underwent repeat ICSI,
22 (85%) achieved fertilization in subsequent cycles

2PN, 2 pronuclei.

From Liu et al., 1995.

azoospermia and vasectomy reversal. However, very few centres had sufficient experience to obtain such good results. Furthermore, many patients with obstructive azoospermia, e.g. congenital absence of the vas deferens (CAVD) were not reconstructable (Silber, 1980, 1988, 1989a,b; Silber & Rodriguez-Rigau, 1981; Silber et al., 1988)

With sperm aspiration and extraction techniques, even if the male were absolutely azoospermic, pregnancy rates could be achieved that were no different from those of a man with a normal sperm concentration (Nagy *et al.*, 1995*b*; Silber *et al.*, 1995*b*). The first successful attempts at sperm aspiration combined with ICSI were reported by Silber and Tournaye in 1994 (Silber *et al.*, 1994; Tournaye *et al.*, 1994). We coined the term 'MESA' for this procedure (microsurgical epididymal sperm aspiration). Conventional *in vitro* fertilization (IVF) with aspirated epididymal spermatozoa, yielded a pregnancy rate of only 9% and a delivery rate of only 4.5%, whereas ICSI with aspirated epididymal spermatozoa in men with CAVD yielded a pregnancy rate of 47% and a delivery rate of 33%. Furthermore, there was no difference in pregnancy rate with retrieved epididymal spermatozoa whatever the cause of the obstruction, be it failed vasoepididymostomy, CAVD, or simply irreparable obstruction (Silber *et al.*, 1995*c*).

It was soon realized that testicular spermatozoa could fertilize as well as epididymal spermatozoa, and also give rise to normal pregnancies (Schoysman *et al.*, 1993; Devroey *et al.*, 1995; Silber *et al.*, 1995*d*). This procedure was called TESE (testicular sperm extraction). TESE truly revolutionized the treatment of infertile couples with azoospermia. Even patients with zero sperm motility in the ejaculate or in the epididymis (or even in men with no epididymis) could still have their own biological child, just so long as

Fig. 10.1. ICSI (intracytoplasmic sperm injection).

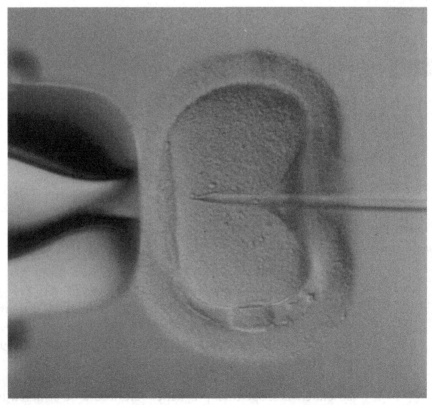

there was normal spermatogenesis. It also meant that surgeons who had no microsurgical skill would be able easily to perform a testicular biopsy, and thus retrieve spermatozoa which could be used for ICSI without the need for microsurgical expertise in performing a conventional MESA procedure.

Next, it was shown that epididymal spermatozoa, despite fairly weak motility, could be frozen and, on thawing, give pregnancy rates that which were no different from those obtained using active (freshly retrieved) epididymal spermatozoa (Devroey *et al.*, 1994). This meant that a man with obstructive azoospermia could undergo a microsurgical reconstruction, without the need to have his partner prepared for simultaneous IVF. Moreover, spermatozoa could be retrieved from the epididymis at the time of the vasoepididymostomy and could be frozen and stored. Thus, frozen stored epididymal spermatozoa could serve as a back-up for future ICSI procedures without the man having to undergo anymore invasive surgeries or aspirations (Silber, 1989*a*,*b*). This also meant that couples did not have to time their MESA cycle exactly with the woman's egg retrieval, and also that men about to undergo chemotherapy and/or radiation for cancer could have just a single ejaculate frozen and thus have no delay in undergoing cancer treatment. This is because one ejaculate would be sufficient for an almost infinite number of IVF-ICSI cycles.

Sperm retrieval for testicular failure

In the majority of cases of patients with testicular failure (caused by maturation arrest, Sertoli cell only syndrome, cryptorchid testicular atrophy, postchemotherapy azoospermia, or even Klinefelter's syndrome), there is usually a very tiny number of spermatozoa or spermatids which can be extracted and utilized for ICSI (Devroey *et al.*, 1995; Silber *et al.*, 1995*a*,*d*, 1996; Silber, 1995). Men who appear to be making no spermatozoa whatsoever could now have their own biological child. This surprising development came out of basic studies in quantitative analysis of testicular biopsy begun by Steinberger and Zuckerman, and finally continued by Silber and Rodriguez-Rigau in the late 1960s and 1970s (Steinberger & Tjioe, 1968; Zuckerman *et al.*, 1978; Silber & Rodriguez-Rigau, 1981). These early studies of the kinetics of spermatogenesis in the testicle demonstrated that there was often a small degree of spermatogenesis present if one looked quantitatively and carefully at a testicular biopsy of men who were azoospermic from non-obstructive testicular failure. However, the significance of this 'threshold' phenomenon was not appreciated until the era of ICSI, when it was realized that these spermatids could be harvested and normal pregnancy rates achieved in the approximately 60% of such patients who had this miniscule degree of spermatogenesis present in otherwise completely deficient testicles (Silber *et al.*, 1995*c*).

The current ability of most men now to father a child no matter how poor the sperm count, even if there appears to be no spermatozoon at all, is dramatic. It appeared that the results of ICSI were not related either to the source of the spermatozoa (whether ejaculated, testicular, or epididymal), or to the quality of the spermatozoa (morphology or motility), whether the spermatozoa have been frozen or obtained fresh, whether they were retrieved with ease (as in the cases of normal spermatogenesis or with ejaculated spermatozoa), or whether they have to be extracted in very small numbers directly from the Sertoli cell after hours of painstaking searching of a testis specimen (see Table 10.3). Interestingly, recent research has indicated that there are significantly higher pregnancy rates in couples with testicular aspiration of spermatozoa from men with normal spermatogenesis compared to men with hypospermatogeneis and germ cell aplasia (see Table 8.2, p. 000). However, the age of the female partner is also a significant factor in determining the success of ICSI (Silber *et al.*, 1995c; and Table 10.4).

The genetics of infertile men about to undergo ICSI

Genetics of oligozoospermia and germinal failure

From 1975 to 1997, in various previous published reports, 7876 infertile men have undergone karyotyping. Of these, 3.8% were found to have sex chromosomal abnormalities and 1.3% were found to have autosomal chromosomal abnormalities, giving a total of 5.1% chromosomal abnormalities in over 7000 men studied and reported. This compares with the incidence in newborn infants of sex chromosomal abnormalities of 0.14%, autosomal chromosomal abnormalities of 0.25%, and of total chromosomal abnormalities in the newborn population of 0.38% (Koulischer & Schoysman, 1974; Chandley, 1979; Abramsson *et al.*, 1982; Zuffardi & Tiepolo, 1982; Gardelle *et al.*, 1983; Matsuda *et al.*, 1989; Dumur *et al.*, 1990; Yoshida *et al.*, 1995; Tables 10.5 and 10.6).

On average, 2% of men with severe oligozoospermia or oligoasthenoteratospermia, exhibited chromosomal defects, five- to six-fold that of a normal population. These chromosomal defects resulted in a higher rate of miscarriage and transmission of paternal chromosomal defects to the offspring. Therefore, in a very small percentage of infertile men (2%), chromosomal abnormalities appear to be able to interfere with spermatogenesis at the meiotic level. However, there are much more subtle genetic defects that appear to be responsible for male factor infertility and will not show up in routine chromosomal analysis.

In a study initiated by David Page and myself in 1992, 89 men with nonobstructive azoospermia caused either by maturation arrest, Sertoli cell only syndrome, or a combination of these two histological defects, underwent detailed sequence-tagged sites mapping of the Y chromosome (Reijo *et al.*, 1995). This study demonstrated microdeletions in 13% of such azoospermic

Table 10.3. ICSI with ejaculated versus epididymal (fresh and frozen) and testicular sperm

	No. of cycles	2PN (%)	Transfer (%)	Clinical pregnancies (%)
Ejaculated	965	70	93	30
Fresh epididymal	43	56	93	30
Frozen epididymal	9	56	100	33
Testicular	17	48	77	39

2PN, 2pronuclei

From Nagy et al., 1995b.

Table 10.4. Obstructive azoospermia – effect of age of wife

Age of wife	No. of cycles	No. of eggs M-II	2PN (%)	Normal cleaved embryos	Ongoing and delivered per cycle
<30	48 (26%)	907	382 (42%)	292 (76%)	22 (46%)
30–36	87 (48%)	1111	610 (55%)	413 (68%)	30 (34%)
37–39	22 (12%)	195	104 (53%)	84 (81%)	3 (14%)
40+	25 (14%)	281	147 (52%)	101 (69%)	1 (4%)
Totals	182 (100%)	2494	1243 (54%)	890 (70%)	56 (31%)

2PN, 2 pronuclei; M-II, meiosis-II.

patients. These microdeletions are located at the distal portion of the euchromatic region of the Y chromosome which is positioned approximately in the middle of the long arm of the Y. These microdeletions are being detected with mapping signposts that presently have a sensitivity of only 20 000 basepairs. Thus, it is possible that many more, much smaller mutations in the Y chromosome, perhaps in this region (*DAZ*), could be responsible for varying degrees of azoospermia and oligozoospermia (Reijo *et al.*, 1995; Silber, 1995; Silber *et al.*, 1995a, 1995c). This is a particularly difficult region of the human genome to sequence accurately because of the presence of so many confusing 'Y-specific repeats'. That is why this region is so easily prone to spontaneous mutations and perhaps why male infertility is very common in human beings.

Even patients with Klinefelter's syndrome (XXY), who were thought never to be able to father children, often have a minute amount of sperm production that can be discovered in the testis. These patients can undergo the TESE-ICSI procedure, develop normal embryos, and live births have been reported (Tournaye *et al.*, 1996). The question arises of whether spermatozoa from these Klinefelter's patients (presumably like those spermatozoa from other severely infertile men, who seem to yield offspring with a higher

Table 10.5. Autosomal abnormalities observed in infertile men (including azoospermic and oligozoospermic males)

Reference	Number	Robertsonian translocation	Reciprocal translocation	Inversion	Extra marker	Total
Total	7876	45 (0.6%)	36 (0.5%)	8 (0.1%)	8 (0.1%)	104 (1.3%)
Newborn studies	94 465	76 (0.08%)	98 (0.10%)	23 (0.02%)	35 (0.04%)	363 (0.38%)

From Van Assche et al., 1996

Table 10.6. Chromosomal abnormalities observed in seven series of infertile men compared to normal newborn population

References	Number	Sex chromosome	Autosomes	Total
Koulischer & Schoysman, 1974	1000	27 (2.7%)	6 (0.6%)	33 (3.3%)
Chandley, 1979	2372	33 (1.4%)	18 (0.7%)	51 (2.1%)
Zuffardi & Tiepolo, 1982	2542	175 (6.9%)	40 (1.6%)	215 (8.6%)
Abramsson et al., 1982	342	6 (1.8%)	4 (1.2%)	10 (2.9%)
de Gardelle et al., 1983	318	13 (4.1%)	7 (2.2%)	20 (6.3%)
Matsuda et al., 1989	295	0 (0)	5 (1.7%)	5 (1.7%)
Yoshida et al., 1995	1007	41 (4.1%)	24 (2.4%)	65 (6.5%)
Total	7876	295 (3.8%)	104 (1.3%)	399 (5.1%)
Newborn infants	94 465	131 (0.14%)	232 (0.25%)	366 (0.38%)

From Van Assche et al., 1996

incidence of sex chromosomal abnormalities) may be a heterogeneous variety (mosaic) consisting of some that are disomic for XX, and some that are disomic for XY, as well as some that are normal haploid Y and normal haploid X. Thus far, the replaceable embryos for the most part do not have sex chromosomal abnormalities, except for one which was a mosaic of XXY and XY (Handyside, 1993; Liu et al., 1994b; Staessen et al., 1996). This matter, therefore, still remains under debate.

Thus, because the ICSI procedure allows us to fertilize the eggs of partners from almost any man, no matter how apparently sterile, we have been able to study and understand better the genetic causes of male infertility, and the possible transference of this male infertility to male offspring generated by the ICSI procedure.

Cystic fibrosis

The genetics of cystic fibrosis and congenital male obstructive sterility have been worked out in great detail thanks to the introduction of ICSI (Silber et al., 1991; Anguiano et al., 1992; Patrizio et al., 1993; and Chillon et al.,

1995). In the past, we never dreamed that congenital absence of the vas might be a genetic condition transmitted via the cystic fibrosis gene. The only clue was the clinical observation that all men with cystic fibrosis also have congenital absence of the vas deferens. However, almost all men appearing in fertility clinics because of azoospermia caused by congenital absence of the vas deferens had normal sweat chloride tests and no clinical signs of cystic fibrosis. Yet when these men were studied genetically, we discovered in 1991 and 1992, that 70% had common cystic fibrosis mutations on one allele, and 10% had common cystic fibrosis mutations on both alleles. In those cases where both alleles were affected, one of the mutations was always an extremely mild one. Now we also see men with frank cystic fibrosis, with both alleles having strong mutations, who are also presenting to our fertility clinic to attempt to get their wives pregnant using MESA-ICSI.

It has now been demonstrated that a splicing error in intron 8 called the T_5 allele was found in patients with congenital bilateral absence of vas deferens (CBAVD) who had either no coding mutations, or none on the opposite allele. Thus, CBAVD patients, who are heterozygous for cystic fibrosis, or in both alleles of those who showed no mutations, each have an intron defect in the cystic fibrosis gene that diminishes cystic fibrosis transmembrane regulator gene (CFTR) protein synthesis. This results in a defective production of CFTR protein which was adequate to prevent cystic fibrosis but inadequate to prevent the development of congenital absence of the vas (Dumur *et al.*, 1990).

Thus, the development of ICSI for treatment of the most severe cases of male factor infertility has led to major molecular genetic discoveries that would never have been anticipated in the era of classical andrology.

References

Abramsson, L., Beckman, G., Duchek, M. & Nordenson, I. (1982). Chromosomal aberrations in male infertility. *Journal of Urology*, **128**, 52–3.

Anguiano, A., Oates, R. D., Amos, J. A., Dean, M., Gerrard, B., Stewart, C. *et al.* (1992). Congenital bilateral absence of the vas deferens: a primarily genital form of cystic fibrosis. *Journal of the American Medical Association*, **267**, 1794–7.

Chandley, A. C. (1979). The chromosomal basis of human infertility. *British Medical Bulletin*, **35**, 181–6.

Chillon, M., Casals, T., Mercier, B., Bassas, L., Lissens, W., Silber, S., Romey, M., Ruiz-Tomero, J., Verlingue, C., Claustres, M., Nunes, V., Ferec, C. & Estivill, X. (1995). Mutations in the cystic fibrosis gene in congenital absence of the vas deferens. *New England Journal of Medicine*, **332**, 1475–80.

Devroey, P., Silber, S., Nagy, Z., Liu, J., Tournaye, H., Joris, H., Verheyen, G. & Van Steirteghem, A. C. (1994). Ongoing pregnancies and birth after intracytoplasmic sperm injection (ICSI) with frozen-thawed epididymal spermatozoa. *Human Reproduction*, **10**, 903–6.

Devroey, P., Liu, J., Nagy, Z., Goossens, A., Tournaye, H., Camus, M., Van

Steirteghem, A. C. & Silber, S. J. (1995). Pregnancies after testicular extraction (TESE) and intracytoplasmic sperm injection (ICSI) in non-obstructive azoospermia. *Human Reproduction*, 10, 1457–60.

Dumur, V., Gervais, R., Rigot, J.-M., Lafitte, J.-J., Manouvrier, S., Biserte, J., Hazeman, E. & Roussel, P. (1990). Abnormal distribution of CF ΔF508 allele in azoospermic men with congenital aplasia of epididymis and vas deferens. *Lancet*, 336, 512–17.

Gardelle, de, G. R., Jaffray, J. Y., Geneix, A. & Malet, P. (1983). Les anomalies due caryotype dans les stérilités hypofertilités masculines. *Pathologica*, 75, 687–91.

Handyside, A. H. (1993). Diagnosis of inherited disease before implantation. *Reproductive Medicine Reviews*, 2, 51–61.

Koulischer, L. & Schoysman, R. (1974). Chromosomes and human infertility. Mitotic and meiotic chromosome studies in 202 consecutive male patients. *Clinical Genetics*, 5, 116–26.

Liu, J., Nagy, Z., Joris, H., Tournaye, H., Devroey, P. & Van Steirteghem, A. C. (1994a). Intracytoplasmic sperm injection does not require a special treatment of the spermatozoa. *Human Reproduction*, 9, 1127–30.

Liu, J., Lissens, W., Silber, S.J., Devroey, P., Liebaers, I. & Van Steirteghem, A. C. (1994b). Birth after preimplantation diagnosis of the cystic fibrosis ΔF508 mutation by polymerase chain reaction in human embryos resulting from intracytoplasmic sperm injection with epididymal sperm. *Journal of the American Medical Association*, 23, 1858–60.

Liu, J., Nagy, Z., Joris, H., Tournaye, H., Smity, J., Camus, M., Devroey, P., & Van Steirteghem, A. (1995). Analysis of 76 total fertilization failure cycles out of 2732 intracytoplasmic sperm injections cycles. *Human Reproduction*, 10, 2630–6.

Matsuda, T., Nonomura, M., Okada, K., Hayashi, K. & Yoshida, O. (1989). Cytogenetic survey of subfertile males in Japan. *Urology International*, 44, 194–7.

Nagy, Z., Liu, J., Joris, H., Verheyen, G., Tournaye, H., Camus, M., Derde, M. P., Devroey, P., & Van Steirteghem, A. C. (1995a). The result of intracytoplasmic sperm injection is not related to any of the three basic sperm parameters. *Human Reproduction*, 10, 1123–9.

Nagy, Z., Liu, J., Janssenwillen, C., Silber, S., Devroey, P. & Van Steirteghem, A. C. (1995b). Comparison of fertilization, embryo development and pregnancy rates after intracytoplasmic sperm injection using ejaculated, fresh and frozen-thawed epididymal and testicular sperm. *Fertility and Sterility*, 63, 808–15.

Palermo, G., Joris, H., Devroey, P. & Van Steirteghem, A. (1992). Pregnancies after intracytoplasmic injection of single spermatozoan into an oocyte. *Lancet*, 340, 17–18.

Patrizio, P., Asch, R. H., Handelin, B. & Silber, S. J. (1993). Aetiology of congenital absence of the vas deferens: genetic study of three generations. *Human Reproduction*, 8, 215–20.

Reijo, R., Lee, T.-Y., Salo, P., Alagappan, R., Brown, L. G., Rosenberg, M., Rozen, S., Jaffe, T., Straus, D., Hovata, O., de la Chapelle, A., Silber, S. & Page, D. C. (1995). Diverse spermatogenic defects in humans caused by Y chromosome deletions encompassing a novel RNA-binding protein. *Nature Genetics*, **10**, 383–93.

Schoysman, R., Vanderzwalmen, P., Nijs, M., Segal, L., Segal-Bertin, G., Geerts, L., van Roosendaal, E. & Schoysman, D. (1993). Pregnancy after fertilisation with human testicular spermatozoa. *Lancet*, **342**, 1237.

Silber, S. J. (1980). Vasoepididymostomy to the head of the epididymis: Recovery of normal spermatozoal motility. *Fertility and Sterility*, **34**, 149–53.

(1988). Pregnancy caused by sperm from vasa efferentia. *Fertility and Sterility*, **49**, 373–5.

(1989*a*). Results of microsurgical vasoepididymostomy: role of epididymis in sperm maturation. *Human Reproduction*, **4**, 298–303.

(1989*b*). Pregnancy after vasovasostomy for vasectomy reversal: a study of factors affecting long-term return of fertility in 282 patients followed for 10 years. *Human Reproduction*, **4**, 318–22.

(1995). What forms of male infertility are there left to cure? *Human Reproduction*, **10**, 503–4.

Silber, S. J.& Rodriguez-Rigau, L. J. (1981). Quantitative analysis of testicle biopsy: determination of partial obstruction and prediction of sperm count after surgery for obstruction. *Fertility and Sterility*, **36**, 480–5.

Silber, S. J., Balmaceda, J., Borrero, C., Ord, T. & Asch, R. H. (1988). Pregnancy with sperm aspiration from the proximal head of the epididymis: a new treatment for congenital absence of the vas deferens. *Fertility and Sterility*, **50**, 525–8.

Silber, S. J., Ord, T., Balmaceda, J., Patrizio, P. & Asch, R. (1991). Cystic fibrosis and congenital absence of the vas deferens. *New England Journal of Medicine*, **323**, 1788–92.

Silber, S. J., Nagy, Z. P., Liu, J., Godoy, H., Devroey, P. & Van Steirteghem, A. C. (1994). Conventional *in-vitro* fertilization versus intracytoplasmic sperm injection for patients requiring microsurgical sperm aspiration. *Human Reproduction*, **9**, 1705–9.

Silber, S. J., Van Steirteghem, A. C. & Devroey, P. (1995*a*). Sertoli cell only revisited. *Human Reproduction*, **10**, 1031–2.

Silber, S. J., Devroey, P., Tournaye, H. & Van Steirteghem, A. C. (1995*b*). Fertilizing capacity of epididymal and testicular sperm using intracytoplasmic sperm injection (ICSI). *Reproduction Fertility and Development*, **7**, 281–93.

Silber, S. J., Nagy, Z., Liu, J., Tournaye, H., Lissens, W., Ferec, C., Liebaers, I., Devroey, P. & Van Steirteghem, A. C. (1995*c*). The use of epididymal and testicular spermatozoa for intracytoplasmic sperm injection: the genetic implications for male infertility. *Human Reproduction*, **10**, 2031–43.

Silber, S. J., Van Steirteghem, A. C., Liu, J., Nagy, Z., Tournaye, H. & Devroey, P. (1995*d*). High fertilization and pregnancy rate after intracytoplasmic sperm injection with sperm obtained from testicle biopsy. *Human Reproduction*, **10**, 148–52.

Silber, S.J., Van Steirteghem, A. C., Nagy, Z., Liu, J., Tournaye, H. & Devroey, P. (1996). Normal pregnancies resulting from testicular sperm extraction and intracytoplasmic sperm injection for azoospermia due to maturation arrest. *Fertility and Sterility*, **55**, 110–17.

Staessen, C., Coonen, E., Van Assche, E., Tournaye, H., Joris, H., Devroey, P., van

Steirteghem, A.C. & Liebaers, I. (1996). Preimplantation diagnosis for X
and Y normality in embryos from three Klinefelter patients. *Human
Reproduction*, **11**, 1650–3.

Steinberger, E. & Tjioe, D. Y. (1968). A method for quantitative analysis of human
seminiferous epithelium. *Fertility and Sterility*, **19**, 960–70.

Tournaye, H., Devroey, P., Liu, J., Nagy, Z., Lissens, W. & Van Steirteghem, A.
(1994). Microsurgical epididymal sperm aspiration and intracytoplasmic
sperm injection: a new effective approach to infertility as a result of congenital bilateral absence of the vas deferens. *Fertility and Sterility*, **61**, 1045–51.

Tournaye, H., Staessen, C., Liebaers, I., Van Assche, E., Devroey, P., Bonduelle, M.
& Van Steirteghem, A. (1996). Testicular sperm recovery in 47,XXY
Klinefelter patients. *Human Reproduction*, **11**, 1644–9.

Van Assche, E., Bonduelle, M., Tournaye, H., Joris, H., Verheyen, G., Devroey, P.,
Van Steirteghem, A. & Liebaers, I. (1996). Cytogenetics of infertile men.
Human Reproduction, **11**, *Suppl.* 4, 1–24; Discussion 25–26.

Van Steirteghem, A. C., Nagy, Z., Joris, H., Liu, J., Staessen, C., Smitz, J., Wisanto,
A. & Devroey, P. (1993). High fertilization and implantation rates after
intracytoplasmic sperm injection. *Human Reproduction*, **8**, 1061–6.

Yoshida, A., Kamayama, T., Nagao, K., Takanami, M., Ishii, N., Miura, K. & Shiria,
M. (1995). A cytogenetic survey of 1,007 infertile males. *Contraception,
Fertility and Sex*, **23**, 103a.

Zuckerman, Z., Rodriguez-Rigau, L. J., Weiss, D. B., Chowdhury, L. J., Smith, K. D.
& Steinberger, E. (1978). Quantitative analysis of the seminiferous epithelium in human testicle biopsies and the relation of spermatogenesis to
sperm density. *Fertility and Sterility*, **30**, 448–55.

Zuffardi, O. & Tiepolo, L. (1982). Frequencies and types of chromosome abnormalities associated with human male infertility. In *Genetic control of gamete
production and function*, ed. P. G Crosignani and B. L. Rubin, pp. 261–73.
Serono Clinical Colloquia on Reproduction, III. London: Academic Press
and Guine and Stratton.

11 The challenge of asthenozoospermia

CHRIS FORD

Introduction

In this review three challenges posed by asthenozoospermia are considered. First, the development of a physiologically and clinically based definition of the condition. Secondly, the identification of the molecular pathology underlying poor sperm motility and, finally, the clinical management of men with asthenozoospermia.

Challenge 1: A physiologically based definition

The first challenge of asthenozoospermia is to decide what precisely it means. The World Health Organization (1992) defined it as 'Fewer than 50% spermatozoa with forward progression . . . or fewer than 25% with category 'a' movement [rapid progressive motility]', but this is a largely qualitative statement. A better definition would be based on objective measurements of sperm concentration and of motility characteristics and their combined relationship to sperm physiology and to clinical outcome. Not all laboratories can make such measurements, but the existence of quantitative criteria would provide a 'Gold Standard' against which more subjective methods could be judged. To develop such definitions, we will need to know what attributes of sperm motility are the most important for predicting fertility under different circumstances. What is required for natural fertility, for instance, may be less important after intra-uterine insemination (IUI) and this may in turn require different attributes from *in vitro* fertilization (IVF). Once parameters have been selected, we must decide how they should be described. For example, is the average velocity in the ejaculate or the concentration of spermatozoa swimming at above or below a given speed the more predictive of fertility? An ejaculate with a high sperm concentration, but a low average velocity, may contain more fast spermatozoa than an ejaculate with a high average velocity but a low sperm concentration. Finally, the conditions of measurement need to be defined. Should we make measurements in seminal plasma or after washing the spermatozoa and resuspending them in a defined medium? What temperature should be used? We must try to measure sperm motion objectively and quantitatively, but how can this best be achieved?

Measurement of sperm motility

Subjective assessment as part of standard semen analysis

It is important that clinical semen analysis is reasonably consistent between different laboratories. Therefore, the analysis should be done according to an agreed protocol, as described in the *WHO Manual* (WHO, 1992). WHO recommend reporting the percentage spermatozoa exhibiting four grades of motility: (a) rapid progressive, (b) slow or sluggish progressive, (c) non-progressive, and (d) immotile. Little guidance is given on how to distinguish grades a and b and the separation is arbitrary. Temperature has a profound effect on sperm motility especially on forward velocity (Fig. 11.1) and measurements should always be made at a constant temperature of 37 °C, otherwise the proportion of vigorously motile sperm will be underestimated. It is also vital for laboratories both to operate internal quality schemes to minimize variation between different technicians and to belong to an external quality control scheme such as that operated by UK NEQAS (National External Quality Assurance Scheme). Computer-assisted semen analysis (CASA) may provide a standard for calibrating the grading of motility (Yeung *et al.*, 1997). Some allowance has to be made for the viscosity of seminal plasma: occasionally the seminal plasma remains extremely viscous, even after prolonged liquefaction and this will decrease the apparent quality of sperm motion.

Objective and quantitative measurements

Various ingenious methods have been devised to make objective measurements of sperm motility. These include laser light-scattering (Lee *et*

Fig. 11.1. Effect of temperature on sperm motility. (Redrawn from Ford *et al.*, 1992*b*.)

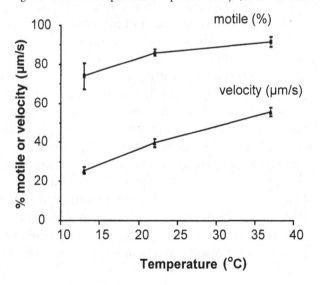

al., 1982), measuring the increase in turbidity as spermatozoa swim from the bottom of a cuvette into the light path (Sokoloski *et al.*, 1977), measuring changes in light-scattering in thick films of spermatozoa (Dott & Foster, 1979) or the rate at which spermatozoa pass through a 5 μm filter (Hong *et al.*, 1981). However, the overwhelming majority of measurements of human sperm motion have been made by tracking individual spermatozoa under the microscope. This has been done by tracking spermatozoa manually, in an image projected onto a digitizing tablet (Hinting *et al.*, 1988), or on a video screen (Holt *et al.*, 1985) or between successive frames of a ciné film (David *et al.*, 1981). Time exposure still photography (Overstreet *et al.*, 1979) was a simple and effective procedure which could be refined by using stroboscopic illumination (Makler, 1978). However, nowadays the methods of choice employ commercial computer systems which automatically track the position of the sperm head in successive video frames and use the stored information to calculate various parameters of sperm motion. The principal parameters derived from CASA are shown in Fig. 11.2. The principles of setting up CASA instruments have been described elsewhere (Davis & Katz, 1992) and the application of CASA has been reviewed (Irvine, 1995; Krause, 1995*a,b*) and discussed by a European Society for Human Reproduction and Embryology (ESHRE) workshop (ESHRE Andrology Special Interest Group, 1996). Discussion here will focus on aspects peculiar to the analysis of asthenozoospermic samples. The chief of these is how best to characterize sperm motion when it may be difficult to find enough motile spermatozoa to achieve statistically precise estimates of their concentration or of other parameters.

It is accepted that the number of cells observed on a slide conforms to a Poisson distribution (Sokal & Rohlf, 1969) in which case, the standard

Fig. 11.2. Principal parameters of sperm motion measured by computer-assisted semen analysis (CASA) machines.

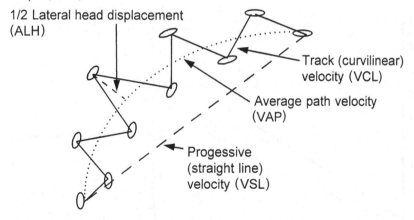

1/2 Lateral head displacement (ALH)

Track (curvilinear) velocity (VCL)

Average path velocity (VAP)

Progessive (straight line) velocity (VSL)

Beat cross frequency (BCF) = no. of times track crosses average path per second
Linearity (LIN) = (VSL/VCL) × 100
Straightness (STR) = (VSL/VAP) × 100

deviation is equal to the square root of the number of spermatozoa observed. Calculated confidence limits for sperm concentration estimated in a single microscopic field of a 20 μm deep chamber with a Hamilton Thorn Version 7 Motility Analyser, set up in line with the manufacturer's instructions according to the number of spermatozoa observed, are shown in Fig. 11.3(*a*). It is evident that the confidence limits are broad and are several times greater than the population concentration, when the concentration and hence the number of spermatozoa observed is low. With oligozoospermic semen it might be possible to increase the sample volume (and the number of spermatozoa observed) by increasing the chamber depth without loss of accuracy. However, asthenozoospermic semen may contain a large number of immotile spermatozoa that would interfere with the imaging of those motile spermatozoa above or below them in deep chambers. This approach cannot therefore be used. The only other approach available (without involving sperm preparation) is to scan more microscope fields. Figure 11.3(*b*) shows the effect of increasing the number of microscope fields on the precision of the estimate of sperm concentration in a semen sample containing 2 million sperm/ml. Precision increases as more fields are included, but remains poor when expressed as the coefficient of variation (which is still >13% after 20 frames). The collection of very large numbers of frames is difficult when operators may have numerous samples to analyse and are, therefore, constrained as to how long they can spend on each one. It also requires care to

Fig. 11.3. Effect of number of sperm observed on the precision of concentration estimation by computer-assisted semen analysis (CASA) calculated using confidence limits for the Poisson distribution (Lentner, 1982): (*a*) sperm concentration and 95% confidence intervals (CI) according to the number of sperm observed in a single microscope field equivalent to a volume of 1.42 nl (Hamilton Thorne Version 7 Motility Analyser, 20 μm deep chamber); (*b*) 95% CI for the estimation of the concentration of a semen sample containing 2×10^6 spermatozoa/ml according to the number of microscope fields examined.

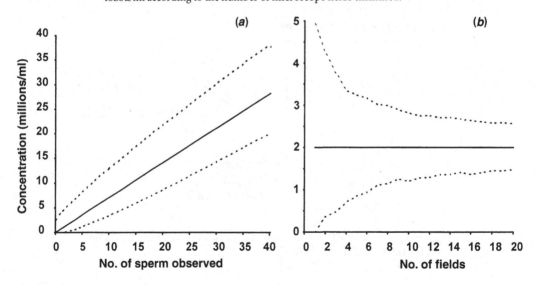

avoid multiple sampling of the same field and possible changes in the characteristics of the population over the observation time. In spite of these problems, we can make quantitative statements of known precision about the
concentration of motile spermatozoa or of spermatozoa with given characteristics of motility in asthenozoospermic semen. Confidence limits will be
wide and fine comparison of different degrees of asthenozoospermia will not
however, be possible. Nevertheless, in the above example, only seven frames
are required to be 95% confident that the sperm concentration lies between
1 million and 3 million/ml. In practice, the usefulness of data of this degree of
precision will depend on how steeply fertility changes as a function of the
motile sperm concentration. If the chance of conception increases by only
2% between the confidence intervals, precision may be sufficient for clinical
purposes, but if the conception rate increased by 15% then precision is clearly
too poor for the test to be of any use.

Similar considerations govern the estimation of continuous parameters
such as velocity. Most machines report these as the mean $\pm$ standard deviation for the spermatozoa observed. This approach has been heavily criti-
cized, because the distribution of many sperm parameters is not normal
(Gladen *et al.*, 1991; ESHRE Andrology Special Interest Group, 1996). This is
particularly striking for asthenozoospermic samples, where the distributions (even of parameters such as velocity, which follow a near normal distribution in highly motile samples) can be highly skewed (Fig. 11.4). If a normal
distribution is assumed, the precision of the estimate of the population
mean depends on the number of spermatozoa in the sample and on standard
deviation of the population (Fig. 11.5). If the population is homogeneous,
that is to say it has a low standard deviation, then a reasonable estimate of the
mean of a parameter can be obtained from 20–40 spermatozoa. However, if
the population is diverse, large numbers of spermatozoa must be sampled to
get a reliable estimate. In view of the wide dispersion of sperm velocities and
their failure to conform to a normal statistical distribution, it is probably best
to express data in terms of the concentrations of spermatozoa with given
characteristics. At least the precision of these estimates can be calculated.

Motility assessment in washed sperm preparations

Many of the problems inherent in measuring sperm motion in asthenozoospermic semen could be circumvented by separating the motile spermatozoa on a Percoll or similar density gradient and then resuspending
them at an increased concentration (Gellert-Mortimer *et al.*, 1988; Ford *et al.*,
1992*a*). Even if this in itself were not sufficient to allow enough spermatozoa
to be studied, the removal of immotile spermatozoa and other debris
should make it possible to use deeper chambers in order to get good statistical precision. It has to be realized that centrifugation through a 'Percoll' or
similar gradient changes the motility of the sperm population in favour of
the faster-swimming spermatozoa with a greater amplitude of lateral head

displacement (ALH) (Fig. 11.6). Such an approach may seem unphysiological. But, it is logical to assess the potential of spermatozoa to succeed in IVF, using the same medium in which the spermatozoa will be mixed with the eggs. Even *in vivo* spermatozoa do not fertilize in seminal plasma and indeed may spend a very short time in this fluid before invading the cervical mucus. It could be argued, therefore, that mucus will select the more motile fraction of a sperm population in the same way as the Percoll gradient does. Therefore, it is possible or even probable that the properties of spermatozoa in Percoll preparations will have as good or better correlation with fertility than the same parameters in semen. Separating spermatozoa on 'Percoll' does not yield a greater number of motile spermatozoa to study. For example, in the 55 ejaculates used for the data shown in Fig. 11.6, 8123 motile spermatozoa were found in semen but only 3996 in the Percoll preparation. The spermatozoa need to be resuspended in a volume smaller than the original volume of semen applied to the gradient and the use of deeper chambers for the purified suspensions has to be considered. Of course, such manoeuvres must be taken into account in the calculations of sperm concentration.

Fig. 11.4. Distribution of average path velocities (VAP) in sperm from 726 ejaculates with >50% of sperm progressively motile (continuous line) and 301 ejaculates with <25% of sperm progressively motile (dashed line). (W. C. L. Ford & E. A. McLaughlin, unpublished data.)

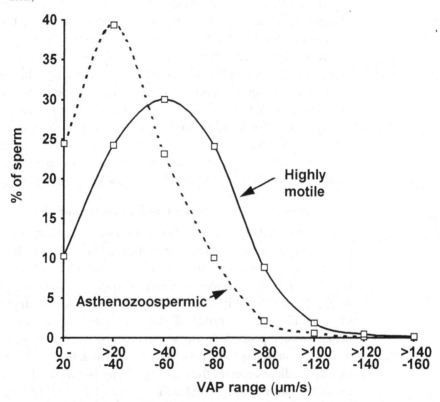

To sum up, it is difficult to get statistically precise data on sperm motility in semen of severely asthenozoospermic men. The problem of numbers can be overcome by collecting data from a large number of microscopic fields (taking care that they are all different and selected at random) or by examining purified preparations in deeper chambers. The increased tendency for parameters in asthenozoospermic samples to exhibit skewed distributions makes it inappropriate to use mean values to describe parameters such as velocity and ALH.

Asthenozoospermia and fertility

It is firmly established that spermatozoa must be motile in order to penetrate cervical mucus (Aitken *et al.*, 1985; Mortimer *et al.*, 1986; Keel & Webster, 1988; Ford *et al.*, 1992*b*). Sperm motility is strongly related to success in the zona-free hamster egg test (Aitken, 1990; Ford *et al.*, 1991). Spermatozoa must generate considerable mechanical force to penetrate the zona pellucida and the development of hyperactivated motility during capacitation is needed to make this possible (Burkman, 1990; Suarez, 1996). We would therefore expect motility to be related to fertility both *in vivo* and *in vitro*.

Fig. 11.5. Effect of number of spermatozoa examined on the reproducibility of estimates of a parameter whose population mean is 40 with standard deviation of 10 (short dashes) or 18 (long dashes). The 'distributions' routine of the Minitab statistical package was used to generate 99 samples of 2 sperm, 99 samples of 3 sperm, and so on, from a normal population as defined above. The means and standard deviations were calculated for each sample size and used to derive the 95% confidence intervals and coefficient of variation.

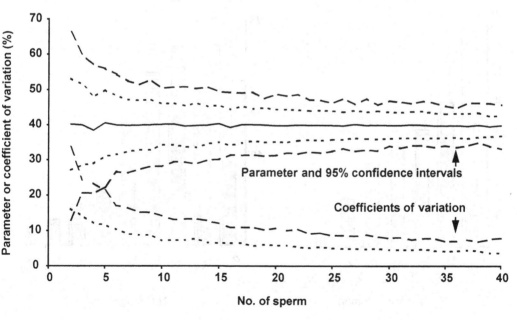

Prediction by conventional seminology

In considering the relationship of motility (or any of any other parameter) to fertility, it is important to realize that few men are totally infertile. The population contains a continuum from men who have a very low probability of impregnating their partners in a cycle (subfertile) to those who have a chance of 50% or more (highly fertile). When the population is divided according to whether they have achieved a pregnancy after 12 months of unprotected intercourse, the group who have succeeded will include subfertile men who have been lucky whereas those who fail will include normally fertile men who have been unlucky. There will therefore be considerable overlap in semen characteristics between the two populations and it is possible to provide a time-limited prognosis of fertility only in the form of a probability. Only in rare cases of complete azoospermia is it possible to advise a man that he is completely infertile.

For natural conception the predictive power of conventional semen parameters is often less than those of age and duration of infertility (Ducot *et al.*, 1988; Dunphy *et al.*, 1989*b*; Duleba *et al.*, 1992; Eimers *et al.*, 1994) and in one large study (Polansky & Lamb, 1988) the World Health Organization (1980) criteria for normal semen had little or no predictive value for fertility. Nevertheless, in other studies motility was related to the chance of conception. Fertility was decreased if <20% of spermatozoa were motile (Jouannet

Fig. 11.6. The distributions of average path velocities (VAP) and amplitude of lateral head displacement (ALH) in 55 asthenozoospermic (<50% motile) ejaculates in semen (light stipple) and after centrifugation through a 40%/80% Percoll gradient and suspension in BWW medium (dark stipple).

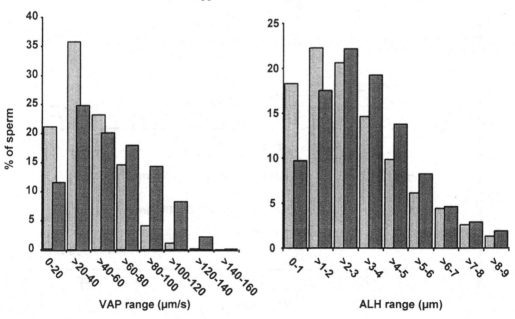

et al., 1988). If <50% of spermatozoa were motile, couples were 30% less likely to conceive in 18 months, or >50% less likely if the concentration of motile spermatozoa was $<5 \times 10^6$/ml (Glazener *et al.*, 1987). The chance of conception was significantly less if the concentration of slow progressive spermatozoa in semen was decreased (Dunphy *et al.*, 1989*a,b*). In this study motility was measured at room temperature and many sluggish spermatozoa may have become rapid at 37 °C. The hazard of becoming pregnant derived from a Cox's regression model was significantly decreased when sperm motility fell below 30%, or progressive motility below 20% (Holland-Morritz & Krause, 1992). The percentage of spermatozoa that were motile was less in a suspected infertile population than in a fertile but a good distinction between the populations could only be made by combining several parameters (Bartoov *et al.*, 1993). In assisted reproduction, the success of donor insemination (DI) depends on the number of motile spermatozoa inseminated, that is up to about 10 million (Fédération CECOS *et al.*, 1993). In IVF the fertilization rate depends on the number of motile spermatozoa available and the risk of failing to obtain at least one embryo increases when fewer than 4×10^6 spermatozoa are recovered whereas the chance of getting four or more embryos decreases (Fig. 11.7). The success of gamete intra-fallopian transfer (GIFT) declines in a similar way (Craft, 1990). Recently, attempts have been made to use receptor operator characteristic curves (ROCC) to define the best cut-off values in predicting fertility from the data

Fig. 11.7. The proportion of couples from whom six or more eggs were collected to achieve ≥4(dark stipple) or ≤1 (light stipple) embryos as a function of the total motile sperm recovered for IVF. (From Joels *et al.*, 1997.)

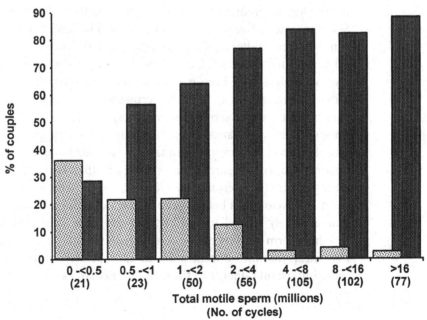

obtained by semen analysis. Comhaire & Vermeulen (1995) proposed that each laboratory should set its own limits of normality based on the 5th centile of a fertile population. They defined three ranges separating probably fertile (F) from probably subfertile (S) and probably infertile (I) semen. Their cut-off to separate group F from S and group S from I were 48 and 14 for % motile (grades a + b) and 21×10^6 and 0.6×10^6/ml for the concentration of motile spermatozoa. Ombelet *et al.* (1997) reported that sperm morphology measured according to strict criteria was the best predictor of fertility, but found that to separate fertile and infertile couples cut-off values for % motility of 28 based on the 10th centile of the fertile population and of 45 based on ROCC were needed. Among 449 husbands of women with tubal disease in our own clinic the 5th and 10th centiles for the percentage of progressively motile spermatozoa (grades a + b) were 18 and 28, respectively.

In conclusion, there is no doubt that men with asthenozoospermia are less fertile than men with good sperm motility. However, the use of motility as a single parameter has limited predictive power although it can be improved by using the concentration rather than the percentage of motile spermatozoa. Attempts to define rational cut-offs have begun, but there is no consensus about what constitutes an acceptable chance of conception per cycle and still less what degree of asthenospermia is compatible with a reasonable probability of achieving it.

Quantitative motility measurements and CASA

There are several studies demonstrating that the parameters of motility of 'infertile' semen are worse than those in 'fertile' semen. But comparatively few investigators have analysed the ability of different parameters to predict fertility with either natural or assisted conception. Seven representative studies are summarized in Table 11.1. Direct comparisons between studies are impossible, because different methods of statistical analysis have been used, a variety of other parameters apart from sperm motion analysis have been measured and results have been obtained from different fertilization systems. Nevertheless, a consensus emerges that the concentration or percentage of motile spermatozoa and their velocity is important for spermatozoa deposited either in the vagina at intercourse or into the cervix by donor insemination. The extra information that can be obtained from other parameters is limited by their correlation with the percentage of motile spermatozoa (Krause, 1995b). This leaves us a long way short of developing a better, quantitative definition of asthenozoospermia that is closely related to fertility. However, the data raise doubts as to whether sperm motility can be considered separately from concentration. It may mean that the concentration of appropriately motile spermatozoa is more important rather than the mean or median values of different parameters.

Table 11.1. Some published studies which relate quantitative measurements of sperm motion to fertility

Reference	System	Statistical method	Parameters selected or equation derived	% variation explained
Krause (1995b)	Natural – CASA	Cox's regression	$h(t) = h_0(t) \times e^{(0.012 \times \%\text{motile} + 0.234 \times \ln(\text{sperm count}))}$ h = hazard of pregnancy in time t; h_0, baseline hazard at time t	
Barratt et al. (1993)	Natural – CASA	Cox's regression	$P = 1 - [0.87]e^{(0.0241 \times \text{VAP} + 0.0025 \times \text{total sperm})}$ P = probability of conceiving within 1 year	72%
Irvine et al. (1994)	Natural – CASA	Cox's regression	Mean head area	
Irvine & Aitken (1986)	DI – time-lapse photography	Multivariate discriminant analysis	Sperm progressively motile (%) Concn motile sperm (0.458) Motile sperm (%) after 3 h + A23187 (0.782) Mean sperm per zona-free hamster egg (0.549) Mean velocity, µm (0.890) Sperm yawing (%) (0.508) Frequency of rotation of progressive sperm (−1.161) (Standardized discriminant function coefficient)	81% correct classification of 'fertile' and 'infertile' ejaculates
Macleod & Irvine (1995)	DI – CASA	Multiple logistic regression	Mean minor axis, µm (−9.86) Mean major axis, µm (−10–74) Mean area, µm² (2.19) Mean ALH, µm (2.69) Mean VAP, µm/s (1.95) (β coefficients)	87% correct classification of 'fertile' and 'infertile' ejaculates
Aitken et al. (1994)	HOPT – CASA on Percoll prep.	Multiple logistic regression	Rapid (>25 µm/s) sperm % (0.482) VAP, µm/s (0.554) STR, (0.347) ALH, µm (−0.613) (β coefficients)	$R^2 = 0.702$
Liu et al. (1991)	IVF – CASA	Multiple logistic regression	Male factor infertility (−1.374) % sperm in insem. med. with VAP 10–20 µm/s (−0.157) LIN in semen (0.046) Tubal disease (0.378) (β coefficients)	

Natural, conception by natural intercourse; DI, donor insemination (intracervical); IVF, *in vitro* fertilization; CASA, computer-assisted semen analysis; HOPT, hamster oocyte penetration test; ALH, amplitude of lateral head displacement; VAP, average path velocity; STR, straightness; LIN, linearity; insem. med., insemination medium.

Challenge 2: defining the causes of asthenozoospermia

Spermatozoa are propelled by active bending of the flagellum. Bends are propagated by sliding between adjacent tubules driven by the hydrolysis of ATP by a dynein ATPase. A sophisticated control mechanism exists to ensure that active sliding between tubules on one side of the axoneme is balanced by opposite sliding on the other side of the axoneme; it also ensures that the frequency and amplitude of binding is appropriate (for reviews, see Bedford & Hoskins, 1990; Tamm, 1994; Tash & Bracho, 1994; Walczak & Nelson, 1994; Lindemann & Kanous, 1997). Poor motility could result from defects in the structure of the flagellum, in its regulatory system or in the metabolic machinery supplying ATP.

Metabolic defects

Restricting ATP production with inhibitors such as the putative male contraceptive α-chlorohydrin will decrease sperm motility (see Ford & Rees, 1990). Moreover, decreases of ATP concentration have been implicated in the anti-motility effect of reactive oxygen species (De Lamirande & Gagnon, 1992). However, if ATP supply were all that was limiting flagellar activity of spermatozoa in the semen of asthenozoospermic men, the axonemes would be expected to function normally if they were demembranated and supplied with adequate ATP in the medium. In practice, the motility of demembranated spermatozoa from asthenozoospermic men, incubated with ATP and cyclic AMP, was closely correlated with the motility of the intact sperm in culture medium (Liu *et al.*, 1987; Yeung *et al.*, 1988), suggesting that their poor motility was due to defects in the axoneme rather than in the supply of ATP. In examining more than 70 men with asthenozoospermia, Ford & Rees (1990) failed to detect any with defective metabolism in the spermatozoa. This suggests that defective ATP production must be a rare cause of poor sperm motility. However, defects in mitochondrial DNA are known to be responsible for many inherited or degenerative human diseases (see Okawa, 1997; Wallace, 1997) and there is some evidence that they may be a cause of sperm dysfunction (Cummins *et al.*, 1994). A patient from a family with four generations of mitochondrial encephalomyopathy caused by reduced activity of enzyme complexes I and IV exhibited reduced sperm motility (Folgero *et al.*, 1993). Spermatozoa from asthenozoospermic patients exhibited shorter midpieces and fewer mitochondrial gyres than spermatozoa from normozoospermic men (Mundy *et al.*, 1995). A high frequency of the 4977 base-pair mitochondrial DNA deletion is associated with asthenozoospermia in a very small number of men (Kao *et al.*, 1995). Inhibition of mitochondrial energy production decreased sperm motility, and spermatozoa from asthenozoospermic men exhibited more mitochondrial DNA deletions when examined by the polymerase chain reaction technique (St John *et al.*, 1997; Chapter 12, this volume).

Defects in the axoneme

Poor sperm motility is associated with a number of defects of the axoneme and of the outer dense fibres, which can be detected by transmission electron microscopy and are distinct from necrozoospermia (see Zamboni, 1987). A well-known example of such a defect is Kartagener's syndrome. Both sperm flagella and epithelial cilia are dysfunctional and the men exhibit frequent respiratory disease as well as infertility (Afzelius *et al.*, 1975; see Bedford & Hoskins, 1990). Characteristically they lack outer dynein arms but other defects have been observed. The disease is controlled by more than one gene and it is possible for sperm flagella to be normal although cilia are defective (Phillips *et al.*, 1995) or for cilia and flagella to demonstrate different defects (Chemes *et al.*, 1990). Several studies suggest that axonemal defects are prevalent in spermatozoa from asthenozoospermic men. Among 400 patients with asthenozoospermia, 3% exhibited a total or partial absence of dynein arms, 23% had a variety of other fine structural defects and 23% were necrospermic. The remainder all had some normal spermatozoa and this was the only group where the couples achieved pregnancies (Ryder *et al.*, 1990). Seven out of ten severely asthenozoospermic patients had axonemal defects (Wilton *et al.*, 1992) and the frequency of axonemal defects was greater in a group of ten asthenozoospermic men than in a group of ten normal men (Hancock & de Kretser, 1992). Sperm tail structural abnormalities were detected in only 42 out of 4231 infertile patients in the course of routine semen analysis (Marmor & Grob-Menendez, 1991) and so electron microscopy is required to detect subtle defects in the axoneme.

Thus, there is good evidence that defects in the flagellum are the underlying cause of asthenozoospermia in many men. Many of these defects are likely to be genetically controlled.

Defects of cell regulation

It has been known for many years that sperm motility is regulated by the second messengers cyclic AMP (cAMP) and Ca^{2+}, through protein phosphorylation. cAMP is required to initiate and to maintain motility but Ca^{2+} increases beat asymmetry and is involved in the regulation of hyperactivation (see Tash & Means, 1983; Tash & Bracho, 1994).

cAMP stimulates phosphorylation of a number of proteins, some of which may be components of the dynein complex and a number of protein kinases may also be involved (Tash & Bracho, 1994; Chaudhry *et al.*, 1995). At the time of writing, attention is focusing on protein tyrosine phosphorylation. The motility of bovine spermatozoa is closely correlated with the extent of phsophorylation of a 55 kilodalton protein that is present in the 100 000 *g* supernatant (Vijayaraghavan *et al.*, 1997*b*). Motility-related tyrosine phosphorylation has been reported for 81 and 105 kilodalton proteins that may also be involved in capacitation (Leclerc *et al.*, 1996). The reactivation of the demembranated human spermatozoon in the presence of cAMP was dependent on the phosphorylation of a number of proteins (Leclerc & Gagnon, 1996). The rate of tyrosine phosphorylation is controlled by the cAMP-dependent Ser/Thr phosphorylation of an unidentified protein which is catalysed by protein kinase A. This protein can be dephosphorylated by protein phosphatases (PP). Spermatozoa contain PP1, PP2A and PP2B. PP2B is calmodulin-dependent and its inhibition affects the motility of human spermatozoa (Ahmad *et al.*, 1995). The activity of PP1 can be controlled by phosphorylation via a glycogen synthase kinase 3-like enzyme (GSK3) and the motility of spermatozoa in the epididymis may be suppressed by a high PP1 activity sustained by a high activity of GSK3. This was six-fold greater in immotile spermatozoa taken from the caput epididymis than in motile spermatozoa from the same region of the epididymis (Smith *et al.*, 1996; Vijayaraghavan *et al.*, 1996). The activity of protein kinase A is also controlled by the fact that the enzyme is bound to the cytoskeleton by anchoring proteins. These proteins may be critical in regulating the specificity of response by confining protein kinase A isoenzymes to specified locations (Pariset & Weinman, 1994; Carrera *et al.*, 1996; Vijayaraghavan *et al.*, 1997*a*).

Thus, it is clear that cAMP regulates sperm motility through protein phosphorylation, and it seems that Ser/Thr phosphorylation of some proteins modulates the tyrosine phosphorylation of others. Calcium modulates this process by influencing the activity of adenylyl cyclase and protein phosphatases and perhaps also, through protein kinase C (Rotem *et al.*, 1990*a*,*b*; Lax *et al.*, 1997). The external signals that regulate these second messengers remain obscure although adenylyl cyclase is influenced by extracellular bicarbonate (Okamura *et al.*, 1985). For example, bicarbonate-induced cAMP-dependent phosphorylation of a 65 kilodalton protein has been demonstrated in mouse spermatozoa (Si & Okuno, 1995). In addition, bicarbonate is high in oviductal fluid (Brackett & Mastroianni, 1975). Both mouse (Fraser & Duncan, 1993) and human spermatozoa (Fenichel *et al.*, 1996) bear type A2 adenosine receptors and adenosine analogues stimulate adenylyl cyclase activity and tyrosine phosphorylation.

There is no direct evidence that defects in these regulatory mechanisms are responsible for asthenozoospermia. However, perhaps the best indication is that phosphodiesterase inhibitors and other pharmacological agents are more effective in stimulating human sperm motility when motility is initially poor (Cummins & Yovich, 1993).

Challenge 3: Treatment of asthenozoospermia

Treatments that so far have been proposed aim to enhance sperm motility by selection or to assist spermatozoa to reach the egg and to penetrate its investments. The second of these approaches has reached its culmination in intracytoplasmic sperm injection (ICSI). ICSI is extremely successful and has transformed the prospects of fatherhood for large numbers of subfertile men. Extremely good success rates, comparable to the best obtained in conventional IVF, are achievable with very small numbers of motile sperm and success is possible with immotile but viable sperm (for a review, see Palermo *et al.*, 1996). ICSI is undoubtedly the treatment of choice for couples with moderate to severe sperm dysfunction, although the possibility that genetic causes of infertility will be passed on to the next generation must be borne in mind (Cummins & Jequier, 1995). For less severe impairment of motility, conventional IVF and even IUI continue to offer a worthwhile chance of success (Hull, 1992, 1994; Ford *et al.*, 1997). Initially encouraging results using the phosphodiesterase inhibitor pentoxifylline to stimulate motility and capacitation (see Yovich, 1993) have not proved to be generally repeatable (Tournaye *et al.*, 1993, 1994) and the ascendancy of ICSI has in any case made this approach of largely historic interest.

Conclusions

The definition of asthenozoospermia remains arbitrary. The quantification of the characteristics of sperm motion in the semen of asthenozoospermic men is imprecise, because of the difficulty of obtaining enough spermatozoa for examination. Because of uncertainties about the distribution of the data, it is probably better to report concentrations of spermatozoa with particular characteristics of motility rather than to use means or medians in a report. The fertility of asthenozoospermic men, as presently defined, probably varies from near normal to near zero and it is likely that multicentre trials will be needed to work out the probability of conception occurring in a given time, associated with specific characteristics of the motility. Very rapid progress is being made in understanding the basic mechanism of sperm motility and of how it is controlled. It is probable that the underlying causes of more (and an increasing number of) cases of asthenozoospermia will be understood within the next decade. This should offer the prospect of better pharmacological methods being used to improve sperm motility.

Acknowledgements

I am grateful for support from Professor M. G. R. Hull and other members of the University of Bristol Reproductive Medicine Group.

References
Afzelius, B. A., Eliasson, R., Johnson, O. & Lindholmer, C. (1975). Lack of dynein arms in immobile human spermatozoa. *Journal of Cell Biology*, **66**, 225–32.
Ahmad, K., Bracho, G. E., Wolf, D. P. & Tash, J. S. (1995). Regulation of human sperm motility and hyperactivation components by calcium, calmodulin, and protein phosphatases. *Archives of Andrology*, **35**, 187–208.

Aitken, R. J. (1990). Motility parameters and fertility. In *Controls of sperm motility: biological and clinical aspects*, ed. C. Gagnon, pp. 175–202. Boca Raton, FL: CRC Press.

Aitken, R. J., Sutton, M., Warner, P. & Richardson. D. W. (1985). Relationship between the movement characteristics of human spermatozoa and their ability to penetrate cervical mucus and zona free hamster oocytes. *Journal of Reproduction and Fertility*, 73, 441–9.

Aitken, R. J., Buckingham, D. & Harkiss, D. (1994). Analysis of the extent to which sperm movement can predict the results of ionophore enhanced functional assays of the acrosome reaction and sperm oocyte fusion. *Human Reproduction*, 9, 1867–74.

Barratt, C. L. R., Tomlinson, M. J. & Cooke, I. D. (1993). Prognostic-significance of computerized motility analysis for in-vivo fertility. *Fertility and Sterility*, 60, 520–5.

Bartoov, B., Eltes, F., Pansky, M., Lederman, H., Caspi, E. & Soffer, Y. (1993). Estimating fertility potential via semen analysis data. *Human Reproduction*, 8, 65–70.

Bedford, J. M. & Hoskins, D. D. (1990). The mammalian spermatozoon: morphology, biochemistry and physiology. In *Marshall's physiology of reproduction*, 4th edn, vol. 2, *Reproduction in the male*, ed. G.E. Lamming, pp. 379–568. Edinburgh: Churchill Livingstone.

Brackett, B. G. & Mastroianni, L. (1975). Composition of oviducal fluid. In *The oviduct and its functions*, ed. A.D. Johnson & C.W. Foley, pp. 133–59. New York: Academic Press.

Burkman, L. J. (1990). Hyperactivated motility of human spermatozoa during *in vitro* capacitation and implications for fertility. In *Controls of sperm motility: biological and clinical aspects*, ed. C. Gagnon, pp. 303–30. Boca Raton, FL: CRC Press.

Carrera, A., Moos, J., Ning, X. P., Gerton, G. L., Tesarik. J., Kopf, G. S. & Moss, S. B. (1996). Regulation of protein-tyrosine phosphorylation in human sperm by a calcium/calmodulin-dependent mechanism – identification of A kinase anchor proteins as major substrates for tyrosine phosphorylation. *Developmental Biology*, 180, 284–96.

Chaudhry, P. S., Creagh, S., Yu, N. & Brokaw, C. J. (1995). Multiple protein-kinase activities required for activation of sperm flagellar motility. *Cell Motility and the Cytoskeleton*, 32, 65–79.

Chemes, H. E., Morero, J. L. & Lavieri, J. C. (1990). Extreme asthenozoospermia and chronic respiratory-disease – a new variant of the immotile cilia syndrome. *International Journal of Andrology*, 13, 216–22.

Comhaire, F. & Vermeulen, L. (1995). Human semen analysis. *Human Reproduction Update*, 1, 343–62.

Craft, I. (1990). Factors affecting the outcome of assisted conception. *British Medical Bulletin*, 46, 769–82.

Cummins, J. M. & Jequier, A. M. (1995). Concerns and recommendations for intracytoplasmic sperm injection (ICSI) treatment. *Human Reproduction*, 10(S1),138–43.

Cummins, J. M. & Yovich, J. M. (1993). Sperm motility enhancement *in vitro*. *Seminars in Reproductive Endocrinology*, 11, 56–71.

Cummins, J. M., Jequier, A. M. & Kan, R. (1994). Molecular biology of human male infertility: links with ageing mitochondrial genetics and oxidative stress. *Molecular Reproduction and Development*, **37**, 345–62.

David, G., Serres, C. & Jouannet, P. (1981). Kinematics of human spermatozoa. *Gamete Research*, **4**, 83–95.

Davis, R. O. & Katz, D. F. (1992). Standardization and comparability of CASA instruments. *Journal of Andrology*, **13**, 81–6.

De Lamirande, E. & Gagnon, C. (1992). Reactive oxygen species and human spermatozoa. II. Depletion of adenosine triphosphate plays an important role in the inhibition of sperm motility. *Journal of Andrology*, **15**, 379–86.

Dott, H. M. & Foster, G. C. A. (1979). The estimation of sperm motility in semen on a membrane slide by measuring the area change frequency with an image averaging computer. *Journal of Reproduction and Fertility*, **55**, 161–6.

Ducot, B., Spira, A., Feneux, D. & Jouannet, P. (1988). Male factors and the likelihood of pregnancy in infertile couples. II. Study of clinical characteristics – practical consequences. *International Journal of Andrology*, **11**, 395–404.

Duleba, A. J., Rowe, T. C., Ma, P. & Collins, J. A. (1992). Prognostic factors in assessment and management of male infertility. *Human Reproduction*, **7**, 1388–93.

Dunphy, B. C., Kay, R., Barratt, C. L. R. & Cooke, I. D. (1989*a*). Female age, the length of involuntary infertility prior to investigation and fertility outcome. *Human Reproduction*, **4**, 527–30.

Dunphy, B. C., Neal, L. M. & Cooke, I. D. (1989*b*). The clinical value of conventional semen analysis. *Fertility and Sterility*, **51**, 324–9.

Eimers, J. M., Tevelde, E. R., Gerritse, R., Vogelzang, E. T., Looman, C. W. N. & Habbema, J. D. F. (1994). The prediction of the chance to conceive in subfertile couples. *Fertility and Sterility*, **61**, 44–52.

ESHRE Andrology Special Interest Group (1996). Consensus workshop on advanced diagnostic andrology techniques. *Human Reproduction*, **11**, 1463–79.

Fédération CECOS, Le Lannou, D. & Lansac, J. (1993). Artificial procreation with frozen donor semen: the French experience of CECOS. In *Donor insemination*, ed. C. L. R. Barratt & I. D. Cooke, pp. 152–69. Cambridge: Cambridge University Press.

Fenichel, P., Gharib, A., Emiliozzi, C., Donzeau, M. & Menezo, Y. (1996). Stimulation of human sperm during capacitation in-vitro by an adenosine agonist with specificity for A2 receptors. *Biology of Reproduction*, **54**, 1405–11.

Folgero, T., Bertheussen, K., Lindal, S., Torbergsen, T. & Oian, P. (1993). Mitochondrial disease and reduced sperm motility. *Human Reproduction*, **8**, 1863–8.

Ford, W. C. L. & Rees, J. M. (1990). The bioenergetics of mammalian sperm motility. In *Controls of sperm motility: biological and clinical aspects*, ed. C. Gagnon, pp. 175–202. Boca Raton, FL: CRC Press.

Ford, W. C. L., Rees, J. M., McLaughlin, E. A., Goddard, R. J. & Hull, M. G. R. (1991). The effect of A23187 concentration and exposure time on the outcome of the hamster egg penetration test. *International Journal of Andrology*, **14**, 127–39.

Ford, W. C. L., McLaughlin, E. A., Prior, S. M., Rees, J. M., Wardle, P. G. & Hull, M. G. R. (1992*a*). The yield, motility and performance in the hamster egg test of human spermatozoa prepared from cryopreserved semen by 4 different methods. *Human Reproduction,* 7, 654–9.

Ford, W. C. L, Ponting, F. A., McLaughlin, E. A., Rees, J. M. & Hull, M. G. R. (1992*b*). Controlling the swimming speed of human sperm by varying the incubation-temperature and its effect on cervical-mucus penetration. *International Journal of Andrology,* 15, 127–34.

Ford, W. C. L., Mathur, R. & Hull, M. G. R. (1997). Intra-uterine insemination. Is it effective treatment for male infertility? *Baillière's Clinical Obstetrics and Gynaecology,* 11, 691–710.

Fraser, L. R. & Duncan, A. E. (1993). Adenosine-analogs with specificity for A2 receptors bind to mouse spermatozoa and stimulate adenylate-cyclase activity in uncapacitated suspensions. *Journal of Reproduction and Fertility,* 98, 187–94.

Gellert-Mortimer, S. T., Hyne, R. V., Clarke, G. N., Johnston, W. I. H. & Baker, H. W. G. (1988). Evaluation of Nycodenz and Percoll density gradients for the selection of motile human spermatozoa. *Fertility and Sterility,* 49, 335–41.

Gladen, B. C., Williams, J. & Chapin, R. E. (1991). Issues in the statistical-analysis of sperm motion data derived from computer-assisted systems. *Journal of Andrology,* 12, 89–97.

Glazener, C. M. A., Kelly, N. J., Weir, M. J. A., David, J. S. E., Cornes, J. S. & Hull, M. G. R. (1987). The diagnosis of male infertility – prospective and time specific study of conception rate related to semen analysis and post-coital sperm mucus penetration in otherwise unexplained infertility. *Human Reproduction,* 2, 665–71.

Hancock, A. D. & de Kretser, D. M. (1992). The axonemal ultrastructure of spermatozoa from men with asthenospermia. *Fertility and Sterility,* 57, 661–4.

Hinting, A., Schoojans, F. & Comhaire, F. (1988). Validation of a single step procedure for the objective assessment of sperm motility characteristics. *International Journal of Andrology,* 11, 277–87.

Holland-Morritz, H. & Krause, W. (1992). Semen analysis and fertility prognosis in andrological patients. *International Journal of Andrology,* 15, 473–84.

Holt, W. V., Moore, H. D. M. & Hillier, S. G. (1985). Computer-assisted measurement of sperm swimming speed in human semen: correlation of results with *in vitro* fertilization assays. *Fertility and Sterility,* 44, 112–19.

Hong, C. Y., Chaput de Saintonge, D. M. & Turner, P. (1981). A simple method to measure drug effects on human sperm motility. *British Journal of Clinical Pharmacology,* 11, 385–7.

Hull, M. G. R. (1992). Infertility treatment: relative effectiveness of conventional and assisted conception methods. *Human Reproduction,* 7, 785–96.

(1994). Effectiveness of infertility treatments – choice and comparative analysis. *International Journal of Gynecology and Obstetrics,* 47, 99–108.

Irvine, D. S. (1995). Computer-assisted semen analysis systems – sperm motility assessment. *Human Reproduction,* 10(S1), 53–9.

Irvine, D. S. & Aitken, R. J. (1986). Predictive value of *in-vitro* sperm function tests in the context of an AID service. *Human Reproduction,* 1, 539–45.

Irvine, D. S., Macleod, I. C., Templeton, A. A., Masterton, A. & Taylor, A. (1994). A prospective clinical study of the relationship between a computer-assisted assessment of human semen quality and the achievement of pregnancy *in vivo. Human Reproduction,* **9**, 2324–34.

Joels, L. A., Ford, W. C. L., Ray, B. & Hull, M. G. R. (1997). Semen parameters for ICSI as a primary choice: probability analysis of treatment outcome by standard IVF. *Human Reproduction,* **12** (abstract book 1), 159.

Jouannet, P., Ducot, B., Feneux, D. & Spira, A. (1988). Male factors and the likelihood of pregnancy in infertile couples. 1. Study of sperm characteristics. *International Journal of Andrology,* **11**, 379–94.

Kao, S. H., Chao, H. T. & Wei, Y. H. (1995). Mitochondrial deoxyribonucleic acid 4977–bp deletion is associated with diminished fertility and motility of human sperm. *Biology of Reproduction,* **52**, 729–36.

Keel, B. A. & Webster, B. W. (1988). Correlation of human sperm motility characteristics with an *in vitro* cervical mucus penetration test. *Fertility and Sterility,* **49**, 138–43.

Krause, W. (1995a). Computer assisted semen analysis systems: comparison with routine evaluation and prognostic value in male fertility and assisted reproduction. *Human Reproduction,* **10**(S1), 60–6.

Krause, W. (1995b). The significance of computer-assisted semen analysis (CASA) for diagnosis in andrology and fertility prognosis. *International Journal of Andrology,* **18** (S2), 32–35.

Lax, Y., Rubinstein, S. & Breitbart, H. (1997). Subcellular distribution of protein kinase C alpha and beta I in bovine spermatozoa, and their regulation by calcium and phorbol esters. *Biology of Reproduction,* **56**, 454–9.

Leclerc, P. & Gagnon, C. (1996). Phosphorylation of triton X-100 soluble and insoluble protein substrates in a demembranated reactivated human sperm model. *Molecular Reproduction and Development,* **44**, 200–11.

Leclerc, P., Delamirande, E. & Gagnon, C. (1996). Cyclic adenosine 3['],5[']-monophosphate-dependent regulation of protein-tyrosine phosphorylation in relation to human sperm capacitation and motility. *Biology of Reproduction,* **55**, 684–92.

Lee, W. I., Gaddum-Rosse, P., Smith, W. D. & Stenchever, M. E. (1982). Laser light scattering study of the effect of washing on sperm motility. *Fertility and Sterility,* **38**, 62–7.

Lentner, C. (1982). *Geigy Scientific Tables,* 8th edn, vol. 2. Basle: CIBA-GEIGY.

Lindemann, C. B. & Kanous, K. S. (1997). Model for flagella motility. *International Review of Cytology – A Survey of Cell Biology,* **173**, 1–72.

Liu, D. Y., Jennings, G. & Baker, H. W. G. (1987). Correlation between defective motility (asthenozoospermia) and ATP reactivation of demembranated human spermatozoa. *Journal of Andrology,* **8**, 349–55.

Liu, D. Y., Clarke, G. N. & Baker, H. W. G. (1991). Relationship between sperm motility assessed with the Hamilton–Thorn motility analyzer and fertilization rates *in vitro. Journal of Andrology,* **12**, 231–9.

Macleod, I. C. & Irvine, D. S. (1995). The predictive value of computer-assisted semen analysis in the context of a donor-insemination programme. *Human Reproduction,* **10**, 580–6.

Makler, A. (1978). A new multiple exposure photography method for objective human spermatozoal motility determination. *Fertility and Sterility,* **30**, 192–9.

Marmor, D. & Grob-Menendez, F. (1991). Male-infertility due to asthenozoospermia and flagellar anomaly – detection in routine semen analysis. *International Journal of Andrology,* **14**, 108–16.

Mortimer, D., Pandya, I. J. & Sawers, R. S. (1986). Relationship between human sperm motility characteristics and sperm penetration into human cervical mucus *in vitro. Journal of Reproduction and Fertility,* **78**, 93–102.

Mundy, A. J., Ryder, T. A. & Edmonds, D. K. (1995). Asthenozoospermia and the human sperm mid-piece. *Human Reproduction,* **10**, 116–19.

Okamura, N., Tajima, Y., Soejima, A., Masuda, H. & Sugita, Y. (1985). Sodium bicarbonate in seminal plasma stimulates the motility of mammalian spermatozoa through the direct activation of adenylate cyclase. *Journal of Biological Chemistry,* **260**, 9699–705.

Okawa, T. (1997). Genetic and functional changes associated with ageing. *Physiological Reviews,* **77**, 425–64.

Ombelet, W., Bosmans, E., Janssen, M., Cox, A., Vlasselaer, J., Gyselaers, W., Vandeput, H., Gielen, J., Pollet, H., Maes, M., Steeno, O. & Kruger, T. (1997). Semen parameters in a fertile versus subfertile population: a need for change in the interpretation of semen testing. *Human Reproduction,* **12**, 987–93.

Overstreet, J. W., Katz, D. F., Hanson, F. W. & Fonseca, J. R. (1979). A simple inexpensive method for objective assessment of human sperm movement characteristics. *Fertility and Sterility,* **31**, 162–72.

Palermo, G. D., Cohen, J. & Rosenwaks, Z. (1996). Intracytoplasmic sperm injection – a powerful tool to overcome fertilization failure. *Fertility and Sterility,* **65**, 899–908.

Pariset, C. & Weinman, S. (1994). Differential localization of 2 isoforms of the regulatory subunit RII-α of cAMP-dependent protein-kinase in human sperm – biochemical and cytochemical study. *Molecular Reproduction and Development,* **39**, 415–22.

Phillips, D. M., Jow, W. W. & Goldstein, M. (1995). Testis factors that may regulate gene-expression – evidence from a patient with Kartagener's syndrome. *Journal of Andrology,* **16**, 158–62.

Polansky, F. F. & Lamb, E. J. (1988). Do the results of semen analysis predict future fertility? A survival analysis study. *Fertility and Sterility,* **49**. 1059–65.

Rotem, R., Paz, G. F., Homonnai, Z. T., Kalina, M. & Naor, Z. (1990*a*). Further studies on the involvement of protein-kinase-C in human sperm flagellar motility. *Endocrinology,* **127**, 2571–7.

(1990*b*). Protein-kinase-C is present in human sperm – possible role in flagellar motility. *Proceedings of the National Academy of Sciences, USA,* **87**, 7305–8.

Ryder, T. A., Mobberley, M. A., Hughes, L. & Hendry, W. F. (1990). A survey of the ultrastructural defects associated with absent or impaired human sperm motility. *Fertility and Sterility,* **53**, 556–60.

Si, Y. M. & Okuno, M. (1995). Activation of mammalian sperm motility by regulation of microtubule sliding via cyclic adenosine 5[']-monophosphate-dependent phosphorylation. *Biology of Reproduction*, **53**, 1081–7.

Smith, G. D., Wolf, D. P., Trautman, K. C., Silva, E. F. D. E., Greengard, P. & Vijayaraghavan, S. (1996). Primate sperm contain protein-phosphatase-1, a biochemical mediator of motility. *Biology of Reproduction*, **54**, 719–27.

Sokal, R. R. & Rohlf, F. J. (1969). *Biometry*, San Francisco: WH Freeman and Co.

Sokoloski, J. E., Blasco, L., Storey, B. T. & Wolf, D. P. (1977). Turbidometric analysis of human sperm motility. *Fertility and Sterility*, **28**, 1337–41.

St John, J. C., Johki, R. P., Barratt, C. L. R. & Cooke, I. D. (1997). The effects of mitochondrial dysfunction on sperm motility. *Journal of the British Fertility Society*, **2**, 15A.

Suarez, S. S. (1996). Hyperactivated motility in sperm. *Journal of Andrology*, **17**, 331–5.

Tamm, S. (1994). Ca^{2+} channels and signalling in cilia and flagella. *Trends in Cell Biology*, **4**, 305–10.

Tash, J. S. & Bracho, G. E. (1994). Regulation of sperm motility: emerging evidence for a major role for protein phosphatases. *Journal of Andrology*, **15** 505–9.

Tash, J. S. & Means, A. R, (1983). Cyclic adenosine 3['],5[']-monophosphate, calcium and protein phosphorylation in flagellar motility. *Biology of Reproduction*, **28**, 75–104.

Tournaye, H., Janssens, R., Camus, M., Staessen, C., Devroey, P. & Vansteirteghem, A. (1993). Pentoxifylline is not useful in enhancing sperm function in cases with previous *in vitro* fertilization failure. *Fertility and Sterility*, **59**, 210–15.

Tournaye, H., Janssens, R., Verhayen, G., Camus, M., Devroey, P. & Van Steirteghem, A. (1994). An indiscriminate use of pentoxifylline does not improve fertilization in poor fertilizers. *Human Reproduction*, **9**, 1289–92.

Vijayaraghavan, S., Stephens, D. T., Trautman, K., Smith, G. D., Khatra, B., Silva, E. F. D. E. & Greengard, P. (1996). Sperm motility development in the epididymis is associated with decreased glycogen-synthase kinase-3 and protein-phosphatase-1 activity. *Biology of Reproduction*, **54**, 709–18.

Vijayaraghavan, S., Goueli, S. A., Davey, M. P. & Carr, D. W. (1997a). Protein kinase A-anchoring inhibitor peptides arrest mammalian sperm motility. *Journal of Biological Chemistry*, **272**, 4747–52.

Vijayaraghavan, S., Trautman, K. D., Goueli, S. A. & Carr, D. W. (1997b). A tyrosine-phosphorylated 55–kilodalton motility-associated bovine sperm protein is regulated by cyclic adenosine 3['],5[']-monophosphate and calcium. *Biology of Reproduction*, **56**, 1450–57.

Walczak, C. E. & Nelson, D. L. (1994). Regulation of dynein driven motility in cilia and flagella. *Cell Motility and the Cytoskeleton*, **27**, 101–7.

Wallace, D. C. (1997). Mitochondrial DNA in ageing and disease. *Scientific American*, **277**(2), 40–7.

Wilton, L. J., Templesmith, P. D. & deKretser, D. M. (1992). Quantitative ultrastructural analysis of sperm tails reveals flagellar defects associated with persistent asthenozoospermia. *Human Reproduction*, **7**, 510–16.

World Health Organization (1980). *WHO laboratory manual for the examination of human semen and sperm–cervical mucus interaction,* 1st edn. Singapore: Press Concern.

World Health Organization (1992). *WHO laboratory manual for the examination of human semen and sperm–cervical mucus interaction,* 2nd edn. Cambridge: Cambridge University Press.

Yeung, C. H., Bals-Pratsch, M., Knuth, U. A. & Nieschlag, E. (1988). Investigation of the cause of low sperm motility in asthenozoospermic patients by multiple quantitative tests. *International Journal of Andrology,* **11**, 289–99.

Yeung, C. H., Cooper, T. G. & Nieschlag, E. (1997). A technique for standardisation and quality control of subjective sperm motility assessments in semen analysis. *Fertility and Sterility,* **67**, 1156–8.

Yovich, J. L. (1993). Pentoxifylline – actions and applications in assisted reproduction. *Human Reproduction,* **8**, 1786–91.

Zamboni, L. (1987). The ultrastructural pathology of the spermatozoon as a cause of infertility – the role of electron-microscopy in the evaluation of semen quality. *Fertility and Sterility,* **48**, 711–34.

12 Molecular techniques for the diagnosis of inherited disorders and male reproductive malfunction

IAN FINDLAY AND JUSTIN ST JOHN

Introduction

Traditionally reproductive medicine has often relied upon whole-sample biochemical assays and scanning procedures to determine genetic disorders and reproductive malfunction. However, in recent years, molecular biological techniques have advanced, resulting in a rapid increase in diagnostic methods that are highly applicable to the assessment and treatment of genetic disorders associated with reproductive medicine. These molecular advances, in combination with assisted-reproductive treatments, such as intracytoplasmic sperm injection (ICSI), have resulted in alternative treatment options and a broadening of our knowledge of reproductive processes.

The aim of this chapter is to give a broad overview of the current methods used to diagnose inherited disorders and male reproductive malfunction and those techniques employed in other fields that could be adopted for these purposes. The diagnostic measures used are discussed first, followed by the diagnosis of inherited disorders and an overview of the different disorders. Then follows a description of how molecular techniques are applied in the investigation of male reproductive malfunction.

Molecular techniques

Karyotyping

Although karyotyping is not a molecular technique as such, its importance in diagnosing inherited disorders cannot be underestimated. Karyotyping involves analysis of cells for their chromosome number and structural anomalies. The cells are arrested in metaphase and stained to reveal characteristic banding patterns that allow the detection of structural defects. Karyotyping still remains the method of choice for diagnosing gross chromosomal abnormalities, especially for some patients who harbour chromosomal abnormalites, for example those with Turner's syndrome.

However, the risk of cytogenetic disorders can arise in either or both of the male and female gametes and can be transmitted to the offspring. Cytogenetic analysis is performed on a number of cell types, but the most common analysis is that of amniocytes and chorionic villus samples. The individuals most likely to be referred are those with advanced maternal age, parental chromosomal abnormality, previous children with cytogenetic abnormality, chromosomal breakage syndromes and some microdeletion syndromes (Charrow *et al.*, 1990).

However, karyotyping, though a valuable diagnostic tool, is limited. The technique often requires lengthy laboratory procedures and is expensive. In addition, cytogenetic analysis is not always possible, particularly when the cell numbers are low, as with prenatal diagnosis, where cell culture fails or where the sample is contaminated. In these instances, molecular techniques such as PCR (polymerase chain reaction) and FISH (fluorescence *in situ* hybridization) are required. Additionally, single-gene defects and most microdeletions require molecular analysis.

PCR techniques

PCR

In recent years, genetic diagnosis has been directed towards investigation of defects directly at the DNA level. Conventional approaches to DNA analysis such as Southern blotting involve the digestion of approximately 5 μg of DNA (approximately 1000 cells). This is followed by electrophoresis, Southern transfer, hybridization to a probe (which is most often radioactively labelled) and exposure of the filters to the film. The whole procedure takes about 4 days and is, in certain circumstances, not sensitive enough. Additionally, very small samples, perhaps containing only one or two cells (the equivalent of only 5–10 pg of DNA) cannot be used for DNA analysis by these techniques and far more sensitive methods must be employed. A method that is now extensively used is PCR, which is perhaps the method of choice for detection or diagnosis of single-gene defects or very low levels of deletion.

In simple terms, PCR is based on the repetitive cycling of three reactions: denaturation, annealing and extension. Denaturation results in the breaking of the bonds of the DNA double helix and the formation of single-stranded DNA. Annealing is the process whereby the primers bind to complementary sequences on the target DNA, one to each 5′ end. The precision of the target-primer annealing gives PCR its specificity. The final step, extension, allows an enzyme, commonly *Taq* polymerase, to synthesize sequences complementary to the original DNA. These new sequences act as templates for subsequent reactions.

PCR is an extremely powerful *in vitro* method for the amplification of specific DNA or RNA sequences. The development of PCR has allowed genetic analysis from a small number of cells (Saiki *et al.*, 1988); in recent years the sensitivity of the method has increased so that even single copies of genes within a single cell can be amplified more than a billion-fold in a fully automated procedure (Li *et al.*, 1988; Arnheim *et al.*, 1990, 1991). Apart from its great sensitivity, a very important advantage of PCR is that DNA fragments can be amplified within a few hours and this allows the product to be visualized through, for example, gel electrophoresis (Fig. 12.1).

However, each reaction requires the use of several components and their optimization is vital to provide as clear a diagnosis as possible. Very careful primer selection is essential for successful PCR, which uses two

Fig. 12.1. PCR amplification of the 5 kilobase deletion in human spermatozoa samples from donors. The samples were divided into 0, 45% and 90% gradients by Percoll centrifugation. Some samples had multiple deletions and/or smaller deletions than predicted. Products were confirmed by restriction enzyme digest. M, *Hinc*II Digest (Pharmacia). Lanes 1, 3, 5: wild-type for donor A, 0, 45% and 90% fractions, respectively. Lanes 2, 4, 6: deleted for donor A, 0, 45% and 90% fractions, respectively. Lanes 7, 9, 11: wild-type for donor B, 0, 45% and 90% fractions, respectively. Lanes 8, 10, 12: deleted for donor B, 0, 45% and 90% fractions, respectively.

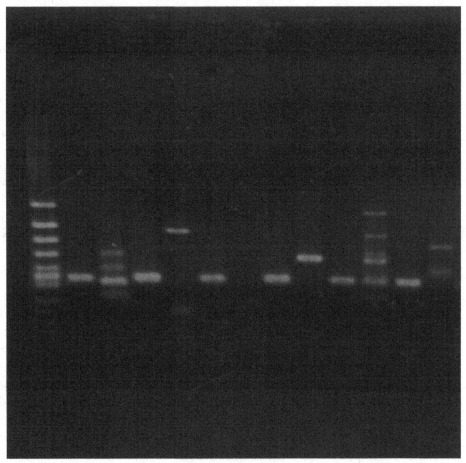

M1   1   2   3   4   5   6   7   8   9   10   11   12

oligonucleotide primers (one forward and one reverse), which are complementary to either strand of the target DNA to be amplified. Primers should ideally be 18–30 bases long and, if possible, span a region of the target sequence that will yield a product of 100–300 base-pairs since this is the optimal range for visualization. Primer length decreases the likelihood of similarity to non-target sequences and, to this extent, should be checked against gene databases for degree of identity. Examples of gene databases include Genbank and others which can be accessed via the Human Genome Project (www.hgmp.mrc.ac.uk).

The method of visualization of PCR products is through either acrylamide or agarose gel electrophoresis. These methods are reliable and accurate only when there is a large amount of product (approximately 1 μg) of a specific known size. Unfortunately, it is often difficult to distinguish the product signal from faint inconsistencies in the gel, particularly when the product yield is low and only a faint signal is seen. This method may be particularly inaccurate when one is distinguishing between allele differences as small as 1 or 2 base-pairs. PCR analysis must also include appropriate controls to ensure that the target product is obtained and is not due to contamination or PCR failure.

Where sample size is low, as with single-cell analysis of the Y chromosome, PCR has two major advantages compared with, for example, Southern blotting:

1   *Sensitivity.* It is possible to detect a single-copy sequence in a single cell or a few cells. A variety of sequences have been amplified from single cells, including human spermatozoa, fibroblasts, human oocytes and polar bodies (Jeffreys *et al.*, 1985; Li *et al.*, 1988; Monk & Holding, 1990).

2   *Speed.* Specific DNA fragments CAN be amplified within a few hours (Saiki *et al.*, 1985, 1988) allowing analysis to be completed within a single day.

The high degree of sensitivity of PCR does, however, present some limitations and difficulties (Findlay *et al.*, 1996*a*). To overcome these difficulties, a variety of modifications and enhancements to the basic technique have been developed and these are discussed below.

Nested PCR amplification

Nested PCR is the second amplification on a small portion of the original PCR product using primers, of which one or both are inside the region mapping the original pair (see Fig. 12.2). This procedure can enhance the sensitivity and specificity of PCR when the amount of starting material is very small, as in single-cell sperm analysis (Li *et al.*, 1988) or the sought after gene defect is extremely low in intensity, especially when specific deleted to wild-type ratio is required, like the 5 kilobase deletion in Alzheimer's disease (Soong & Arnheim, 1996).

As a PCR plateau is usually limited by reagent depletion and PCR product competition, some of the product can be transferred from the first reaction to a second reaction using fresh reagents for further cycling. Typically, a larger fragment is produced in this first round with the outer flanking primers and then a small aliquot is added to a fresh reaction mix for further cycling (see Fig. 12.2). These additional cycles increase the amount of product. Nested PCR is also used when the first round of amplification results in non-specific as well as specific products (Mullis & Faloona, 1987). In this case, the first round of nested PCR will increase the relative proportion of target to non-specific contaminant and the second round of PCR, using more specific primers, will further increase the yield and accuracy. Indeed, the specificity of this technique allows detection of every molecule in the reaction.

The main disadvantage of nested PCR, is however, contamination, for example by DNA aerosol. This can easily occur when the product is transferred from the first reaction to the second and loading of the samples may necessitate use of a PCR-dedicated area in the laboratory or a fume cupboard.

Multiplex PCR

Multiplex PCR involves a reaction containing several different probes. These various probes can identify deletions, at several different loci on one or more chromosomes, associated with a single disease. For example the amplification of nine regions of the Duchenne muscular dystrophy (DMD) gene in a single reaction (Chamberlain *et al.*, 1988) enabled the detection of 81% of all the DMD deletions. Alternatively, several different single-gene defect diseases can be screened in one reaction. Other examples of gene defects involving multiplex PCR screening are cystic fibrosis, trisomy 21 and Y chromosome deletions.

Multiplex PCR is a sophisticated technique that requires exacting reaction conditions to allow each probe to amplify equally. Very careful design of the primers and PCR conditions are critical so that artefacts formed between

Fig. 12.2. Nested PCR. Primers MT1A, MT2 and MT3 are used to amplify the 5 kilobase deletion in mitochondrial DNA. (*a*) MT1A and MT3 are used for an initial round of 25 cycles of PCR; (*b*) 1 to 5 μl of the product from the initial round provides a further template for a second round of PCR employing primers MT1A and MT2.

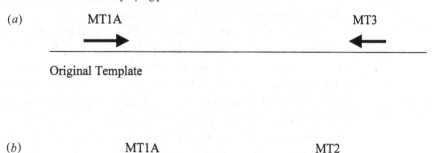

the primers and non-specific amplification are avoided. The primers must also generate products that are of different sizes to facilitate interpretation.

Fluorescent PCR

In the last few years, PCR analysis has been automated by modifications in PCR technology. One such modification is fluorescent PCR. This system uses fluorescent primers and an automated DNA sequencer to detect the reaction products (McBride & O'Neill, 1991), resulting in improved accuracy and sensitivity of the method (Zeigle et al., 1992; Kimpton et al., 1993).

Fluorescent PCR is essentially very similar to conventional PCR except that each primer is tagged with a fluorescent dye. This produces a fluorescent product, which is detected in a different way. The fluorescent product is electrophoresed on a gel passing under a scanning laser beam, which makes the product fluoresce. Using a photomultiplier and computer enhancement technology, the fluorescent dye is detected at a much lower threshold than conventional agarose or polyacrylamide gel analysis. This system, therefore, allows highly accurate and reliable detection of the signal, even when the signal is very weak or many times lower (to approx. 1%) than that of the other allele. Fluorescent PCR has also been shown to be approximately 1000 times more sensitive than conventional polyacrylamide gel analysis (Hattori et al., 1992).

An ultrasensitive fluorescent DNA sequencer is then used to separate, detect, and analyse the fluorescently labelled PCR products. One such example of a DNA sequencer is the 373A DNA sequencer with 362 Genescanner software (Applied Biosystems, Warrington, UK). A DNA sequencer has the additional advantage that it can also be used for gene sequencing, a major tool in molecular genetics. The computer analyses these signals and constructs a representation of the gel from which electrophoretograms are generated. These signals enable different primer products to be easily differentiated by their distinct emission wavelengths. In addition, the quantity of the products can be determined by the relative intensities of their fluorescence. Stored data can be analysed to provide product sizes and the relative amount of product in each sample.

A further advantage of fluorescent PCR is that several primers, including as many as eight sets, can be multiplexed together, because different fluorescent dyes can be simultaneously determined, even if the product ranges overlap each other (Kimpton et al., 1993). These different coloured dyes allow identification of one product from the other even if the product sizes are within 1–2 base-pairs of each other.

Fluorescent PCR has already been successfully applied to genetic screening for cystic fibrosis (Cuckle et al., 1996), Down's syndrome (Pertl et al., 1994), muscular dystrophy (Schwartz et al., 1992; Mansfield et al., 1993a) and Lesch–Nyhan syndrome (Mansfield et al., 1993b).

Quantitative PCR

Quantitative PCR is where the amount of PCR product from each allele or the ratio of wild-type to deleted DNA is compared, allowing a calculation of the relative number of molecules. In some disease states, for example Kearns–Sayre syndrome (KSS) and chronic progressive external ophthalmoplegia (CPEO), the intensity of the deleted product when compared to wild-type is critical to diagnosis. Indeed, KSS is considered to be a milder form of CPEO because the mutant to wild-type ratio is lower. Understanding of the intensity of the disorder is thus vital for both treatment available today and possible gene therapy in the future. Various different quantitative PCR methods have been developed: serial dilution, kinetic PCR, competitive PCR and fluorescent PCR. Trisomies have been detected by employing both fluorescent PCR and polymorphic small tandem repeats (STRs) (for a review, see Adinolfi *et al.*, 1995). This allows peak ratios of abundance of one allele to the other to be calculated. STRs can also be used to determine the origin of the extra chromosome and, if maternally derived, whether the extra chromosome is derived during meiosis-I or meiosis-II (Kotzot *et al.*, 1996).

Four main types of STR signal are obtained depending on trisomy status (Fig. 12.3, a single homozygous peak is not shown). Trisomic samples produce either a triallelic signal (three peaks of similar size) seen in Fig. 12.3(*a*); a diallelic or double-dose signal (two peaks, one of which is double the size of the other) seen in Fig. 12.3(*b*); or a homozygous signal (single peak which would be regarded as uninformative). Disomic samples produce either a homozygous signal (single peak) or a heterozygous signal (double peaks of equal size) (Fig. 12.3(*c*)).

Although this method was first described in the early 1990s (Mansfield *et al.*, 1993*a*), there have been only a few reports of this technique being applied clinically to trisomy detection in prenatal diagnosis (Eggeling *et al.*, 1993; Pertl *et al.*, 1994; Adinolfi *et al.*, 1995). This has been due mainly to the relatively high numbers of cells required and in many cases can be time consuming and difficult to interpret. Difficulties in interpretation occur for two reasons: diagnoses may have to be deduced from potential double doses and there are difficulties caused by preferential amplification.

The other quantitative PCR methods, especially kinetic PCR and competitive PCR, are excellent techniques for providing accurate analysis. Kinetic PCR involves the labelling of either the primers or dNTPs with a radioisotope and the ratio of wild-type to deleted molecules is determined using densitometry readings. Competitive PCR employs the use of a plasmid with an insert of similar size and gene content as the target template and the two templates compete for the same reaction components. The difference between the two templates is that the plasmid template contains an extra common restriction enzyme site introduced by site-directed mutagensis. The PCR products are then cut with a restriction enzyme and the different-sized products are quantified either through densitometry or through imaging analysis. Competitive PCR is particularly effective in the quantification of various types of mitochondrial DNA disease (see Chen *et al.*, 1995).

Primer extension preamplification (PEP)

Another method that has been used for amplification of low copy numbers is whole genome amplification (Zhang *et al.*, 1992; Xu *et al.*, 1993;

Fig. 12.3. Quantitative PCR of D21 small terminal repeats in trisomic and disomic samples. Trisomic samples produce either a triallelic signal (three peaks of similar size) seen in (*a*), a diallelic or double-dose signal (two peaks, one of which is twice the size of the other) seen in (*b*), or a homozygous signal (single peak not shown which would be regarded as uninformative). (*c*) Disomic samples produce either a homozygous signal (single peak, now shown) or a heterozygous signal (double peaks of similar size). (From Findlay *et al.*, 1998.)

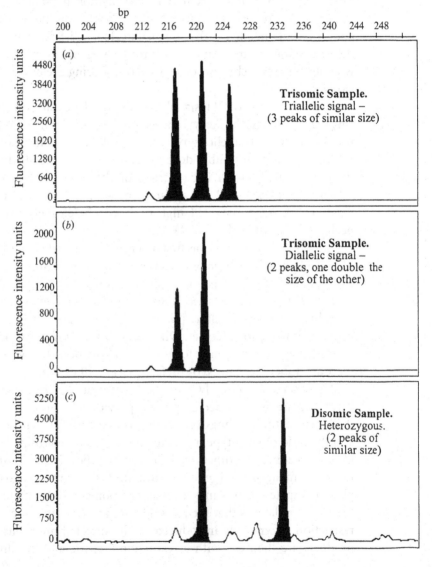

Snabes *et al.*, 1993, 1994; Kristjansson *et al.*, 1994). This method is more correctly termed PEP. In theory, the entire genome is amplified using PCR and,
in this way, the amount of template available for subsequent PCR reactions
increases from 1 copy to 50–100 copies. PEP is essentially a prediagnostic
PCR treatment because the PCR product derived from PEP is then used in a
further PCR reaction to amplify the specific gene of interest. Many aliquots
can be removed from the reaction mix and multiple diagnoses can be run in
parallel.

Although the entire genomic DNA from one cell should be amplified into
the DNA of 50–100 cells, PEP unfortunately has two major disadvantages,
particularly at the single-cell level, where it would be of most value.

1 The time taken for the diagnosis, usually 8–12 h for the PEP and the subsequent approx. 5–10 h for the diagnostic PCR and analysis, makes it difficult
to perform a diagnosis in a single day.

2 Although the whole genome can be amplified, the amplification appears to
be random and in practice only approx. 80% of the genome is effectively
amplified. The remaining 20% of the genome, which may contain the gene
of interest, may not be amplified at all. This problem is particularly important in the diagnosis of heterozygotes, where misdiagnosis could result.

Notwithstanding, this technique has been successfully employed in preimplantation genetic diagnosis (Kristjansson *et al.*, 1994), though it required
longer than 14 h to perform. Furthermore, the technique has been further
refined, with a shorter protocol, to examine several loci of interest in human
genetic diseases with good amplification efficiency (Sermon *et al.*, 1996).

Long PCR

Conventional PCR allows the reliable amplification of short fragments (50–1000 base-pairs). However, with fragments that are above 1000
base-pairs, the technique is limited. Nevertheless, an important advance,
along with that of quantification, has been the extension of PCR for amplifying long fragments, a process known as long PCR (LPCR). The technique has
been used to amplify up to 22 kilobases from human genomic DNA. LPCR
has also been employed to identify multiple somatic mitochondrial DNA
(mtDNA) deletions in a variety of diseases such as those in polymyalgia
rheumatica (Reynier *et al.*, 1994), cardiac tissue (Li *et al.*, 1995), and multiple
deletions associated with partial duplications in KSS and CPEO (Fromenty
et al., 1996).

To date, although LPCR has not been used effectively for screening
patients for specific disease types in the diagnostic laboratory, one particular
application has been the preamplification of long fragments of target DNA,
with the product in turn employed as the template for multiplex PCR. This
reduces the sequence complexity arising from multiplex PCR primer design
(Li & Vijg, 1996). LPCR has also been used to investigate tandem duplications
within the fibrillin 1 gene (Siracusa *et al.*, 1996) and to determine somatic
deletions in the testis of obstructive azoospermic men (St John *et al.*, 1997a).

Reverse transcriptase -PCR (RT-PCR)

PCR can be combined with reverse transcription of messenger RNA (mRNA). mRNA transfers genetic information from the nucleus to the ribosomes in the cytoplasm and also acts as the template for the synthesis of polypeptides. RNA is more difficult to work with than DNA due to its increased lability and the necessity of examining the tissue in which the mRNA is expressed. Once the mRNA has been reversibly transcribed into complementary DNA (cDNA), the resulting single-stranded cDNA molecule can then be employed as the starting template for PCR. This is necessary for the construction of a cDNA library, for the testis, say, which could be employed for screening gene expression. The advantage of analysing mRNA is that the gene can be detected and analysed only if it has been transcribed from genomic DNA and expressed prior to analysis. Reverse transcription of the gene of interest ensures, for the researcher, that the sequence of interest is transcribed, and is not junk DNA contained in the introns. This has been clearly demonstrated by Lahn & Page (1997) in identifying novel genes on the Y chromosome. Quantification of the cDNA PCR product can be performed as described above. Clinically, RT-PCR has been employed for prenatal diagnosis and expression of endometrial genes. Of relevance to the andrologist is the application of RT-PCR to detect human immunodeficiency virus infection in human spermatozoa (Lasheeb *et al.*, 1997). These authors were able to demonstrate, through quantitative RT-PCR, that washing of spermatozoa (see Semprini *et al.*, 1992) was efficient but not comprehensive enough to prevent transmission to the mother and subsequently to the offspring.

In situ hybridization (ISH)

This technique was originally developed by Pardue & Gall (1970) and consists of two basic steps. First, a DNA probe and the metaphase chromosomes on a slide are denatured, thus separating the double-stranded DNA into two separate strands. Secondly, the probe and chromosomal DNA are allowed to hybridize, resulting in the probe finding its specific counterpart in the chromosomes.

There are two main difficulties of ISH. First, the probes may fail to hybridize with the nuclei. Secondly, the time required to arrest the majority of cells in metaphase is more than 12 h, so that a further 24 h is required for the detection of hybridization. These difficulties have been partially overcome by using fluorescent methods for detecting ISH. This technique is termed fluorescence *in situ* hybridization (FISH). FISH can be carried out within one day and has the added advantages of increased specificity and sensitivity. In addition, the simultaneous detection of several probes is possible using different fluorescent labels (Nederlof *et al.*, 1989).

FISH

FISH is a recent modification of ISH (reviewed by Joos *et al.*, 1994; Flaherty *et al.*, 1997) and involves the hybridization of biotin- or digoxigenin-labelled DNA probes to denatured metaphase chromosomes. These probes are visualized using fluorochrome-conjugated reagents. Thus, both single- and multi-coloured probes can be employed. Minor variations of the basic procedure, such as varying hybridization protocols, allow successful visualization of single-copy probes or of whole chromosome 'painting'. In principle, the DNA sequence that is to be used as a probe is modified chemically or enzymically with a reporter molecule. This reporter molecule can then be detected by a reporter binding protein coupled to a fluorochrome and the resulting fluorescent signal can be visualized using a fluorescence microscope. The use of special microscopic equipment, such as the confocal laser microscope with a digital imaging system, can further improve signal detection (Koch *et al.*, 1989; Lichter *et al.*, 1990). Non-radioactive *in situ* hybridization techniques are generally rapid, results being obtained within a few days, whilst new protocols have dramatically reduced the time taken for analysis to only a few hours (Griffin *et al.*, 1991).

FISH has been used to detect aneuploidies and chromosomal rearrangements. Specifically, FISH can detect chromosomal abnormalities in human spermatozoa. Examples include disomy sperm nuclei (Guttenbach & Scmid, 1991; Blanco *et al.*, 1996); analysis of reciprocal translocation carriers (Goldman & Hulten, 1993; Spriggs & Martin, 1994; Spriggs *et al.*, 1995); aneuploidy (Bischoff *et al.*, 1994; MacDonald *et al.*, 1994; Martin & Rademaker, 1995); and non-dysjunction (Williams *et al.*, 1993). Recently, it has been used to detect gene activation, using comparative genome hybridization. Many other probes, including monoclonal antibodies, can also be used and multiple hybridizations can be carried out at the same time using different coloured labels. In addition, FISH now makes it possible to identify specific chromosomes when the cells are in interphase. In the last few years, FISH has been applied to trisomy diagnosis from blastomeres biopsied from human embryos for preimplantation genetic diagnosis (Verlinsky *et al.*, 1996).

Post-PCR analysis

PCR analysis can provide details about the presence and quantity of an amplified fragment. However, it is often vital to determine that the amplified fragment is indeed the fragment that is sought. To this extent, two techniques can be employed: restriction enzyme digest and DNA sequencing.

Restriction enzymes

Restriction enzymes (also known as restriction endonucleases), and in particular type II restriction enzymes, are those most commonly used. PCR products can be digested with the appropriate restriction enzyme, which has one or more identifiable sites within the amplified sequence. Following digestion, the bands can be visualized on an electrophoretic gel. The presence of the expected number of bands at the correct molecular weight will confirm that the sought-after fragment has been amplified.

However, should the correct number of bands fail to appear or bands of differing sizes be visualized then one of two possibilities could have arisen. Either the amplified fragment contains a mutation, or the primer is not specific enough to the region required.

In addition, when amplifying a region of DNA suspected of containing point mutations, PCR on its own cannot confirm that the mutation is present. An ideal technique is to introduce a base change into the target DNA that on its own does not create a new restriction site. This can be performed by creating a mismatch primer. However, should the mutation be present, then the combination of the two base changes will result in the formation of a new restriction enzyme site (see Hutchin & Cortopassi, 1995; Hutchin *et al.*, 1997). If the second base change is present, the enzyme will cut at the specific site and the mutation will thus be identified.

DNA sequencing

Restriction enzyme analysis is a simple and efficient method of product identification and confirmation of mutagenesis. However, often when single-base-pair identification is required due to heteroplasmy (presence of both wild-type and diluted molecules), as in the case of mitochondrial DNA point mutations, DNA sequencing is required. Sequencing of DNA can be carried out using two methods, chemical or enzymic, and technological advances have led to the development of DNA sequencers. For each base analysed, a peak is recorded on a sequence data sheet that is very similar in format to the data retrieved following fluorescent PCR (see p. 218). Here, the peaks will specifically indicate the presence of the mutation, identified by the colour representation for each dNTP after labelling. Additionally, this is an important tool for the identification of a complete or partial gene sequence that might be larger in size than a point mutation.

Furthermore, for the researcher investigating the expression of novel genes, it is vital to determine the sequence of this gene. The data arising from the sequence can shed valuable light on the potential homology of this new gene to genes expressed similarly in other species, thus explaining evolutionary development, and may also help to explain the function of the protein that it transcribes. Additionally, the sequence can be analysed to investigate which particular bases encoded by the DNA might be vital to the function of the protein that the gene encodes and would thus allow site-directed mutagenesis to be performed in experimental systems.

Future techniques

The techniques described above are those which are either currently employed in a diagnostic capacity in genetic laboratories or are being developed to enhance those already established. In this section, we wish to highlight the potential clinical relevance of three techniques that are either used in other areas of research or are still very much in the developmental stage in reproductive medicine, particularly male reproductive malfunction.

Comparative genomic hybridization (CGH)

CGH is a relatively new technique that is primarily an extension of FISH and has the advantage of being capable of detecting gene activation. To date, it has been employed mainly in detecting chromosomal aberrations in cancers (see Wolff *et al.*, 1997) and is extremely sensitive. An example of its sensitivity showed that chromosomal imbalances, not detectable by cytogenetic analysis, could be detected by CGH (Dierlamm *et al.*, 1997). The confirmation of these observations required both FISH and Southern blot analysis, thus substantiating the sensitivity and diversity of this technique. The transfer of this technique to screen for reproductive and inherited disorders at the level of the gene and for larger chromosomal abnormalites could be of great clinical diagnostic benefit, especially in improving cytogenetic analysis.

Recombinant protein expression

The *in vivo* expression of recombinant proteins is vital to many areas of molecular biology. There is frequently a requirement to express and purify cloned gene products in prokaryotic and eukaryotic systems for studies of protein structure and function, protein–protein and protein–DNA interactions, antibody interactions and mutagenesis.

An example of the use of recombinant expression systems is that for ZP3, one of a family of glycoproteins located within the zona pellucida. Complementary receptor molecules exist on both the head of spermatozoa and the zona and interaction between these two molecules is understood to be necessary for sperm binding and the subsequent acrosome reaction. Recently, the recombinant zona binding assay (ZBA) was developed as a sperm function test. This technique is an *in vitro* assay mimicking the process that initiates fertilization and requires the attachment of recombinant zona proteins, produced using an *in vitro* transcription and translation system, to agarose beads (Whitmarsh *et al.*, 1996). Motile spermatozoa then attach to these beads via the head region. Although the successful expression of biologically active recombinant human ZP3 has been reported (see Barratt & Hornby, 1995; Brewis *et al.*, 1996; Chapman *et al.*, 1998), complications in expressing this protein currently restrict the use of this assay in a clinical environment (Barratt & St John, 1998).

Recombinant protein expression has also been employed in the design of contraceptive vaccines. Recombinant fertilin subunits produced in a bacterial expression system have been employed to test fertilin as an immunocontraceptive and demonstrated that high levels of circulating sperm-reactive anti-fertilin antibodies do not sufficiently hinder infertility (Hardy *et al.*, 1997). A further example involves the cDNA for a sperm antigen, fertilization antigen (FA-1), which was subcloned into the pGEX-2T vector and expressed in a glutathione S-transferase gene fusion system to obtain the recombinant protein (Zhu & Naz, 1997). The recombinant protein reacted specifically with ZP3 from mouse oocyte and its affinity-purified antibodies completely blocked sperm–zona interaction.

Analysis of DNA damage

The role that DNA damage, in either of the gametes, plays in fertilization outcome has become increasingly debated and the subject of much research. Two prime sources of DNA damage are smoking and environmental toxins and either of these may be involved in the formation of reactive oxygen species (ROS). The hydroxyl radical (OH·) is the most destructive of the ROS and, when it complexes with deoxyguanosine (dG), produces 8-hydroxydeoxyguanosine (8-OH-dG). The formation of this complex results in the separation of the double strands of DNA, a precursor to DNA fragmentation (Ozawa, 1995). Shen *et al.* (1997) found that DNA from the spermatozoa of smokers contained a significantly higher amount of 8-OH-dG than that from non-smokers, and that the level of 8-OH-dG was closely correlated with the concentration of seminal cotinine. Additionally, paternal preconception smoking has been related to a significantly elevated risk of childhood cancers especially acute leukaemia and lymphoma (Ji *et al.*, 1997).

Environmental toxins such as polychlorinated biphenyls and cadmium have been implicated in Sertoli cell damage and, when administered to Sertoli cells in culture, produce morphological changes (Syed *et al.*, 1997), although the Sertoli cells did maintain viability. Additionally, following mRNA differential display, a number of novel cDNAs were detected, suggesting changes in gene expression associated with these morphological changes.

DNA damage can be assessed primarily through three techniques.

Comet assay

The comet assay or single-cell gel electrophoresis resolves DNA break frequencies of up to a few thousand per cell so the distances between breaks are of the order of 10^9 Da, beyond the range of fragment size suitable for conventional electrophoresis. The body of the non-damaged DNA fragment is about 1 mm in diameter and the length of the comet tail, the damaged DNA, is a few hundredths of this (Collins *et al.*, 1997). Preliminary work has been conducted on spermatozoa (McKelvey-Martin *et al.*, 1997), though considerable refinement is necessary. Potentially this tool could be predictive of fertilization outcome, as fertilization rates are considerably lower for spermatozoa with damaged DNA (Sun *et al.*, 1997). The disadvantage of this assay is that it demonstrates end-point damage to DNA and does not indicate what the precursors to this damage might be.

Chromomycin A3 and in situ nick translation

The process of spermiogenesis sees the replacement of nuclear histones with protamines in mammalian chromatin. This results in the highly condensed nature of DNA in mature spermatozoa. However, defects in the chromatin organization can account for subfertility in some men (Manicardi *et al.*, 1995).

Two methods have been developed to assess sperm chromatin quality. The first employs the guanosine-cytosine-specific flourochrome, chromomycin A_3 (CMA_3). This flourochrome assesses the packaging quality of the chromatin in human spermatozoa and provides an indirect visualization of protamine deficiency of nicked or partially denatured DNA (Bianchi *et al.*, 1993). This method is supported by a second technique, *in situ* nick translation, which determines the existence of endogenous nicks in the DNA of ejaculated spermatozoa (Bianchi *et al.*, 1993). Indeed, a strong correlation exists between these two techniques in human spermatozoa (Manicardi *et al.*, 1995) and together provide the clinician with an effective diagnostic tool.

Recent studies involving ICSI indicate lower fertilization rates for spermatozoa with higher CMA_3 positivity (Sakkas *et al.*, 1996). This could arise from poor chromatin packaging and/or damaged DNA and may result in the inability of spermatozoa to decondense following ICSI, with fertilization failure an end result. Also of consequence is ROS, an inducer of infertility. ROS may result either from endogenous nicks or from loosely packaged chromatin that causes DNA damage making certain spermatozoa more susceptible to further damage.

TUNEL assay

The percentage of sperm DNA fragmentation can be also be analysed by employing the method of terminal deoxynucleotidyl transferase-mediated dUTP-biotin end-labelling (TUNEL) and fluorescence-activated cell sorting. An example of this technique is given in the study of Sun *et al.* (1997), which demonstrated a negative correlation between the percentage of DNA fragmentation and the motility, morphology and concentration of ejaculated spermatozoa. A negative correlation was also found between the percentage of spermatozoa with DNA fragmentation and fertilization rate ($p =$ 0.008) and embryo cleavage rate ($p = 0.01$).

Again, it must be emphasized that these three techniques measure endpoint damage, and not what happens prior to this. The measurement of mitochondrial membrane permeability, mtDNA disruption, or caspase activity could be clear indicators of the activation pathway to this kind of damage and indicate whether the damage is apoptotic or necrotic.

Diagnosis of inherited disorders

Inherited disorders

Inherited disorders are often of great concern to the couple who either have recently conceived or want to. This is especially the case for those who have a familial trait or regard themselves or their partner as a potential carrier. The three main groups of inherited disorders are classed as chromosomal abnormalities, sex-linked diseases and mitochondrial disease.

Chromosomal abnormalities

Trisomies account for 17% of all fetal deaths and approx. 53% of all chromosome abnormalities in early fetal deaths (Hook, 1992). The most common single trisomies are 16, 21, 22, 2 and 18, of which only 21 and 18 are generally seen in live births (although other trisomies such as trisomy 13 have been infrequently observed).

Trisomy 21, Down's syndrome, is the most common trisomy seen in live births, with an incidence of about 1 in 700. Trisomy 21 causes varying degrees of mental retardation, a high risk of congenital heart disease, and other multiple malformations. In more than 90% of cases, the additional chromosome 21 is derived from the mother. Trisomy 18 (Edwards's syndrome) is seen in 1 in 1000 live births. This trisomy manifests as severe mental retardation, multiple malformation and is generally fatal before one year of age. Trisomy 13 (Patau's syndrome) is the most severe viable trisomy, with an incidence of 1 in 5000 births, and results in severe mental retardation and death a few hours after birth.

Carriers of translocation and certain inversions have the highest risk of chromosomally abnormal offspring. The most common form of translocation is a robertsonian translocation, which involves an exchange between acrocentric chromosomes in the centromeric region. The most frequent translocation is between chromosomes 21 and 14 and results in Down's syndrome. Reciprocal translocation carriers are at a high risk of transmitting trisomies to their children as these translocations reflect breakage and recombination between two or more chromosomes. Most reciprocal translocations are unique to the family involved and risk factors must be calculated from the pedigree.

Sex-linked diseases

Diseases caused by genes on one of the sex chromosomes are known as sex-linked or X-linked diseases, since the majority of the genes are located on the X rather than the Y chromosome. As yet, only a few genes of significance appear to be on the Y chromosome (Skinner, 1990). Over 480 X-linked diseases have been described (McKusick, 1994) and, although many, such as haemophilia and muscular dystrophy, are well known, the majority are relatively rare. These disorders are usually recessive and typically affect only males.

A few X-linked diseases have now been characterized at the molecular level and detection of the specific defect can be achieved at the prenatal stage. However, prenatal diagnosis is very restricted or impossible for many other X-linked diseases, since they have not been fully characterized at the molecular level. For couples at risk of such an X-linked disease, identification of the sex of the embryo and selective abortion of a potentially affected male fetus is often the only option available if the disease cannot be detected prenatally.

Fragile (X) is inherited as an X-linked disease and is characterized by mental retardation and hyperactivity. The mutation involves the amplification of a trinucleotide repeat $(CCG)_n$ and it is this increased amplification in the number of repeats in successive generations that is responsible for the higher penetrance observed. The relationship between copy number and phenotype is now the main method used to predict the phenotype in prenatal diagnosis (Fu *et al.*, 1991).

Single-gene defects

Well-known genetic diseases caused by single-gene defects include cystic fibrosis, Huntington's disease, haemophilia, the muscular dystrophies, and the inborn errors of metabolism. The incidence of single-gene defects has been the subject of many investigations. Although individually they are relatively rare, there are very many of them and this group constitutes an important cause of genetic disease. The incidence may have been underestimated, since some of the disorders do not manifest themselves until later in life and they are often misdiagnosed.

Of the 8252 known single-gene defects (or variants), 7686 are autosomal, 483 X-linked and 23 Y-linked (McKusick, 1994). Autosomal diseases affect both males and females with equal frequency and can be either dominant or recessive. Unlike autosomal dominant diseases, autosomal recessives manifest only when the mutated gene is present in the homozygous state. Affected individuals have parents who, although generally healthy, are both heterozygous (carriers) for the gene. Carrier individuals have a 25% chance of having a homozygous affected child, a 50% chance of having a heterozygous carrier child and a 25% chance of having a homozygous unaffected child.

Cystic fibrosis (CF) and Huntington's disease are both diseases where diagnosis has been attempted from either small numbers of cells or single cells. CF is the most common serious autosomal recessive condition in Caucasian populations and is caused by a deletion in the cystic fibrosis transmembrane regulator (CFTR) gene on the long arm (q) of chromosome 7 (Kerem *et al.*, 1989). It affects approximately 1 in 2500 live births and, until recently, life expectancy rarely exceeded 30 years. The frequency and analysis of this gene is discussed in Chapter 9. This mutation causes the deletion of a single amino acid, phenylalanine, at position 508; has thus been designated DF508 and screening for this mutation is commonly performed using PCR.

Mitochondrial point mutations

Although the majority of known genetic diseases are caused by gene mutations in the nucleus of cells, some are also inherited in a non-Mendelian fashion and result from defects in DNA located in mitochondria. The mitochondrial genome produces 13 of the polypeptides associated with the electron transport chain, which produces ATP. However, mitochondrial replication requires interaction with transcription and regulatory factors exported from the nucleus. Mutations in mtDNA may result in disease, but this is dependent on the wild-type to mutant ratio and above a certain threshold, which is specific to each cell type, the mutation can prove life theatening. A 19-year-old deceased cardiomyopathy patient was reported to have an 84% mutant to wild-type ratio (Katsumata *et al.*, 1994).

Mitochondrial disorders can be divided into four groups:

1 Maternally inherited point mutations, either base substitution (e.g. Leber hereditary optic neuropathy (LHON) and Alzheimer's disease) or protein synthesis mutations (e.g. neurogenic muscle weakness, ataxia and refinitis pigmentosum (NARP)).

2 Autosomally dominant mutations involving interactions with nuclear transfer factors and the mitochondrial transcription-regulating region (D-loop).

3 Single sporadic deletions or duplications (e.g. KSS).

4 Multiple somatic deletions (cardiomyopathy, polymyalgia rheumatica and Alzheimer's disease).

Mitochondria carry several copies of mtDNA and, for maternally inherited diseases, this type of inheritance is distinguished by transmission of the mutation through the oocyte of an affected mother to all her children regardless of sex. However, only the daughters would pass this trait to subsequent generations. The maternal inheritance of mtDNA is likely to be a result of evolutionary divergence as various degrees of biparental transmission have been recorded in other species, for example mussels (Fisher & Skibinski, 1990; Hoeh *et al.*, 1991).

PCR can be employed as a diagnostic tool to assess whether deletions are present. This is essential to the detection of both point mutations and multiple somatic deletions. In particular, amplification of the whole mitochondrial genome using LPCR provides a clear picture of the types of deletion present (St John *et al.*, 1997*a*). In addition, use of PCR quantification techniques will determine whether the particular patient harbours sufficient deleted molecules to account for disease onset.

Prenatal diagnosis

Couples who are at high risk of having a child with a genetic disorder are offered prenatal diagnosis. Prenatal diagnosis currently involves sampling of fetal cells by one of amniocentesis, chorionic villus sampling (CVS) or coelocentesis. Analysis of the biopsied material is by cytogenetic, biochemical or molecular methods.

Amniocentesis involves the removal of amniotic fluid which contains fetal cells at 15 to 16 weeks of gestation. These cells are generally cultured for 2–4 weeks to provide a karyotype (Charrow *et al.*, 1990). This means that affected pregnancies are terminated at 17–20 weeks. A further difficulty is a miscarriage rate of between 0.5% and 3.5%, though these rates are lower if the technique is performed by a trained experienced operator. However, amniocentesis is particularly useful in some twin pregnancies, since sampling of both fetuses is not possible with CVS, or in circumstances when CVS is contraindicated.

Coelocentesis is an alternative method (Jauniaux *et al.*, 1991; Wathan *et al.*, 1991), providing sampling and diagnosis within the first trimester. The coelomic cavity is an extra-embryonic cavity which surrounds the foetus and reaches maximum volume at approximately 7–9 weeks gestation, then subsequently disappearing at around 13 weeks gestation. Fluid from the coelomic cavity also contains embryonic cells (Jurkovic *et al.*, 1993, 1995) although the exact origin of these cells has yet to be established.

These embryonic cells have been used to determine fetal sex using both FISH and PCR technologies (Jurkovic *et al.*, 1993; Findlay *et al.*, 1996b) and diagnose single-gene defects such as sickle-cell anaemia (Jurkovic *et al.*, 1995) using a modified single-cell conventional PCR protocol (Sheardown *et al.*, 1992) and cystic fibrosis (Findlay *et al.*, 1996a). Diagnosis of autosomal trisomies (Findlay *et al.*, 1998) and DNA-fingerprints (Findlay *et al.*, 1996b, 1997) can also be determined. However, the relative safety of coelocentesis remains to be evaluated.

CVS permits fetal cells to be biopsied via the cervix or transabdominally at about 9–12 weeks of gestation, and cytogenetic analysis from CVS samples can be obtained from 2 days to 2 weeks. However, performing CVS prior to 11 weeks of pregnancy is not practised due to the increased risk of fetal limb defects (Firth *et al.*, 1991; Burton *et al.*, 1992).

Finally, transcervical cell (TCC) samples have been shown to contain fetal cells amenable to molecular analysis (Griffith-Jones *et al.*, 1992; Delhanty *et al.*, 1995; Tutschek *et al.*, 1995). These cells can be obtained from the cervix by lavage, aspiration, or cytobrush between 6 and 13 weeks of gestation and analysed using FISH or PCR. However, the potential of this technique and its safety require full evaluation.

If the prenatal tests indicate that the fetus is affected, the couple face the difficult and traumatic choice of whether or not to terminate the pregnancy. This decision is more difficult if it is made at a relatively late stage of pregnancy. Currently, the only hope for starting a pregnancy that is known to be unaffected is to be able to diagnose a potentially affected oocyte or embryo prior to implantation (preimplantation genetic diagnosis) and so reduce the need for abortion. Alternatively, the parents may choose not to have any children, to adopt, or to use reproductive technologies such as artificial insemination or *in vitro* fertilization (IVF) with gamete donation.

One particular technique that could be employed to eliminate some inherited disorders is the selection of either Y- or X-bearing spermatozoa. However, the choice of method is vital in this instance. Sufficient data exist to suggest that albumin and Percoll gradients, Sephadex columns and swim-up procedures do not satisfactorily enrich the purified sample in favour of either X- or Y-bearing spermatozoa. The protocol of choice would be flow cytometry, which can yield clinically significant enrichment of X or Y spermatozoa (Johnson *et al.*, 1993). This method of separation is based on DNA content. The selection of X-bearing spermatozoa prior to fertilization would, through flow cytometry for example, reduce the possibility of conceiving a child with a sex-linked disorder. This does not, however, eliminate the possibility of an affected child, since Turner's syndrome, where only one X-chromosome is present, could occur.

If defects can be identified during the early stages of embryonic development before implantation, then only those embryos that are shown to be unaffected by the disease could be implanted. This process, preimplantation genetic diagnosis (PGD), eliminates the need for termination in these cases. The introduction of IVF has allowed human embryos to undergo clinical PGD. This has been demonstrated by Handyside *et al.* (1989) for X-linked diseases and by Verlinsky *et al.* (1990) for autosomal recessive diseases.

Currently, two methods are employed for PGD: FISH for diagnosis of sex and trisomies and PCR for the detection of single-gene defects. Both these methods require one or more cells to be biopsied from the oocyte or embryo.

Diagnosis of male reproductive malfunction

The role of basic semen analysis is well established as a method of assessing male fertility (see Chapters 0–00) and a strong case for its continued use can still be made (Barratt & St John, 1998). Even the increasing demand for new techniques in assisted reproduction, such as IVF and ICSI, does not exclude the requirement for semen analysis. However, it must be recognized as only one of several modes of investigation of the infertile male. Other investigations, such as molecular assays, could and should be used in the diagnosis of azoospermia, asthenozoospermia, teratozoospermia or other male factor defects. This is also true for detecting inheritable genetic disorders and their effects.

ICSI has increased the awareness for genetic analysis of patients who wish to undergo assisted-reproductive treatment. Some genetic disorders may be passed on from generation to generation and these also include some categories of male reproductive malfunction.

Semen analysis

A meaningful interpretation of the semen picture is complicated and by no means easy. Many reports have indicated a relationship between a low sperm count and decreases in male fertility, whilst others have shown none (for a discussion, see Lipshultz, 1996). The importance of sperm pleiomorphism, sperm motility patterns and adequate liquification of seminal plasma, not to mention seminal plasma constituents, are all subject to different interpretation. Not only is this true, but UK NEQAS (External

Quality Assessment Scheme) reports also show that there are serious differences in quantification both between and within laboratories. The World Health Organization Manual (1992) has attempted to standardize semen analysis, but only computer-assisted sperm analysis (CASA) can be relied upon for fully reproducible results. Even with this, differences in interpretation remain a problem and the wrong parameters might be chosen as a measure of functional efficiency in spermatozoa.

Testicular biopsy techniques

In the past, failure to detect spermatozoa in an ejaculate resulted in donor insemination (DI) being the main treatment option. However, ICSI has allowed these patients the possibility to father their own genetic children. In this case, testicular biopsy (testicular sperm extraction (TESE)) is undertaken to determine whether spermatozoa are present. However for non-obstructive cases, such as congenital absence of the vas deferens (CAVD), microsurgical epididymal sperm aspiration (MESA) may be performed and, if unsuccessful, followed by TESE.

As a diagnostic tool for clinical decision making in azoospermia, Tournaye *et al.* (1997) found that no marker (such as semen analysis, maximum testicular volume and levels of serum follicle-stimulating hormone) was predictive and that there were no overall strong predictors for testicular sperm recovery except for testicular histopathology. However, for both obstructive and non-obstructive azoospermic patients, genetic screening is strongly recommended, since subfertility can be acquired either somatically or through mendelian transmission. Two specific examples have been described: CBAVD (congenital bilateral absence of vas deferens) associated with obstructive azoospermia, and microdeletions on the Y chromosome associated with non-obstructive azoospermia. The former is caused mainly by mutations in the cystic fibrosis region and can be screened by PCR. Screening for a panel of up to 30 exon mutations by PCR has been used to advise couples of the simple mendelian risk of having offspring with CF (Silber *et al.*, 1995). However, other applications are currently being considered (see Mak *et al.*, 1997). PCR screening of the Y chromosome is also essential for microdeletions, as karyotyping or any of the other cytogenetic tools are only efficient at detecting large multiple deletions spanning much of the long arm of the Y chromosome.

Y chromosome microdeletions

To date, several azoospermia factors have been mapped to region Yq11 (Ma *et al.*, 1992; Vogt *et al.*, 1992, 1996; Nagafuchi *et al.*, 1993; Reijo *et al.*, 1995), although specificity in terms of the actual pathology of severe oligozoospermia and azoospermia still needs to be verified. Microdeletions in these putative azoospermic factors can, however, be detected through the sequence-tagged site – polymerase chain reaction (STS-PCR) (Kobayashi *et al.*, 1994; Reijo *et al.*, 1995; Stuppia *et al.*, 1996) and the presence of any of these microdeletions could indicate the choice of treatment (i.e. ICSI versus the use of donor gametes) for non-obstructive azoospermia. One of the major problems facing these patients is whether or not they would be transmitting deleted chromosomes to their male offspring (should they succeed in reproducing) and thus rendering the offspring infertile also.

However, evidence from recent reports now demands the screening of sperm DNA as well as that of blood DNA (see Kent-First *et al.*, 1996; Reijo *et al.*, 1996). Reijo *et al.* (1996) reported two severely oligozoospermic men harbouring Y chromosome microdeletions that were not present in the leukocytes of their fathers. In one of these patients, they analysed sperm DNA and demonstrated the same Y chromosome deletion seen in the leukocytes, suggesting the presence of *de novo* mutations. The problem arises, as Reijo *et al.* (1996) argued, that these patients may be mosaic for the Y chromosome, in which case the patients would carry one intact set from their fertile fathers and one set with *de novo* deletions.

Kent-First *et al.* (1996) have reported *de novo* deletions that arose through the germ cell lineage of the fertile parental generation, one common deletion in one father–son pair being recorded. Additionally, two further cases in the same study indicated the presence of microdeletions in the AZF region of ICSI-derived sons that were not detected in the blood of their infertile fathers. This suggests that mosaicism consisting of an intact Y spermatozoon and a microdeleted Y spermatozoon was present, resulting in a failure to detect them in the blood of the infertile generation, as well as the possibility that the son will inherit a mosaic sperm population. The significance of this analysis presents further problems as spermatozoa genetically screened cannot then be used for treatment. The only satisfactory outcome for the couple would be to undertake preimplantation genetic diagnosis to differentiate between Y-deleted and Y-intact embryos.

An additional complication in the interpretation of conventional and multiplex PCR is that they rely on the use of already well-established sequences on the chromosome to detect the presence or loss of the gene. However, between each STS there is DNA-coded information that has not been previously identified and could contain repeat copies of the sought-after gene. Lahn & Page (1997) have recently demonstrated the presence of 12 novel genes, 7 of which demonstrated multiple repeats, on the Y chromosome. Furthermore, through the use of LPCR, multiple copies of the *Daz* gene have been identified (J. St John, unpublished data). The diagnostic as well as experimental screening of these genes through conventional or multiplex PCR could result in the failure to detect the active copy of the sought-after gene, thus affecting the assessment of the frequency of the gene and its deletion within the population. In diagnostic terms, the repeat of the gene in the inactive form could mask the absence of the active copy and thus incorrectly inform ICSI candidate patients of their potential to pass the deletion(s) on to their male offspring. Thus, until the entire coding region of the Y chromosome is mapped and understood, tools such as LPCR are required to support multiplex diagnosis.

Cytoplasmic disorders and ICSI

Spermatozoa and mitochondrial mutations

The heteroplasmic segregation of mitochondrial disease is well established (for a review, see Zeviani & Antozzi, 1997). Specifically to asthenozoospermia, the heteroplasmic segregation of a point mutation that is maternally inherited has been demonstrated in a patient with encephalomyopathy and sperm dysfunction (Folgero *et al.*, 1993). A further report analysing the segregation of maternally inherited sporadic deletions associated with Kearns-Sayre syndrome has demonstrated that these particular deletions were heteroplasmically segregated during embryogenesis (Lestienne *et al.*, 1997). Thus, for male patients suffering from a maternally inherited mitochondrial disease and sperm dysfunction, PCR screening of a sperm sample, using quantitative LPCR, should be performed to assess the overall level of deletion against wild-type to determine whether this defect would affect their fertility.

Many reports have implicated the role of ROS in sperm dysfunction and, in terms of multiple somatic deletions, ROS are considered to be a major cause of these deletions. There are several common deletions indicative of overall mtDNA deletion rate, of which the 5 and 7.4 kilobase are the most frequently analysed. Mimicking of the 5 kilobase deletion with mtDNA inhibitors demonstrates that the presence of this deletion in spermatozoa could indeed be a cause of poor motility (St John *et al.*, 1997*b*) and a patient with such a deletion could be categorized as asthenozoospermic.

The data obtained from analysing the 5 kilobase deletion has been mixed. The deletion has been detected in semen samples, although the origins (spermatozoa or leukocytes) were not established (Kao *et al.*, 1995). Other studies have detected and analysed the 5 kilobase deletion (St John *et al.*, 1997*c*) and the 7.4 kilobase deletion (J. St John *et al.*, unpublished data) in human ejaculated spermatozoa, but the prevalence of these deletions does not mirror the level of motility. However, preliminary studies employing LPCR indicate the presence of multiple deletions which, in sperm samples from asthenozoospermic patients, demonstrate a large mutant to wild-type ratio (St John *et al.*, 1997*d*).

Although there is little research on the role of mtDNA deletions in sperm motility, it has also been suggested that mtDNA deletions could be associated with the apoptotic state of spermatozoa (St John *et al.*, 1997*d*) and that loss of metabolic activity might not be merely a marker of poor motility but could also denote cell suicide. This has been suggested for the testis, where mtDNA deletions in some azoospermic patients have levels of mtDNA deletion correlated with the number of spermatozoa recovered following testicular biopsy (St John *et al.*, 1997*a*).

ICSI and paternal mtDNA inheritance

Since the introduction of ICSI, modifications have been made to this treatment, resulting in round spermatids being injected. In this respect, a live birth has been reported in the UK (Fishel *et al.*, 1997). Recently, Cohen *et al.* (1997) reported a successful birth following the transfer of anucleate donor oocyte cytoplasm into recipient eggs along with a spermatozoon using ICSI. The consequences of such a technique could result in the offspring being the recipient of three genomes: the nuclear complements from the mother and father and some or all mitochondrial complement from the donor (St John & Barratt, 1997).

At the time of writing, few researchers have concentrated on the effects that ICSI can have on the transmission of mitchondrial disease and whether or not the elimination of paternal mtDNA is in fact the norm. ICSI bypasses some of the selective barriers imposed by the oocyte, namely sperm–zona binding and sufficient evidence exists to suggest that intracellular signalling following sperm injection is very different (Tesarik *et al.*, 1994). In this instance, we need to establish whether the selective measures for elimination of paternal mtDNA are being bypassed.

The technique of ICSI overrides many of the processes required of a fit spermatozoa to enter an oocyte. Spermatozoa contain high levels of mtDNA mutations and deletions. Should the nuclear control regulating elimination of sperm mitochondria either fail or be bypassed as a result of the ICSI, the consequence would be an increased risk of possible mitochondrial disease in the offspring.

Allen (1996) has argued that, in humans, the oocyte is dormant, at a low metabolic rate, thus preserving its mitochondria. It is then the intact, under-utilized maternal mtDNA that is transmitted, while paternal mtDNA is sacrificed. However, experimental evidence suggests that deleted mtDNA are seen in oocytes, although with an increase of female mtDNA deletions with age (Keefe *et al.*, 1995). Significantly, Chen *et al.* (1995) reported up to 0.1% transmission of defective mtDNA in oocytes harbouring the 5 kilobase deletion in KSS and CPEO patients. This rate is high considering that the 5 kilobase deletion would be a marker and could be representative of up to 235 different mtDNA deletions (Ozawa, 1995).

It has been argued that in the ageing oocyte, where mtDNA deletions are higher, a fault in the genetic filter that would normally exclude deleted mtDNA could result either in the transmission of deleted molecules or the possibility of paternal leakage (St John *et al.*, 1997*b*). Such possibilities exist in cases of donor cytoplasmic transfer (Cohen *et al.*, 1997), where success at ICSI requires nuclear interaction with the cytoplasm of a third party.

The consequences for humans of paternal mtDNA inheritance are immense. First, an increase in the prevalence of known inherited disorders would arise because of the higher paternal mtDNA mutation rate. Secondly, there would be a greater probability of new inherited disorders arising owing to heteroplasmic segregation of mtDNA during embryogenesis, as demonstrated by Chen *et al.* (1995). For example, a cardiomyopathy that arises through multiple somatic large deletions could become inherited by the offspring and, depending on the segregation of that particular copy or copies, would result in mitochondrial disease. It is therefore imperative that the mtDNA of the individuals involved in ICSI and its derivative treatments should be screened using a PCR assay.

Other chromosomal abnormalities

Chromosomal abnormalities associated with subfertility are 47,XXY, aneuploidy and structural rearrangements. The most common chromosome anomaly detected in azoospermic men is the 47,XXY aneuploidy condition associated with Klinefelter's syndrome (Chandley, 1979). These men require not only effective screening analysis but also counselling. Even though they normally have no spermatozoa present in their ejaculate, the possibility of detecting small numbers from a biopsy sample is becoming more likely as the techniques of sperm recovery become increasingly refined. In this instance, the use of disomic spermatozoa in ICSI would thus lead to 47,XXY in offspring sons.

Approximately 4% of azoospermic and oligozoospermic men are heterozygous for structural rearrangements, for example, reciprocal translocation, insertion, inversion, or ring chromosome aberrations (for a review, see Chandley, 1988). The oligozoospermic men would harbour chromosomally unbalanced spermatozoa in their ejaculate. Again the problem arises of the somatic karyotype being normal, but with chromosomal errors arising from the germ line of men with impaired spermatogenesis. Thus, the use of disomic spermatozoa in ICSI will probably lead to trisomy in the fetus, with the possibility of survival to term for viable trisomics (for a discussion, see Chandley & Hargreave, 1996).

Suggestions and predictions

As geneticists, reproductive biologists and clinicians, we are able to offer today increasingly more techniques to achieve a pregnancy outcome. In addition, genetic disorders are enhanced by some of these reproductive technologies. In order that a couple can conceive and be aware of the consequences that face them and their offspring, both genetic counselling and screening are vital to the patients' assessment for treatment. We suggest that all ICSI candidate fathers should be screened using karyotyping, PCR analysis for deletion of the Y chromosome and CF, and multicoloured FISH (and potentially CGH) to assess the possible aneuploidy of spermatozoa in oligozoospermic men. Indeed, these techniques should be applied to both blood and spermatozoa. If one or more of these criteria demonstrate abnormalities then the patient should receive counselling and be warned of the consequences.

With the possible onset of human cloning as a treatment for infertile patients, molecular and genetic screening techniques assume considerably greater importance. Human cloning could be justified on the basis that the offspring does not descend from the mother, but from her ovary, suggesting that the body is merely an evolutionary vehicle for the gene (for a discussion, see Ridley, 1994).

However, the interactions between the cellular components involved in cloning need to be clearly understood. The effects of an older nucleus in an oocyte cytoplasm must be investigated. Cytoplasmic gene replication is partly regulated by exported nuclear factors. In this case, an age-associated decrease in regulation can result in a decrease in mitochondrial replication and promote mitochondrial disease.

In the case of cloning, screening of somatic cells is vital as genetic disease is more likely to arise in the somatic line, for example some cancers, and the roles of X-inactivation, genetic imprinting and the regulator functions of tumour suppressor genes might be overridden. However, cloning, like IVF or ICSI, would require embryo transfer and thus reduce the transmission of genetic disease, as the patient could be offered the assurity that PGD would answer the genetic causes of concern in the offspring. If we manage to provide the patient with the necessary assurance through our skills to screen correctly, the offspring of tomorrow will not be saying as we now do: 'we can't choose our parents' but more likely 'we can't choose the somatic cell from which we are derived'.

References

Adinolfi, M., Sherlock J. & Pertl, B. (1995). Rapid detection of selected aneuploidies by quantitative fluorescent PCR. *Bioessays*, **17**, 661–4.

Allen, J. F. (1996). Separate sexes and the mitochondrial theory of aging. *Journal of Theoretical Biology*, **180**, 135–40.

Arnheim, N., Li, H. H. & Cui, X. F. (1990). PCR analysis of DNA-sequences in single cells – single sperm gene-mapping and genetic-disease diagnosis. *Genomics*, **8**, 415–19.

Arnheim, N., Li, H., Cui, X. & Navidi, W. (1991). Single sperm PCR analysis – implications for preimplantation genetic disease diagnosis. In *Preimplantation genetics*, ed. Y. Verlinsky & A. M. Kuliev, pp. 121–30. New York: Plenum Press.

Barratt, C. L. R. & Hornby, D. P. (1995). Induction of the acrosome reaction by rhuZP3. In *Human sperm acrosome reaction*, ed. P. Fenichel & J. Parinaud *Colloque INSERM/John Libbey Eurotext*, **326**, 105–22.

Barratt, C. L. R. & St John, J. C. (1998). Diagnostic tools in male infertility. *Human Reproduction*, in press.

Bianchi, P. G., Manicardi, G. C. Bizzaro, D. & Sakkas, D. (1993). Effect of DNA pro-
tamination on fluorochrome staining and in situ nick-translation of
murine and human mature spermatozoa. *Biology of Reproduction*, **49**,
1038–43.

Bischoff, F. Z., Nguyen, D. D., Burt, K. J. & Shaffer, L. G. (1994). Estimates of aneuploidy using multicolor fluorescence in situ hybridization on human
sperm. *Cytogenetics and Cell Genetics*, **66**, 237–43.

Blanco, J., Egozcue, J. & Vidal, F. (1996). Incidence of chromosome 21 disomy in
human spermatozoa as determined by fluorescent in-situ hybridization.
Human Reproduction, **11**, 722–6.

Brewis, I. A., Clayton, R., Barratt, C. L. R., Hornby, D. P. & Moore, H. D. M. (1996)
Characterisation of the calcium influx and the acrosome reaction in
human spermatozoa in response to recombinant ZP3. *Molecular Human
Reproduction*, **2**, 583–9.

Burton, B. K., Schulz, C. J., Burd & L. I. (1992). Limb anomalies associated with
chorionic villus sampling. *Obstetrics and Gynecology*, **79**, 726–30.

Chamberlain, J. S., Gibbs, R. A., Ranier, J. E., Nguyen, P. N. & Caskey, C. T. (1988).
Deletion screening of the Duchenne muscular dystrophy locus via multiplex DNA amplification. *Nucleic Acids Research*, **23**, 1141–56.

Chandley, A. C. (1979). The chromosomal basis of male infertility. *British Medical
Bulletin*, **35**, 181–6.

(1988). Meiosis in man. *Trends in Genetics*, **4**, 79–84.

Chandley, A. C. & Hargreave, T. B. (1996). Genetic anomaly and ICSI. *Human
Reproduction*, **11**, 930–2.

Chapman, N. R., Kessopoulou, E., Andrews, P. D., Hornby, D. P. & Barratt, C. L. R.
(1998). The polypeptide backbone of recombinant human zona pellucida
glycoprotein-3 initiates acrosomal exocytosis in human spermatozoa *in
vitro*. *Biochemical Journal*, **330**, 839–45.

Charrow, J., Nadler, H. L. & Evans, M. I. (1990). Prenatal diagnosis and therapy. In
Principles and practice of medical genetics ed. A. E. H. Emery & D. L.
Rimoin, pp. 1959–94. New York: Churchill Livingstone.

Chen, X., Prosser, R., Simonetti, S., Sadlock, J., Jagiello, G. & Schon, E. A. (1995).
Rearranged mitochondrial genomes are present in human oocytes.
American Journal of Human Genetics, **57**, 239–47.

Cohen, J., Scott, R., Schimmel, T., Levron, J. & Willadsen, S. (1997). Birth of infant
after transfer of anucleate donor oocyte cytoplasm into recipient eggs.
Lancet, **350**, 186–7.

Collins, A. R., Dobson, V. L., Dusinska, M., Kennedy, G. & Stetina, R. (1997). The
comet assay: what can it really tell us? *Mutation Research – Fundamental
and Molecular Mechanisms of Mutagenesis*, **375**, 183–93.

Cuckle, H., Quirke, P., Sehmi, I., Lewis, F., Murray, J., Cross, D., Cuckle, P. &
Ozols, B. (1996). Antenatal screening for cystic-fibrosis. *British Journal of
Obstetrics and Gynaecology*, **103**, 795–9.

Delhanty, J., Adinolfi, M.,Sherlock, J., Tutschek, B., Halder, A. & Rodeck, C.
(1995). Detection of fetal cells in transcervical samples and prenatal diagnosis of chromosomal abnormalities. *Prenatal Diagnosis*, **15**, 943–9.

Dierlamm, J., Rosenberg, C., Stul, M., Pittaluga, S., Wlodarska, I., Michaux, L.,

Dehaen, M., Verhoef, G., Thomas, J., de Kelver, W., Bakker Schut, T., Cassiman, J. J., Raap, A. K., De Wolf Peeters, C., Van den Berghe, H. & Hagemeijer, A. (1997). Characteristic pattern of chromosomal gains and losses in marginal zone B cell lymphoma detected by comparative genomic hybridization. *Leukemia*, 11, 747–58.

Eggeling, F., Freytag, M., Fahsold, R., Horsthemke, B. & Claussen, U. (1993). Rapid detection of trisomy 21 by quantitative PCR. *Human Genetics*, 91, 567–70.

Findlay, I., Quirke, P., Hall, J. & Rutherford, A. J. (1996a). Fluorescent PCR: a new technique for PGD of sex and single-gene defects. *Journal of Assisted Reproduction and Genetics*, 13, 96–103.

Findlay, I., Atkinson, G., Chambers, M., Quirke, P., Campbell, J. & Rutherford, A. (1996b). Rapid genetic diagnosis at 7–9 weeks' gestation: diagnosis of sex, single gene defects and DNA fingerprint from coelomic samples. *Human Reproduction*, 11, 2548–53.

Findlay, I., Taylor, A., Quirke, P., Frazier, R. & Urquhart, A. (1997). DNA fingerprinting from single cells. *Nature*, 389, 555–6.

Findlay, I., Tóth, T., Matthews, P., Marton, T., Quirke, P. & Papp, Z. (1998). Rapid trisomy diagnosis using fluorescent PCR and short tandem repeats: applications for prenatal diagnosis and preimplantation genetic diagnosis. *Journal of Assisted Reproduction and Genetics*, 15, 265–74.

Firth, H. V., Boyd, P. A., Chamberlain, P., McKenzie, I. Z., Liedenbaum, R. H. & Husan, S. M. (1991). Severe limb abnormalities after chorion villus sampling at 56 days gestation. *Lancet*, 337, 726–63.

Fishel, S., Green, S., Hunter, A., Lisi, F., Rinaldi, L., Lisi, R. & McDermott, H. (1997). Human fertilization with round and elongated spermatids. *Human Reproduction*, 12, 336–40.

Fisher, C. & Skibinski, D. O. F. (1990). Sex-biased mitochondrial DNA heteroplasmy in the marine mussel *Mytilus*. *Proceedings of the Royal Society, London B*. 242, 149–56.

Flaherty, S. P., Michalowska, J., Swann, N. J., Dmowski, W. P., Matthews, C. D. & Aitken, R. J. (1997). Albumin gradients do not enrich Y-bearing human spermatozoa. *Human Reproduction*, 12, 938–42.

Folgero, T., Bertheussen, K., Lindal, S. Torbergsen & Oian, P. (1993). Mitochondrial disease and reduced sperm motility. *Human Reproduction*, 8, 1863–8.

Fromenty, B., Manfredi, G., Sadlock, J., Zhang, L., King, M.P. & Schon, E. A. (1996). Efficient and specific amplification of identified partial duplications of human mitochondrial-DNA by long PCR. *Biochimica. et Biophysica Acta*, 1308, 222–30.

Fu, Y. H., Kuhl, D. P., Pizzuti, A., Sutcliffe, J. S., Richards, S., Verkerk, A. J., Holden, J. J., Fenwick, R. G. & Warren, S. T. (1991). Variation of the CGG repeat at the fragile X site results in genetic instability: resolution of the Sherman paradox. *Cell*, 67, 1–20.

Goldman, A. S. & Hulten, M. A. (1993). Analysis of chiasma frequency and first meiotic segregation in a human male reciprocal translocation heterozygote, t(1;11)(p36.3;q13.1), using fluorescence in situ hybridisation. *Cytogenetics and Cell Genetics*, 63, 16–23.

Griffin, D. K., Handyside, A. H., Penketh, R. J. A., Winston, R. M. L. & Delhanty, J.

D. A. (1991). Fluorescent in-situ hybridization to interphase nuclei of human preimplantation embryos with X and Y chromosome specific probes. *Human Reproduction*, **6**, 101–5.

Griffith-Jones, M. D., Miller, D., Lilford, R. J., Scott, J. & Bulmer J. (1992). Detection of fetal DNA in trans-cervical swabs from 1st trimester pregnancies by gene amplification – a new route to prenatal diagnosis. *British Journal of Obstetrics and Gynaecology*, **99**, 508–11.

Guttenbach, M. & Scmid, M. (1991). Non-isotopic detection of chromosome 1 in human meiosis and demonstration of disomic sperm nuclei. *Human Genetics*, **87**, 261–5.

Handyside, A. H., Penketh, R. J. A., Winston, R. M. L., Pattison, J. K., Delhanty, J. D. A. & Tuddenham, E. G. D. (1989). Biopsy of human preimplantation embryos and sexing by DNA amplification. *Lancet*, **8634**, 347–9.

Hardy, C. M., Clarke, H. G., Nixon, B., Grigg, J. A., Hinds, L. A. & Holland, M. K. (1997). Examination of the immunocontraceptive potential of recombinant rabbit fertilin subunits in rabbit. *Biology of Reproduction*, **57**, 879–86.

Hattori, M., Yoshioka, K. & Sakaki, Y. (1992). Highly-sensitive fluorescent DNA sequencing and its application for detection and mass-screening of point mutations. *Electrophoresis*, **13**, 560–5.

Hoeh, W. M., Blakley, K. H. & Brown, W. M. (1991). Heteroplasmy suggests limited biparental inheritance of *Mytilus* mitochondrial DNA. *Science*, **251**, 1488–90.

Hook, E. B. (1992). Chromosome abnormalities. In *Prenatal diagnosis and screening*, ed. D. J. H. Brock, C. H. Rodek and M. A. Ferguson-Smith. Edinburgh: Churchill Livingstone.

Hutchin, T. P. & Cortopassi, G. (1995). A mitochondrial DNA clone is associated with increased risk for Alzheimer's disease. *Proceedings of the National Academy of Sciences, USA*, **92**, 6892–5.

Hutchin, T. P., Heath, P. R., Pearson, R. C. & Sinclair, A. J. (1997). Mitochondrial DNA mutations in Alzheimer's disease. *Biochemical and Biophysical Research Communications*, **241**, 221–5.

Jauniaux, E., Jurkovic, D., Gulbis, B., Gervy, C., Ooms, H.A. & Campbell, S. (1991). Biochemical composition of exocoelomic fluid in early human pregnancy. *Obstetrics and Gynaecology*, **78**, 1124–8.

Jeffreys, A. J., Wilson, V. & Thein, S. L. (1985). Individual specific fingerprints of human DNA. *Nature*, **316**, 76–9.

Ji, B. T., Shu, X. O., Linet, M. S., Zheng, W., Wacholder, S., Gao, Y. T., Ying, D. M. & Jin, F. (1997). Paternal cigarette smoking and the risk of childhood cancer among offspring of nonsmoking mothers. *Journal of the National Cancer Institute*, **89**, 238–44.

Johnson, L. A., Welch, G. R., Keyvanfar, K., Dorfmann, A., Fugger, E. F. & Schulman, J. D. (1993). Gender preselection in humans? Flow cytometric separation of X and Y spermatozoa for the prevention of X-linked diseases. *Human Reproduction*, **8**, 1733–9.

Joos, S., Fink, T. M., Ratsch, A. & Lichter, P. (1994). Mapping and chromosome analysis: the potential of fluorescence in situ hybridisation. *Journal of Biotechnics*, **35**, 135–53.

Jurkovic, D., Jauniaux, E., Campbell, S., Pandya, P., Cardy, D. L. & Nicolaides, K.

H. (1993). Coelocentesis: a new technique for early pre-natal diagnosis. *Lancet*, **341**, 1623–4.

Jurkovic, D., Jauniaux, E., Campbell, S., Mitchell, M., Lees, C. & Layton, M. (1995). Detection of sickle-cell by coelocentesis in early pregnancy: a new approach to prenatal diagnosis of single gene disorders. *Human Reproduction*, **10**, 1287–9.

Kao, S. H., Chao, H. T. & Wei, Y. H. (1995). Mitochondrial deoxyribonucleic acid 4977 bp deletion is associated with diminished fertility and motility of human sperm. *Biology of Reproduction*, **52**, 729–36.

Katsumata, K., Hayakawa, M., Tanaka, M., Sugiyama, S. & Ozawa, T. (1994). Fragmentation of human heart mitochondrial DNA associated with pre-mature aging. *Biochemical and Biophysical Research Communications*, **202**, 102–10.

Keefe, D. L., Niven-Fairchild, T., Powell S. & Buradagunta, S. (1995). Mitochondrial deoxyribonucleic acid deletions in oocytes and reproductive ageing in women. *Fertility and Sterility*, **64**, 577–83.

Kent-First, M. G., Kol, S., Muallem, A., Blazer, S. & Itskovitzeldor, J. (1996). Infertility in intracytoplasmic sperm injection derived sons. *Lancet*, **348**, 332.

Kerem, B. S., Rommens, J., Buchanon, J. A., Markiewicz, D., Cox, T. K., Chakravarti, A., Buchwald, M. & Tsui, L. C. (1989). Identification of the cystic fibrosis gene: genetic analysis. *Science*, **245**, 1073–80.

Kimpton, C. P., Gill, P., Walton, A., Urquhart, A., Millican, E. S. & Adams, M. (1993). Automated DNA profiling employing multiplex amplification of short tandem repeat loci. *PCR Methods and Applications*, **3**, 13–22.

Kobayashi, K., Mizuno, K., Hida, A., Komaki, R., Tomita, K., Matsushita, I., Namiki, M., Iwamoto, T., Tamura, S., Minowada, S., Nakahori, Y. & Nakagome, Y. (1994). PCR analysis of the Y chromosome long arm in azoospermic patients – evidence for a 2nd locus required for spermatogenesis. *Human Molecular Genetics*, **3**, 1965–7.

Koch, K. E., Kolvraa, S., Petersen, K. B., Gregersen, N. & Bolund, L. (1989). Oligonucleotide-priming methods for the chromosome-specific label of alpha satellite DNA in situ. *Chromosoma*, **98**, 259–65.

Kotzot, D., Bundscherer, G., Bernasconi, F., Brecevic, L., Lurie, I. W. & Basaran, S., (1996). Isochromosome 18P results from maternal meiosis-II nondisjunction. *European Journal of Human Genetics*, **4**, 168–74.

Kristjansson, K., Chong, S. S., Vandenveyver, I. B., Subramanian, S., Snabes, M. C. & Hughes, M. R. (1994). Preimplantation single cell analysis of dystrophin gene deletions using whole genome amplification. *Nature Genetics*, **6**, 19–23.

Lahn, B. T. & Page, D. C. (1997). Functional coherence of the human Y chromosome. *Science*, **24**, 675–80.

Lasheeb, A. S., King, J., Ball, J. K., Curran, R., Barratt, C. L. R., Afnan M. A. M. & Pillay D. (1997). Semen characteristics in HIV-1 positive men and the effect of semen washing. *Genitourinary Medicine*, **73**, 303–5.

Lestienne, P., Reynier, P., Chretien, M. F., Penisson-Besnier, I., Malthiery, Y. & Rohmer, V. (1997). Oligoasthenospermia associated with multiple mito-chondrial DNA rearrangements. *Molecular Human Reproduction*, **3**, 811–14.

Li, A., Gyllensten, U. B., Cui, X., Saiki, R. K., Erlich, H. A. & Arnheim, N. (1988). Amplification and analysis of DNA sequences in single human sperm and diploid cells. *Nature*, **335**, 414–19.

Li, D. & Vijg, J. (1996). Multiplex co-amplification of 24 retinoblastoma gene exons after pre-amplification by long-distance PCR. *Nucleic Acids Research*, **24**, 538–9.

Li, Y.-Y., Hengstenberg, C. & Maisch, B. (1995). Whole mitochondrial genome amplification reveals basal level multiple deletions in mtDNA of patients with dilated cardiomyopathy. *Biochemical and Biophysical Research Communications*, **210**, 211–18.

Lichter, P., Tang, C. J., Call, K., Hermanson, G., Evans, G. A., Housman, D. & Ward, D. C. (1990). High-resolution mapping of human chromosome 11 by in situ hybridization with cosmid clones. *Science*, **247**, 64–9.

Lipshultz, L. I. (1996). The debate continues – the continuing debate over the possible decline in semen quality. *Fertility and Sterility*, **65**, 909–11.

Ma, K., Sharkey, A., Kirsch, S., Vogt, P., Keil R., Hargreave, T. B., McBeath, S. & Chandley, A. C. (1992). Towards the molecular localisation of the AZF locus: mapping of microdeletions in azoospermic men within 14 subintervals of interval 6 of the human Y chromosome. *Human Molecular Genetics*, **1**, 29–33.

MacDonald, M., Hassold, T. & Harvey, J. (1994) The origin of 47,XXY and 47,XXX aneuploidy heterogeneous mechanisms and role of aberrant recombination. *Human Molecular Genetics*, **3**, 1365–71.

Mak, V., Jarvi, K. A., Zielenski, J., Durie, P. & Tsui, L. C. (1997). Higher proportion of intact exon 9 CFTR mRNA in nasal epithelium compared with vas deferens. *Human Molecular Genetics*, **6**, 2099–107.

Manicardi, G. C., Bianchi, P. G., Pantano, S., Azzoni, P., Bizzaro, D., Bianchi, U. & Sakkas, D. (1995). Underprotamination and nicking of DNA in ejaculated human spermatozoa are highly related phenomena. *Biology of Reproduction*, **52**, 864–7.

Mansfield, E. S., Blasband, A., Kronick, M. N., Wrabetz, L., Kaplan, P., Rappaport, E., Sartore, M., Parrella, T., Surrey, S. & Fortina, P. (1993a). Fluorescent approaches to diagnosis of Lesch–Nyhan syndrome and quantitative analysis of carrier status. *Molecular and Cellular Probes*, **7**, 311–24.

Mansfield, E. S., Robertson, J. M., Lebo, R. V., Lucero, M. Y., Mayrand, P. E., Rappaport, E., Parrella, T., Sartore, M., Surrey, S. & Fortina, P. (1993b). Duchenne–Becker muscular-dystrophy carrier detection using quantitative PCR and fluorescence-based strategies. *American Journal of Medical Genetics*, **48**, 200–8.

Martin, R. H. & Rademaker, A. (1995). Reliability of aneuploidy estimates in human sperm: results of fluorescence in situ hybridization studies using two different scoring criteria. *Molecular Reproduction and Development*, **42**, 89–93.

McBride, L. & O'Neill, M. D. (1991). Automated analysis of mutations responsible for genetic diseases in humans. *American Laboratory*, November 1991.

McKelvey-Martin, V. J., Melia, N., Walsh, I. K., Johnston, S. R., Hughes, C. M., Lewis, S. E. M. & Thompson, W. (1997). Two potential clinical applications of the alkaline single cell gel electrophoresis assay: (1) human bladder

washings and transitional cell carcinoma of the bladder; and (2) human
    sperm and male infertility. *Mutation Research*, **375**, 93–104.

McKusick, V. A. (1994). *Mendelian inheritance in man*. 11th edn. Catalogs of
    human genes and genetic disorders. Baltimore, MD: Johns Hopkins
    University Press.

Monk, M. & Holding, C. (1990). Amplification of a beta-hemoglobin sequence in
    individual human oocytes and polar bodies. *Lancet*, **335**, 985–8.

Mullis, K. B. & Faloona, F. A. (1987). Specific synthesis of DNA *in vitro* via a poly-
    merase-catalysed chain reaction. *Methods in Enzymology*, **155**, 335–50.

Nagafuchi, S., Namiki, M., Nakahori, Y., Kondoh, N., Okuyama, A. & Nakagome,
    Y. (1993). A minute deletion of the Y-chromosome in men with azoosper-
    mia. *Journal of Urology*, **150**, 1155–7.

Nederlof, P. M., Robinson, D., Abuknesha, R., Wiegant, J., Hopman, A. H. N.,
    Tanke, H. J. & Raap, A. K. (1989). 3-Color fluorescence in situ hybridization
    for the simultaneous detection of multiple nucleic-acid sequences.
    Cytometry, **10**, 20–7.

Ozawa, T. (1995). Mechanism of somatic mtDNA mutations associated with age
    and diseases. *Biochimica et Biophysica Acta*, **1271**, 177–89.

Pardue, M. L. & Gall, J. G. (1970). Chromosomal localization of mouse satellite
    DNA. *Science*, **168**, 1356–8.

Pertl, B., Yau, S. C., Sherlock, J., Davies, A. F., Mathew, C. G. & Adinolfi, M. (1994).
    Rapid molecular method for prenatal detection of Down's syndrome.
    Lancet, **343**, 1197–8.

Reijo, R., Lee, T. Y., Salo, P., Alagappan, R., Brown, L. G., Rosenberg, M., Rozen, S.,
    Jaffe, T., Straus, D., Hovatta, O., de la Chapelle, A., Silber, S. & Page, D. C.
    (1995). Diverse spermatogenic defects in humans caused by Y-chromo-
    some deletions encompassing a novel RNA binding protein gene. *Nature
    Genetics*, **10**, 383–93.

Reijo, R., Alagappan, R. K., Patrizio, P. & Page, D. C. (1996). Severe oligozoosper-
    mia resulting from deletions of azoospermia factor gene on Y-chromo-
    some. *Lancet*, **347**, 1290–3.

Reynier, P., Pellissier, J.-F., Harle, J.-R. & Malthiery, Y. (1994). Multiple deletions of
    the mitochondrial DNA in polymyalgia rheumatica. *Biochemical and
    Biophysical Research Communications*, **205**, 375–80.

Ridley, M. (1994). *The red queen*. London: Penguin Books.

Saiki, R., Scharf, S., Faloona, F., Mullis, K., Hom, G., Erlich, H. & Arnheim, N.
    (1985). Enzymatic amplification of beta-globin genomic sequences and
    restriction site analysis for diagnosis of sickle cell anemia. *Science*, **230**,
    1350–4.

Saiki, R. K., Gelfand, D. H., Stoffel, S., Scharf, S. J., Higuchi, R., Horn, G. T.,
    Mullis, K. B. & Erlich, H. A. (1988). Primer-directed enzymatic
    amplification of DNA with a thermostable DNA polymerase. *Science*, **239**,
    487–91.

Sakkas, D., Urner, F., Bianchi, P. G., Bizzaro, D., Wagner, I., Jaquenoud, N.,
    Manicardi, G. C. & Campana, A. (1996). Sperm chromatin anomalies can
    influence decondensation after intracytoplasmic sperm injection. *Human
    Reproduction*, **11**, 837–43.

Schwartz, L. S., Tarleton, J., Popovich, B., Seltzer, W. K. & Hoffman, E. P. (1992). Fluorescent multiplex linkage analysis and carrier detection for Duchenne/Becker muscular dystrophy. *American Journal of Human Genetics*, **51**, 721–9.

Semprini, A. E., Levi-Setti, P., Bozzo, M., Ravizza, M., Taglioretti, A., Sulpizio, P., Albani, E., Oneta, M. & Pardi, G. (1992). Insemination of HIV-negative women with processed semen of HIV-positive partners. *Lancet*, **340**, 1317–19.

Sermon, K., Lissens, W., Joris, H., Van Steirteghen, A. & Liebaers, I. (1996). Adaptation of primer extension pre-amplification (PEP) reaction for pre-implantation diagnosis: single blastomere analysis using short PEP protocol. *Molecular Human Reproduction*, **2**, 209–12.

Sheardown, S. A. Findlay, I., Turner, A., Greaves, D., Bolton, V., Mitchell, M., Layton, D. M. & Muggleton-Harris, A. L. (1992). Preimplantation diagnosis of a human β-globin transgene in biopsied trophectoderm cells and blastomeres in the mouse embryo. *Human Reproduction*, **7**, 1297–1304.

Shen, H. M., Chia, S. E., Ni, Z. Y., New, A. L., Lee, B. L. & Ong, C. N. (1997). Detection of oxidative DNA damage in human sperm and the association with cigarette smoking. *Reproductive Toxicology*, **11**, 675–80.

Silber, S. J., Nagy, Z., Liu, J., Tournaye, H., Lissens, W., Ferec, C., Liebaers, I., Devroey, P. & Van Steirteghem, A. C. (1995). The use of epididymal and testicular spermatozoa for intracytoplasmic sperm injection, the genetic implications for male infertility. *Human Reproduction*, **10**, 2031–43.

Siracusa, L. D., McGrath, R., Ma, Q., Moskow, J. J., Manne, J., Christner, P. J., Buchberg, A. M. & Jimenez, S. A. (1996). A tandem duplication within the fibrillin 1 gene is associated with the mouse tight skin mutation. *Genome Research*, **6**, 300–13.

Skinner, R. (1990). Unifactorial inheritance. In *Principles and practice of medical genetics*, ed. A. E. H. Emery & D. L. Rimoin, pp. 95–106. New York: Churchill Livingstone.

Snabes, M. C., Subramanian, S., Kristjansson, K., Chong, S., Cota, J. & Hughes, M. R. (1993). Whole genome amplification in preimplantation genetic diagnosis. *American Journal of Human Genetics*, **53**, 90.

Snabes, M. C., Chong, S. S., Subramanian, S. B., Kristjansson, K., Disepio, D. & Hughes, M. R. (1994). Preimplantation single-cell analysis of multiple genetic loci by whole geneome amplification. *Proceedings of the National Academy of Sciences, USA*, **91**, 6181–5.

Soong, N. W. & Arnheim, N. (1996). Detection and quantification of mitochondrial DNA deletions. *Methods in Enzymology*, **264**, 421–31.

Spriggs, E. L. & Martin, R. H. (1994). Analysis of segregation in a human male reciprocal translocation carrier, t(1;11) (p36.3;q13.1), by two-colour fluorescence in situ hybridization. *Molecular Reproduction and Development*, **38**, 247–50.

Spriggs, E. L., Rademaker, A. W. & Martin, R. H. (1995). Aneuploidy in human sperm: results of two-and three-color fluorescence in situ hybridization using centromeric probes for chromosomes 1, 12, 15, 18, X, and Y. *Cytogenetics and Cell Genetics*, **71**, 47–53.

St John, J. C. & Barratt, C. L. R. (1997). Use of anucleate donor oocyte cytoplasm in recipient egg. *Lancet*, **350**, 961–2.

St John, J. C., Cooke I. D. & Barratt, C. L. R. (1997a). Detection of multiple deletions in the mitochondrial DNA of human testicular tissue from azoospermic and severe oligozoospermic patients. In *Genetics of male fertility*, ed. C. L. R. Barratt, C. De Jonge, D. Mortimer, J. Parinaud, pp. 333–47. Paris: EDK.

St John, J. C., Jokhi, R. P., Barratt, C. L. R. & Cooke, I. D. (1997b). The effects of mitochondrial dysfunction on sperm motility. *Human Reproduction*, **12**, SS, p.P11 (Abstract).

St John, J. C., Jokhi, R. P., Barratt, C. L. R. & Cooke, I. D. (1997c) The association between mitochondrial DNA deletions and free radicals. *Serono Symposia USA: XIV Testis Workshop: Germ Cell Development, Division, Disruption and Death*, 19 to 22 February, 1997, (Abstract).

St John J. C., Cooke I. D. & Barratt C. L. R. (1997d). Mitochondrial mutations and male infertility. *Nature Medicine*, **3**, 124–5.

Stuppia, L., Mastroprimiano, G., Calabrese, G., Peila, R. Tenaglia, R. & Palka, G. (1996). Microdeletions in interval-6 of the Y-chromosome detected by STS-PCR in 6 of 33 patients with idiopathic oligospermia or azoospermia. *Cytogenetics and Cell Genetics*, **72**, 155–8.

Sun, J. G., Jurisicova, A. & Casper, R. F. (1997). Detection of deoxyribonucleic acid fragmentation in human sperm: correlation with fertilization *in vitro*. *Biology of Reproduction*, **56**, 602–7.

Syed, V., Gu, W. & Hecht, N. B. (1997). Sertoli cells in culture and mRNA differential display provide a sensitive early warning assay system to detect changes induced by xenobiotics. *Journal of Andrology*, **18**, 264–73.

Tesarik, J., Sousa, M. & Testart, J. (1994). Human ovary activation after intracytoplasmic sperm injection. *Human Reproduction*, **9**, 511–18.

Tournaye, H., Verheyen, G., Nagy, P., Ubaldi, F., Goossens, A., Silber, S., Van Steirteghem, A. C. & Devroey, P. (1997). Are there any predictive factors for successful testicular sperm recovery in azoospermic patients? *Human Reproduction*, **12**, 80–6.

Tutschek, B., Sherlock, J., Halder, A., Delhanty, J., Rodeck, C. & Adinolfi, M. (1995). Isolation of fetal cells from transcervical samples by micromanipulation – molecular confirmation of their fetal origin and diagnosis of fetal aneuploidy. *Prenatal Diagnosis*, **15**, 951–60.

Verlinsky, Y., Ginsberg, N., Lifchez, A., Valle, J., Moise, J. & Strom, C. M. (1990). Analysis of the first polar body: preconceptual genetic analysis. *Human Reproduction*, **5**, 826–9.

Verlinsky, Y., Cieslak, J., Ivakhnenko, V., Lifchez, A., Strom, C., Kuliev, A., Freidine, M., White, M., Wolf, G., Moise, J., Valle, J., Kaplan, B. & Ginsberg, N. (1996). Birth of healthy children after preimplantation diagnosis of common aneuploidies by polar body fluorescent in-situ hybridization analysis. *Fertility and Sterility*, **66**, 126–9.

Vogt, P., Chandley, A. C., Hargreave, T. B., Keil, R., Ma, K. & Sharkey, A. (1992). Microdeletions in interval 6 of the Y-chromosome of males with idiopathic sterility point to disruption of AZF, a human spermatogenesis gene. *Human Genetics*, **89**, 491–6.

Vogt, P. H., Edelmann, A., Kirsch, S., Henegariu, O., Hirschmann, P., Kiesewetter, F., Kohn, F. M. Schill, W. B., Farah, S., Ramos, C., Hartmann, M., Hartschuh, W., Meschede, D., Behre, H. M., Castel, A., Nieschlag, E., Weidner, W., Grone, H. J., Jung, A., Engel, W. & Haidl, G. (1996). Human Y chromosome azoospermia factors (AZF) mapped to different subregions in Yq11. *Human Molecular Genetics*, **5**, 933–44.

Wathan, N. C., Cass, P. L., Campbell, D. J., Kitau, M. J. & Chard, T. (1991). Early amniocentesis: alphafetoprotein levels in amniotic fluid, extraembryonic coelomic fluid and maternal serum between 8 and 13 weeks. *British Journal of Obstetrics and Gynaecology*, **98**, 866–70.

Whitmarsh, A. J., Woolnough, M. J., Moore, H. D. M., Hornby, D. P. H. & Barratt, C. L. R. (1996). Biological activity of recombinant human ZP3 produced *in vitro*: potential for a sperm function test. *Molecular Human Reproduction*, **2**, 911–19.

Williams, B., Ballenger, C. & Malter, H. (1993). Non-disjunction in human sperm: results of fluorescence in situ hybridization studies using two and three probes. *Human Molecular Genetics*, **2**, 1929–36.

Wolff, E., Liehr, T., Vorderwulbecke, U., Tulusan, A. H., Husslein, E. M. & Gebhart, E. (1997). Frequent gains and losses of specific chromosome segments in human ovarian carcinomas shown by comparative genomic hybridization. *International Journal of Oncology*, **11**, 19–23.

World Health Organization (1992). *WHO laboratory manual for the examination of human semen and semen-cervical mucus interaction*, 3rd edn. Cambridge: Cambridge University Press.

Xu K. P, Tang, Y. X., Grifo, J. A., Rosenwaks, Z. & Cohen, J. (1993). Primer extension preamplification for detection of multiple genetic-loci from single human blastomeres. *Human Reproduction*, **8**, 2206–10.

Zeviani, M. & Antozzi, C. (1997). Mitochondrial disorders. *Molecular Human Reproduction*, **3**, 133–48.

Zhang, L., Cui, X. F., Schmitt, K., Hubert, R., Navidi, W. & Arnheim, N. (1992). Whole genome amplification from a single cell: implications for genetic analysis. *Proceedings of the National Academy of Sciences, USA*, **89**, 5847–51.

Zhu, X. & Naz, R. K. (1997). Fertilization antigen-1: cDNA cloning, testis specific expression, and immunocontraceptive effects. *Proceedings of the National Academy of Sciences, USA*, **89**, 5847–51.

Ziegle, J. S., Su, Y., Corcoran, K. P., Nie, L., Mayrand, P. E., Hoff, L. B., McBride, L. J., Kronick, M. N. & Diehl, S. R. (1992). Application of automated DNA sizing technology for genotyping microsatellite loci. *Genomics*, **14**, 1026–31.

13 Gazing into the crystal ball: future diagnosis and management in andrology

JIM CUMMINS AND ANNE JEQUIER

Introduction

We have been given the extremely difficult task of looking into the future of andrology. One only has to consider how intracytoplasmic sperm injection (ICSI) has revolutionized our treatment of the infertile male over the past five years to realize the daunting task facing any would-be soothsayers. The first experiments in micro-assisted fertilization were in rodent models in the 1970s (Uehara & Yanagimachi, 1976), but out of these exploded the present spectrum of techniques starting in 1992 with Palermo *et al.*'s report of successful pregnancies following ICSI. What was regarded as incurable male infertility a decade ago is now routinely treatable by the average clinic. Only a handful of visionaries ten years ago could have foretold such a rapid application of basic research to the human arena (Yanagimachi, 1995).

In this chapter we review briefly the history of andrology and attempt to identify key areas that we think will advance our understanding. We are also a bit provocative and argue that the medicalization of human infertility may be a late twentieth century aberration. Is infertility simply an inevitable by-product of our recent evolution, albeit perhaps made worse by our deteriorating human environment? Such a biological perspective may help us to resolve some of the ethical, religious and legal tensions that surround reproductive technology. It may even help infertile couples to an understanding and acceptance of their condition, because we also need to recognize that there may be ethical, economic and medical limits to the development of andrological techniques. This is particularly relevant in situations where we may be asked to apply techniques to a man whose infertility is caused by a genetic defect that will be transmitted to his sons, and that can only be 'cured' by the controversial application of germline gene therapy. Finally, we draw attention to the urgent need for specialist medical training in both male and female infertility. Andrology is a term frequently used as though it refers solely to semen analysis and sperm function testing. These applied laboratory aspects of the discipline are, of course, important. However, they cannot be a substitute for good clinical practice, which should be attempting to define and understand the causes of infertility as opposed to merely treating the symptoms. The history of reproductive technology reflects a see-saw between basic sciences and the humanistic application of medicine. At present, we argue, science and technique are in the ascendancy, but diagnostic medicine urgently needs to catch up.

History

A discussion of the past as well as the future of this branch of medicine is timely. The term 'andrology' was first coined over 100 years ago by the Congress of American Physicians and Surgeons to differentiate the study of the male from the field of gynaecology. It disappeared from view, only to be reinvented in Germany in the twentieth century (Niemi, 1987). Andrology is defined by Dorland's medical dictionary (Friel, 1985) as the 'scientific study of the masculine constitution and of the diseases of the male sex; especially the study of diseases of the male organs of generation'.

The first true clinical andrologist was Edward Martin (Jequier, 1991). He was the first to describe and define the difference between the two major forms of azoospermia, namely ductal obstruction and primary testicular disease (Martin *et al.*, 1902). He also pointed out the need for the analysis of a sample of semen in couples complaining of childlessness. The first major cause of male infertility to be treated surgically was ductal obstruction and Martin and notable successors such as Hagner (1936), Bayle (1952) and Schoysmann (1981) obtained results from their macrosurgical procedures of which many prominent microsurgeons of today would be justifiably proud. However, over the last 100 years the causation of ductal obstruction seems to have changed (Jequier, 1986), making it a condition that today is much more difficult to remedy surgically.

The huge advances that were made in the 1930s in the field of reproductive endocrinology, together with the description of the pituitary–gonadal feedback system by Moore & Price (1932) greatly aided our understanding of the male genital system and its pathology. The award at this time of the Nobel Prize for Chemistry to the German biochemist Adolf Butenandt for his discovery and synthesis of testosterone (Butenandt & Hansch, 1935) added lustre to much of this work. By mid century, the importance of semen analysis was being emphasized with the publication of a book devoted to this subject which was written by the eminent reproductive physician Hotchkiss (1947).

Andrology thus has a well-defined history. However, today it is almost exclusively used to describe the laboratory techniques for treating semen and sadly many clinicians working in infertility are ill equipped to deal with the causes, as opposed to the symptoms, of male infertility. We return to this theme later.

Diagnosis

In so far as science is 'the systematic observation of natural phenomena for the purpose of discovering laws governing those phenomena' (Friel, 1985), then andrology in the 1990s is profoundly inconsistent. That is because, although we have very effective techniques for treating the symptoms of male infertility – or at least resolving the distress associated with it, which is the inability to be a biological father – we are very far from understanding the complex roots of the disorders that cause it.

The commonest cause of infertility in the male is primary testicular disease (Jequier & Holmes, 1993). Its treatment – or perhaps what is more important, its prevention – is impossible, because we do not understand the underlying cause or causes. Because of this deficiency, we continue to treat the resulting infertility by manipulation of the spermatozoa, but there is no virtue in this glaring gap in our knowledge (Cummins & Jequier, 1994).

Because the changes in semen that occur in many different forms of infertility are probably non-specific, the 'treatment' of the spermatozoa by techniques such as ICSI cannot be based on any rational diagnostic criteria. Thus it is impossible to examine differences in the effectiveness of the treatment in relation to cause.

The seduction of ICSI

We now know that there are many different and varied causes of infertility in the male and the advances that have been made in the whole subject of imaging in medicine have greatly enhanced our understanding of this subject. However, there is no doubt that the greatest advance in treatment made over the past 100 years involves the use of *in vitro* fertilization (IVF) and ICSI. ICSI has been stunningly successful in overcoming almost every form of male infertility, whether it be a severe reduction in sperm production, obstruction of the duct system or many of the disorders of ejaculation that can result in infertility. It allows us to use immotile sperm retrieved from the testis as well as sperm aspirated from areas of the excurrent duct system that are proximal to sites of obstruction. This obviates the need for any remedial surgery, whose results in any case give no guarantee of fertility (Silber *et al.*, 1996). Using ICSI, it is now possible to offer treatment in some cases of Klinefelter's syndrome (Tournaye *et al.*, 1996) and even immotile cilia (Kartagener's syndrome; (Nijs *et al.*, 1996), conditions that were previously untreatable.

However, the success of ICSI in the treatment of male infertility has had one clear adverse affect. It has spread the idea among clinicians that it is so effective that investigation of a patient or even a definition of the cause of his infertility is no longer necessary or economically viable (Hamberger & Janson, 1997). This is a worrying trend, for without a thorough understanding of the causes of infertility we can do little to prevent it. Indeed, there is a widespread view that as long as a few sperm can be identified for use in an ICSI procedure, no clinical evaluation of the patient nor any other investigation apart from routine semen analysis (which is of limited diagnostic value) is necessary. This makes for dangerous medicine and, frequently, for the unnecessary application of complex procedures such as IVF to patients' problems. Paradoxically, ICSI and IVF have, if anything, enhanced our ability to diagnose specific causes of male infertility today, which makes a *laissez-faire* attitude all the more remiss. Despite these advances and despite public warnings, poor clinical evaluation of men in cases of infertility is likely to persist until and unless market forces push clinicians towards a change of outlook (Cummins & Jequier, 1994, 1995; Cummins, 1997a; Jequier & Cummins, 1997).

Future management

How will the management of male infertility advance in the next century? There are several changes in clinical andrology that will probably happen over the next 20–30 years. The first change – which may already be happening – is a possible increase in the overall incidence of male infertility. The reduction in the sperm count that has been claimed in the human (Carlsen *et al.*, 1992) could render male infertility a more common and distressing medical problem than it has been regarded hitherto. Whether this is already happening is, of course, controversial and is compounded by other demographic factors such as reductions in the dizygotic twinning rate (James, 1997).

Why this apparent reduction in human sperm numbers has occurred is uncertain, because no such change can be identified in domestic animals that share our environment (Setchell, 1997). However, there is increasing evidence that many commonly used chemicals such as pesticides have potent endocrine effects (Gray *et al.*, 1997). Many of these substances are anti-androgens that act by competitive binding to the androgen receptor and thus reducing androgenization. Others act as oestrogen mimics. These may reduce the sperm count in the adult but they can also produce profound effects on genital development, if a developing fetus *in utero* should happen to be exposed to them. Any increases in the incidence of testicular cancer, and in genital anomalies such as hypospadias and cryptorchidism, over the last generation could be examples of the effects of such pollutants on the human fetus (Jensen *et al.*, 1995). If these trends prove significant they will add yet another problem to the management of male infertility in the future. However, at least the world is now much more aware of the damage that chemical pollution can do to humans as well as to many species of wildlife (Kelce & Wilson, 1997) and the use of these agents is starting to be much more tightly controlled. Nevertheless, the long-lived nature and bioaccumulation of these compounds, such as DDT, would pose a grave threat to all lifeforms well into the next century even if their use were to be stopped immediately. Rachel Carson's prescient book *Silent spring* (1963) is quite chilling.

Genetics of male infertility

The genetic causation of male infertility is now being actively explored worldwide and it will become a very important part of the evaluation of the infertile male well into the next century. The demonstration of the presence of microdeletions at interval 6 on the long arm of the Y chromosome among men with oligozoospermia or azoospermia (Vogt *et al.*, 1996) has clearly demonstrated that male infertility can have a genetic basis. However, analysis is made difficult by the inherent instability of the Y chromosome, by multiple gene copies on the chromosome itself and by the presence of copies of genes controlling spermatogenesis on autosomes (Graves, 1995; Ruggiu *et al.*, 1997). Moreover, the mutations may occur during spermatogenesis, so that the sperm population may be heterogeneous for Y deletions or mutations even in a genetically normal man. It is also clear that this genetic anomaly may be transmitted to the male offspring of the infertile man (Kent-First *et al.*, 1996). Thus male infertility in the next generation may be increased by treating men who, without such assistance, would be sterile. This is a dilemma for infertility clinics. Where does the right to reproduce end and responsibility for the interests of the child (as yet not conceived) begin? Who decides? This debate will undoubtedly continue into the next century.

Spermatogenesis is a complex and continuous process of mitotic and meiotic cell proliferation within a supportive framework of Sertoli cells. Undoubtedly, the complete mapping of the human genome will bring a deeper understanding of the genetic mechanisms controlling spermatogenesis. Many of the genes are already mapped, although assigning functions to them is still at an early stage (Elliott & Cooke, 1997). The recognition that mature spermatozoa carry a spectrum of messenger RNAs derived from genes activated during spermatogenesis offers the exciting prospect of identifying those genes and of pinpointing where spermatogenic lesions may occur (Miller, 1997). Techniques such as differential RNA display may allow us to differentiate the genes that are switched on and off during spermatogenesis (Catalano *et al.*, 1997). Ultimately, we could even consider the possibility of germline gene therapy on men with genetically determined infertility, but, of course, this is currently banned in most countries. Even more radical would be the prospect of transplanting fertile donated germ cells into the testis of an infertile man (Brinster & Avarbock, 1994), but this would not necessarily relieve problems caused by autosomal genes, such as endocrinopathy or androgen insensitivity (Brinkmann *et al.*, 1996).

'Cures' for the infertile man will pose troubling problems for those administering public health and for the taxpayers and consumers paying for services. Just as the incidence of other genetic disorders such as diabetes mellitus continues to increase due to good care and good blood sugar control in pregnancy, it is possible that over the next 20–30 years that we will see an increase in genetically determined infertility in humans. This will put pressure on the health services which are already struggling to meet the needs of an ageing population. Much of human variation is driven by mutations that preferentially accrue in the testis (Short, 1997), and infertility is probably only one manifestation of this. The paradox here is that infertility clinics may be creating or transmitting new forms of infertility that only they can cure. The analogy with the management of diabetes is clear and we need to be open and consistent in our public policy debates. The United Nations Declaration of Human Rights certainly avers the right to bear children, but when it was drafted the authors had probably not even dreamed that one day we would be 'curing' infertility at the expense of creating a new generation of infertile or sickly children. Paradoxically, many infertile couples today are so fixated on having a child that they discount this risk. This child-as-solution attitude may be a late twentieth century aberration of the intensely self-centred postwar 'Me-generation'.

While clinics are generally at pains to defend their record, it is clear at least to us that awareness of potential risks and dangers must be raised from within the discipline, otherwise we run the very real risk of limitations imposed on clinics by political forces (Cummins, 1997a; Cummins & Jequier, 1994, 1995; Tournaye & Van Steirteghem, 1997). Already many aspects of the advanced techniques, such as immature germ cell injection, are banned in countries such as the Netherlands and the UK. Whilst there is as yet little convincing evidence that the techniques are dangerous, many consider them to be ethically unsound as they are not based on appropriate animal models.

The concern that morphologically abnormal spermatozoa selected for ICSI may be genetically abnormal has only a weak foundation. There is little evidence that sperm morphology reflects the haploid genome it carries, and there have been births of normal mouse young after the injection of grossly abnormal spermatozoa (Burruel *et al.*, 1996). However, rodent models may not be entirely appropriate as certain types of abnormal human sperm injected into mouse oocytes show increased levels of chromosomal anomalies (Lee *et al.*, 1996). All of these observations point out the need for continuous vigilance as we test the limits of reproductive forces that have been set in place over billions of years of evolution, and that we are far from understanding.

Epigenetic factors in fertilization

Fertilization is not merely the transfer of paternal genes into the oocyte. The human spermatozoon carries with it the centrosome that acts as a template for the first cleavage spindle of the embryo, and failure of this process is now recognized as one cause of male infertility (Asch *et al.*, 1995). The spermatozoon also carries mitochondria with their own mitochondrial DNA (mtDNA), which do not normally persist in the zygote. The reasons for this remain a mystery (Ankel-Simons & Cummins, 1996). One concern is that the use of very immature germ cells could by-pass the normal elimination processes and allow the inoculation of abnormal mtDNA into the oocyte, thereby leading to bioenergetic diseases in the offspring (Cummins, 1997*b*). The spermatozoon also triggers activation of the oocyte by transmission of a soluble factor associated with the head (Wilding & Dale, 1997). One candidate for this initiator of Ca^{2+} fluxes has been named oscillin (Swann & Lai, 1997), but the sperm head also carries transcription factors (Herrada & Wolgemuth, 1997) and mRNAs (Miller, 1997) that could play roles in modifying fertilization and early embryonic development. As yet we have little understanding of how these epigenetic factors are involved in male infertility, but this area promises to be a rich source of future research.

Laboratory training and quality control

Enormous advances have been made in the andrology laboratory, with much emphasis on standardizing techniques and developing external and independent quality assurance schemes. Almost every phase of the life-cycle of spermatozoa, from motility and hyperactivation to the acrosome reaction and zona penetration, is now amenable to routine laboratory testing, using a variety of molecular biological and other tools (Mortimer, 1994; Jeremias & Witkin, 1996). This is a necessary stage in the maturation of the discipline that can only advance as laboratory andrology moves from *ad hoc* training to more formal tertiary and transnational qualifications. Societies such as Alpha and the Australian group Scientists in Reproductive Technology are rapidly moving to ensure that such standards are imposed in all pathology laboratories involved in seminology. Unfortunately this maturation has not yet been mirrored in the clinical field.

The development of computer-assisted image analysis of sperm movement (CASA) has contributed to some understanding of the pathology and physiology of sperm movement, and may well develop further as new algorithms for tracking and analysing flagellar movement are developed (Mortimer, 1997). Areas that are rapidly advancing include the use of fluorescence microscopy, flow cytometry, and single-cell gel electrophoresis to study the structure and composition of the sperm nucleus and to identify DNA damage (Aravindan *et al.*, 1997). This is important because we know that sperm DNA damage (cigarette smoking being a possible cause) can result in increased levels of disease and cancer in the next generation (Ji *et al.*, 1997). Chromosomal anomalies can now easily be studied in spermatozoa that are permitted to decondense and proceed to metaphase in mouse or hamster eggs (Martin *et al.*, 1996), and many anomalies can be detected *in vitro* by fluorescence *in situ* hybridization (Downie *et al.*, 1997).

Demographic factors in male infertility

What of other trends that will affect andrology in the next century? There is a range of environmental, epigenetic and genetic factors that influence human fertility, development and life expectancy and we anticipate that these will soon be unravelled and further understood. Increasing paternal age, for example, has an influence on certain genetic diseases and even on life expectancy in offspring through increasing mutation rates in the testis (Gavrilov *et al.*, 1997). Transgenerational effects of parental age are demographically complex. In the USA, mean paternal age has dropped from a high of 36.9 years to 28.5 years over the period 1876–1981 (Riccardi, 1988). By contrast, maternal age at first pregnancy is currently increasing – indeed advancing maternal age is a major factor in the increased demand for infertility services (Mosher & Pratt, 1991). Paternal genes are known to modify embryonic growth rates through gene imprinting (Haig, 1996) and, of course, birth weight (or more strictly fetal placental weight ratios) is a powerful predictive element in determining health in later life (Robinson *et al.*, 1994). The recognition that minor disturbances in embryo culture conditions can have a marked effect on birth weight is a continuing concern, especially as birth weights are known to be low for babies conceived through reproductive technology (Seamark & Robinson, 1995). The epidemiologists' concerns that ICSI may lead to increased genetic defects in offspring will not be resolved until several thousand children are born (Kurinczuk & Bower, 1997), but so far it seems unlikely.

Diagnostics – the future?

An important question for the future is whether there will be any improvement in diagnosis as the basis for the management of male infertility. The new techniques of molecular biology are making rapid inroads into our ability to detect reproductive tract disease, autoimmune problems, defects in sperm and egg receptor–ligand interactions and alterations to nuclear and mitochondrial DNA (Jeremias & Witkin, 1996). We anticipate that many of these techniques will eventually become standard in male infertility clinic work-up.

Improvement in surgical imaging, especially with computer enhancement of images, is likely to be of great help diagnostically. Magnetic resonance imaging (MRI) and the generation of three-dimensional and real-time selectively enhanced images will provide immense improvements in our judgements on all areas of the male genital tract (McClure, 1986). It will reduce our need for surgical (or indeed endoscopic) assessment of the male genital tract considerably. This technology will probably be of greatest value in determining those pathologies that may be present in the excurrent duct system of the testis (Jequier, 1986). The use of MRI will also allow the renal tract to be examined concurrently with the genital tract. As renal and genital tract anomalies frequently coexist, such a system will be of considerable diagnostic help to the clinician.

The use of assisted conception is likely to increase greatly over the next decade. The techniques are likely to change substantially in the future and it is hoped that they will be associated with much improved pregnancy rates. The use of primordial follicles, perhaps even from ovarian tissue cryopreserved while the mother-to-be is in her prime fertile years (Gosden et al., 1997) and their in vitro maturation before fertilization, is likely to replace the standard IVF procedure of today, with all its concomitant risks to women who have been subjected to ovarian hyperstimulation. The principle of freezing gametes in the early years of life as an 'insurance' against future use seems a logical consideration for both sexes, although how this would be administered in practice is not clear.

Computers, artificial intelligence and the Internet

One area of human endeavour that will undoubtedly have a major impact on andrology is the development of computer expert systems and artificial intelligence for diagnosis, coupled with the vast resources of the World Wide Web (WWW). There has been some speculatation that, by the mid twentieth century, the rate of change of information technology and 'nanotechnology' will reach an asymptote that is almost impossible to see beyond (Broderick, 1997). Presently, the use of electronic mail, specialist mailing lists such as Androlog and SperMail, electronic publishing, and graphical real-time interactions using virtual reality tools and WWW browsers means that we can now disseminate information around the world vastly more rapidly and more effectively than even a decade ago. Much of this information is of course available to infertile couples, who now actively use the Internet to exchange information and to 'shop around' for the best clinics and treatment. Of course, these communication facilities can also be used to spread misinformation and mischief (Cummins, 1997c). The human mind is strongly attracted to irrationality and mysticism and it is clear that there is a powerful move away from Western science-based medicine to 'alternative' therapies (Sagan, 1996). The challenge for andrologists in the next decade is to challenge this 'New Age' move with good, evidence-based medicine. Indeed we suspect that market forces may well impel clinicians into more effective training. Specialists treating infertile couples will be obliged to become accurate diagnosticians, since they will increasingly encounter patients who are not only very knowledgeable about their own problems but who may indeed know more than the clinician!

Infertility – an evolutionary perspective

Turning now from a rather focused technical view of infertility to a more speculative vision, we might ask what lessons can be learned about human infertility from an evolutionary perspective?

Variability and human origins

All extant human groups derive from a limited set (about 10 000) of ancestors that probably first emerged in Africa around a quarter of a million years ago and expanded rapidly into the remaining land masses except for Antarctica. This population superseded pre-existing hominids in Europe and Asia. This process of primary expansion culminated in the peopling of the Pacific islands and New Zealand around 1000 years ago (Diamond, 1991; Kingdom, 1993). This picture was crystallized by a comparative study of mtDNA (Cann *et al.*, 1987) and received the tabloid label of 'African Eve', based on a supposed common female ancestor (actually a statistical artefact). Although the molecular biologists' assumptions of strict maternal inheritance of mtDNA are oversimplistic (Birky, 1995; Ankel-Simons & Cummins, 1996), the estimate of a recent African origin for *Homo sapiens* is confirmed by a study of the paternally inherited Y chromosome (Hammer, 1995) and by craniometric data (Relethford & Harpending, 1994). While genetic variability is greatest in Africa, as would be expected (the lineage is longest there), there seems little doubt that the spread and radiation of humans into a diverse range of habitats have resulted in the development of very wide phenotypic variations in features such as skin and hair pigmentation and body size (Diamond, 1991). The establishment of phenotypic and cultural diversity is strongly reinforced, perhaps even driven, by sexual competition and mate preference. In this process variation is largely generated by mutations accumulating in the male germ cells (Short, 1997).

This rapid expansion of the 'third chimpanzee' (Diamond, 1991) has been paralleled by an apparent reduction in the intensity of selective pressures that could affect and reinforce fertility. This is difficult to quantify. However, a comparative study of primate testes in relation to body mass, sperm output and breeding system suggests that humans and gorillas are only moderately polygynous. We have relatively small testes compared to our highly promiscuous cousins, the chimpanzees (Møller, 1988; Short, 1997). This is backed up by a survey of 849 human societies, indicating that the majority (83%) are normally or occasionally polygynous, only 16% are monogamous and only 4 (0.5%) are polyandrous (Murdock, 1967, cited in Daly & Wilson, 1983). Even in ostensibly monogamous societies the longer reproductive life of men, as compared with women who enter the menopause well before the biological limit of their life-span, frequently results in serial monogamy as resource-rich men re-marry younger women. As Short (1997) puts it, 'the net result is that more men will have children by more than one wife than women will have children fathered by more than one husband. In other words, serial monogamy effectively results in a polygynous mating system'.

Like gorillas, men have highly pleiomorphic spermatozoa (Seuanez *et al.*, 1977). This is a feature that commonly turns up in species where the intensity of sperm competition is low, such as thoroughbred stallions, koalas, cheetahs and other large felids (Cummins, 1990). Even fertile human males produce sperm with high levels of immature or poorly condensed nuclei marked by incomplete replacement of histones with protamines (Dadoune, 1995). Moreover there are clear geographical differences in semen parameters between human populations (Auger *et al.*, 1995; Auger & Jouannet, 1997) and wide variations in semen parameters even in fertile men (Mallidis *et al.*, 1991). All of these observations confirm human male reproduction as being only weakly driven by selective pressures for high fertility. As mentioned in Chapter 3 of this book human infertility therefore may simply reflect an extreme on the distribution curve of fecundity.

Can we prevent or delay the onset of male infertility?

As we point out at length below, most clinicians seeing infertile couples either do not or cannot make a diagnosis of male infertility, so it is rather premature to think of prevention when we cannot understand what the causes are in the first place. Much male infertility presents as stereotypical seminal pathology: oligozoospermia, teratozoospermia, asthenozoospermia, or various combinations of all three. Most of the damage to sperm function seems to be based on oxidative damage mediated by reactive oxygen species (ROS) (Aitken, 1995, 1997) and dietary antioxidants have given encouraging results on sperm performance criteria in patients with high levels of reactive oxygen in their semen (Kessopoulou *et al.*, 1995). Certainly antioxidant therapy can probably do little harm, especially where one can identify a known and avoidable source of oxidative stress such as smoking or zinc deficiency (Fraga *et al.*, 1996; Oteiza *et al.*, 1996). Other forms of therapy such as the use of kallikrein, or angiotensin-inhibiting agents have reported occasional improvements in semen parameters but the basis for this is obscure (Schill *et al.*, 1994; Schill, 1995).

Many instances of male infertility undoubtedly have a partial cause in trauma, and it is interesting that in at least one survey, over 9% of boys reported non-sexual genital assault, of which about a quarter involved injury of some form (Finkelhor & Wolak, 1995). We have pointed out elsewhere the vulnerability of the human testis to ischaemic damage and oxidative stress (Cummins *et al.*, 1994). Many avoidable cases of trauma undoubtedly occur in a sporting context, but apart from education and the wearing of suitable protective devices there is probably little we can do once an injury has occurred, apart from the obvious use of ice to reduce oxygen demand and hence the possibility of ischaemic damage.

Training of andrologists

One unfortunate aspect that emerges from the above concerns is that of effective training for clinical andrologists. This needs to be addressed urgently. Traditionally, the management of male infertility is undertaken by male gynaecologists. Few gynaecologists have ever had any proper training in the examination of the male genital tract. Indeed many clinicians working with infertility today never even bother to take a history from an infertile male, let alone carry out a clinical examination. It is, therefore, not very surprising that so much less is known about the aetiology of infertility in the male than in the female. If so few clinicians bother to attempt a diagnosis, then little will be learnt about aetiology. In practice, the treatment of the male is often left to laboratory scientists. Occasionally one may see comments on semen analysis reports such as 'this patient will need ICSI'. Scientists, no matter how competent, are not and should not be in a position to make such comments. In the words of Carl Schirren (1996), 'this is a disastrous development that has to be stopped'. It is totally unacceptable that infertile men should be subjected to treatment without a full examination by a medical specialist trained in the field (Jequier & Cummins, 1997). The treatment of a patient without at least making an attempt at a diagnosis is not only unethical but lays the clinician open to a successful medico-legal challenge should the use of IVF and/or ICSI later be found to have been unnecessary. This is especially true if the woman is normal but has had to submit to invasive and life-threatening procedures on her partner's behalf. We suspect that there will indeed be major problems for clinicians in this area in the future as couples and the general public become more aware of this dangerous avoidance of clinical responsibility.

It is frequently argued that infertility is a problem of a couple, not of an individual. An interactive relationship between infertility in the male and the female has been known for many years (Steinberger & Rodrigues-Rigau, 1983). This truism can be and is trotted out to justify subjecting normal women to life-threatening procedures to resolve the problem of their infertile partners. However, it continues to be made by the very gynaecologists who ignore even a perfunctory examination of the male genitalia. The complete clinician treating an infertile couple should be able to examine and make a diagnosis in both partners, and to manage the male as well as the female causes of their infertility.

We have long argued that special attention should be given to the training in andrology of all clinicians involved in the management of infertility (Jequier, 1990; Jequier & Cummins, 1997). At present infertile couples, especially where there is a male problem present, tend to be treated by a 'committee' of clinicians made up of different specialists. The responsibility for the overall care of the couple is thus diluted and good treatment, together with the confidence of the couple in that treatment, is consequently eroded.

We believe that all specialists treating infertility should have specialist training in both gynaecology and urology. Indeed many causes of male infertility can have a urological basis. Understanding urological pathologies and treating them is, therefore, essential for the proper management of male infertility. If the basic training of an individual is in gynaecology, then an adequate period should also be spent in urology, and vice versa. The well-rounded infertility specialist will also require training in basic laboratory techniques, including endocrinology and, of course, semen analysis. There would obviously have to be close cooperation between the specialties for such a scheme to be successful. However, just such an interrelationship is currently being forged among the gynaecological oncologists, and a similar arrangement could easily be made for the training of clinicians in infertility. The German Society of Andrology has put forward very similar specific targets for the training of clinical andrologists as a one–year postgraduate course in a department of andrology, or in a functional andrology unit in a teaching hospital (Schirren, 1996). Such a training scheme will of course be unpopular with the present generation of clinicians who want to achieve specialist status in the shortest possible time. One way of achieving this goal is to educate referring general practitioners so that they refer infertile couples only to clinics that have such complete specialists.

We urge that such training and education schemes should be made high priorities for the specialist national and international infertility societies. This is being optimistic. In reality the success of ICSI in dealing with male problems has already led to calls for a shift in resource allocation away from diagnosis to treatment (Hamberger & Janson, 1997). In our view this is short sighted.

Conclusions

In this vision of the future we have examined present trends in andrology and attempted to extrapolate to the next century. There have been remarkable technical achievements in treating the infertile male. Unfortunately these technical advances have not been accompanied by a corresponding increase in diagnostic capacity or specialist medical training. This, we feel, is a major challenge for the next century. We also argue that infertility in many ways seems to be inextricably linked with our evolutionary history. One could even argue that by freeing individuals or couples from the need to invest in child-raising, humanity as a whole could benefit by an acceptance of infertility rather than defining it as a pathological condition.

References
Aitken, R. J. (1995). Free radicals, lipid peroxidation and sperm function. *Reproduction, Fertility and Development*, 7, 659–68.
(1997). Molecular mechanisms regulating human sperm function. *Molecular Human Reproduction*, 3, 169–73.

Ankel-Simons, F. & Cummins, J. M. (1996). Misconceptions about mitochondria and mammalian fertilization – implications for theories on human evolution. *Proceedings of the National Academy of Sciences, USA*, **93**, 13859–63.

Aravindan, G. R., Bjordahl, J., Jost, L. K. & Evenson, D. P. (1997). Susceptibility of human sperm to *in situ* DNA denaturation is strongly correlated with DNA strand breaks identified by single-cell electrophoresis. *Experimental Cell Research*, **236**, 231–7.

Asch, R., Simerly, C., Ord, T., Ord, V. A. & Schatten, G. (1995). The stages at which human fertilization arrests – microtubule and chromosome configurations in inseminated oocytes which failed to complete fertilization and development in humans. *Human Reproduction*, **10**, 1897–906.

Auger, J. & Jouannet, P. (1997). Evidence for regional differences of semen quality among fertile French men. *Human Reproduction*, **12**, 740–5.

Auger, J., Kunstmann, J. M., Czyglik, F. & Jouannet, P. (1995). Decline in semen quality among fertile men in Paris during the past 20 years. *New England Journal of Medicine*, **332**, 281–5.

Bayle, H. (1952). Azoospermia of excretory origin. *Proceedings of the Society for the Study of Fertility*, **4**, 30–8.

Birky, C. W. (1995). Uniparental inheritance of mitochondrial and chloroplast genes: mechanisms and evolution. *Proceedings of the National Academy of Sciences, USA*, **92**, 11331–8.

Brinkmann, A., Jenster, G., Risstalpers, C., Van der Korput, H., Bruggenwirth, H., Boehmer, A. & Trapman, J. (1996). Molecular basis of androgen insensitivity. *Steroids*, **61**, 172–5.

Brinster, R. L. & Avarbock, M. R. (1994). Germline transmission of donor haplotype following spermatogonial transplantation. *Proceedings of the National Academy of Sciences, USA*, **91**, 11303–7.

Broderick, D. (1997). *The spike. Accelerating into the unimaginable future.* Kew, Victoria: Reed Books.

Burruel, V. R., Yanagimachi, R. & Whitten, W. K. (1996). Normal mice develop from oocytes injected with spermatozoa with grossly misshapen heads. *Biology of Reproduction*, **55**, 709–14.

Butenandt, A. & Hansch, G. (1935). Über testosteron. Undwandlung des dehydro-testosteron in androstendiol und testosteron; ein weg zur darstellung des testosteron aus cholesterin. *Zeitschrift für Physiologische Chemie*, **257**, 89–97.

Cann, R. L., Stoneking, M. & Wilson, A. (1987). Mitochondrial DNA and human evolution. *Nature*, **325**, 31–6.

Carlsen, E., Giwercman, A., Keiding, N. & Skakkebaek, N. E. (1992). Evidence for decreasing quality of semen during past 50 years. *British Medical Journal*, **305**, 609–13.

Carson, R. (1963). *Silent spring.* London: Hamish Hamilton.

Catalano, R. D., Vlad, M. & Kennedy, R. C. (1997). Differential display to identify and isolate novel genes expressed during spermatogenesis. *Molecular Human Reproduction*, **3**, 215–21.

Cummins, J. M. (1990). Evolution of sperm form: levels of control and competition. In *Fertilization in mammals*, eds. B. D. Bavister, J. M. Cummins & E. R. S. Roldan, pp. 51–64. Norwell, MA: Serono Symposia.

(1997a). Controversies in Science: ICSI may foster birth defects. *Journal of NIH Research*, **9**, 38–42.

(1997b). Mitochondrial DNA: implications for the genetics of human male infertility. In *Genetics of human male fertility*, ed. C. Barratt, C. De Jonge, D. Mortimer and J. Parinaud pp. 287–307. Paris: EDK.

(1997c). Reproductive resources on the Internet: information and misinformation. In *Fertility Society of Australia – Annual Scientific Meeting, Adelaide*. http://numbat.murdoch.edu.au/spermatology/fsa97.html

Cummins, J. M. & Jequier, A. M. (1994). Treating male infertility needs more clinical andrology, not less. *Human Reproduction*, **9**, 1214–19.

(1995). Concerns and recommendations for intracytoplasmic sperm injection (ICSI) treatment. *Human Reproduction*, **10**, 138–43.

Cummins, J. M., Jequier, A. M. & Kan, R. (1994). Molecular biology of human male infertility – links with aging, mitochondrial genetics, and oxidative stress? *Molecular Reproduction and Development*, **37**, 345–62.

Dadoune, J. P. (1995). The nuclear status of human sperm cells. *Micron*, **26**, 323–45.

Daly, M. & Wilson, M. (1983). *Sex, evolution and behavior*. Boston, MA: PWS Publishers.

Diamond, J. (1991). *The rise and fall of the third chimpanzee*. London: Radius.

Downie, S. E., Flaherty, S. P. & Matthews, C. D. (1997). Detection of chromosomes and estimation of aneuploidy in human spermatozoa using fluorescence-in-situ hybridization. *Molecular Human Reproduction*, **3**, 585–98.

Elliott, D. J. & Cooke, H. J. (1997). The molecular genetics of male infertility. *Bioessays*, **19**, 801–9.

Finkelhor, D. & Wolak, J. (1995). Nonsexual assaults to the genitals in the youth population. *Journal of the American Medical Association*, **274**, 1692–7.

Fraga, C. G., Motchnik, P. A., Wyrobek, A. J., Rempel, D. M. & Ames, B. N. (1996). Smoking and low antioxidant levels increase oxidative damage to sperm DNA. *Mutation Research – Fundamental and Molecular Mechanisms of Mutagenesis*, **351**, 199–203.

Friel, J. P. (ed.) (1985). *Dorland's illustrated medical dictionary*, 26th edn. Philadelphia, PA: W.B. Saunders.

Gavrilov, L. A., Gavrilova, N. S., Kroutko, V. N., Evdokushkina, G. N., Semyonova, V. G., Gavrilova, A. L., Lapshin, E. V., Evdokushkina, N. N. & Kushnareva, Y. E. (1997). Mutation load and human longevity. *Mutation Research*, **377**, 61–2.

Gosden, R., Krapez, J. & Briggs, D. (1997). Growth and development of the mammalian oocyte. *Bioessays*, **19**, 875–82.

Graves, J. A. M. (1995). The origin and function of the mammalian Y chromosome and Y-borne genes – an evolving understanding. *Bioessays*, **17**, 311–20.

Gray, L. E., Jr, Kelce, W. R., Wiese, T., Tyl, R., Gaido, K., Cook, J., Klinefelter, G., Desaulniers, D., Wilson, E., Zacharewski, T., Waller, C., Foster, P., Laskey, J., Reel, J., Giesy, J., Laws, S., McLachlan, J., Breslin, W., Cooper, R., Di Giulio, R., Johnson, R., Purdy, R., Mihaich, E., Safe, S., Colborn, T. & *et al.* (1997). Endocrine Screening Methods Workshop report: detection of estrogenic and androgenic hormonal and antihormonal activity for chemicals that act via receptor or steroidogenic enzyme mechanisms. *Reproductive Toxicology*, **11**, 719–50.

Hagner, F. R. (1936). The operative treatment of sterility in the male. *Journal of the American Medical Association*, **107**, 1851–5.

Haig, D. (1996). Altercation of generations – genetic conflicts of pregnancy. *American Journal of Reproductive Immunology*, **35**, 226–32.

Hamberger, L. & Janson, P. O. (1997). Global importance of infertility and its treatment – role of fertility technologies. *International Journal of Gynecology & Obstetrics*, **58**, 149–58.

Hammer, M. F. (1995). A recent common ancestry for human Y chromosomes. *Nature*, **378**, 376–8.

Herrada, G. & Wolgemuth, D. J. (1997). The mouse transcription factor Stat4 is expressed in haploid male germ cells and is present in the perinuclear theca of spermatozoa. *Journal of Cell Science*, **110**, 1543–53.

Hotchkiss, R. S. (1947). *Fertility in men.*, Portsmouth, N.H: William Heinemann.

James, W. H. (1997). Secular trends in monitors of reproductive hazard. *Human Reproduction*, **12**, 417–21.

Jensen, T. K., Toppari, J., Keiding, N. & Skakkebaek, N. E. (1995). Do environmental estrogens contribute to the decline in male reproductive health. *Clinical Chemistry*, **41**, 1896–901.

Jequier, A. M. (1986). Obstructive azoospermia: a study of 102 patients. *Clinical Reproduction and Fertility*, 3, 21–36.

(1990). Andrology: a new sub-specialty. *British Journal of Obstetrics and Gynaecology*, **97**, 969–72.

(1991). Edward Martin (1859–1938). The founding father of modern clinical andrology. *International Journal of Andrology*, **14**, 1–10.

Jequier, A. M. & Cummins, J. M. (1997). Attitudes to clinical andrology – a time for change. *Human Reproduction*, **12**, 875–6.

Jequier, A. M. & Holmes, S. C. (1993). Primary testicular disease presenting as azoospermia or oligozoospermia in an infertility clinic. *British Journal of Urology*, **71**, 731–5.

Jeremias, J. & Witkin, S. S. (1996). Molecular approaches to the diagnosis of male infertility. *Molecular Human Reproduction*, **2**, 195–202.

Ji, B. T., Shu, X. O., Linet, M. S., Zheng, W., Wacholder, S., Gao, Y. T., Ying, D. M. & Jin, F. (1997). Paternal cigarette smoking and the risk of childhood cancer among offspring of nonsmoking mothers. *Journal of the National Cancer Institute*, **89**, 238–44.

Kelce, W. R. & Wilson, E. M. (1997). Environmental antiandrogens: developmental effects, molecular mechanisms, and clinical implications. *Journal of Molecular Medicine*, **75**, 198–207.

Kent-First, M. G., Koi, S., Muallem, A., Blazer, S. & Itskovitz-Eldor, J. (1996). Infertility in intracytoplasmic-sperm-injection-derived sons. *Lancet*, **348**, 332.

Kessopoulou, E., Powers, H. J., Sharma, K. K., Pearson, M. J., Russell, J. M., Cooke, I. D. & Barratt, C. L. R. (1995). A double-blind randomized placebo cross-over controlled trial using the antioxidant vitamin E to treat reactive oxygen species associated male infertility. *Fertility and Sterility*, **64**, 825–31.

Kingdom, J. (1993). *Self-made man and his undoing*. London: Simon & Schuster.

Kurinczuk, J. J. & Bower, C. (1997). Birth defects in infants conceived by intracytoplasmic sperm injection – an alternative interpretation. *British Medical Journal*, **315**, 1260–5.

Lee, J. D., Kamiguchi, Y. & Yanagimachi, R. (1996). Analysis of chromosome constitution of human spermatozoa with normal and aberrant head morphologies after injection into mouse oocytes. *Human Reproduction*, **11**, 1942–6.

Mallidis, C., Howard, E. J. & Baker, H. W. (1991). Variation of semen quality in normal men. *International Journal of Andrology*, **14**, 99–107.

Martin, E., Benton, Carnett, J., Levy, J. V. & Pennington, M. E. (1902). The surgical treatment of sterility due to obstruction of the epididymis together with a study of the morphology of human sperm. *Therapeutics Gazette*, March, 1–14.

Martin, R. H., Spriggs, E. & Rademaker, A. W. (1996). Multicolor fluorescence in situ hybridization analysis of aneuploidy and diploidy frequencies in 225 846 sperm from 10 normal men. *Biology of Reproduction*, **54**, 394–8.

McClure, R. D. (1986). Magnetic resonance imaging: its application to male infertility. *Urology*, **27**, 91–8.

Miller, D. (1997). RNA in the ejaculate spermatozoon – a window into molecular events in spermatogenesis and a record of the unusual requirements of haploid gene expression and post-meiotic equilibration. *Molecular Human Reproduction*, **3**, 669–76.

Møller, A. P. (1988). Ejaculate quality, testis size and sperm competition in primates. *Journal of Human Evolution*, **17**, 489–502.

Moore, C. R. & Price, D. (1932). Gonad hormone functions and the reciprocal influence between gonads and hypophysis with its bearing on sex hormone antagonism. *American Journal of Anatomy*, **50**, 13–71.

Mortimer, D. (1994). The essential partnership between diagnostic andrology and modern assisted reproductive technologies. *Human Reproduction*, **9**, 1209–13.

Mortimer, S. T. (1997). A critical review of the physiological importance and analysis of sperm movement in mammals. *Human Reproduction Update*, **3**, 403–29.

Mosher, W. D. & Pratt, W. F. (1991). Fecundity and infertility in the United States: incidence and trends. *Fertility and Sterility*, **56**, 192–3.

Niemi, M. (1987). Andrology as a specialty–its origin. *Journal of Andrology*, **8**, 201–2.

Nijs, M., Vanderzwalmen, P., Vandamme, B., Segalbertin, G., Lejeune, B., Segal, L., Vanroosendaal, E. & Schoysman, R. (1996). Fertilizing ability of immotile spermatozoa after intracytoplasmic sperm injection. *Human Reproduction*, **11**, 2180–5.

Oteiza, P. L., Olin, K. L., Fraga, C. G. & Keen, C. L. (1996). Oxidant defense systems in testes from zinc-deficient rats. *Proceedings of the Society for Experimental Biology and Medicine*, **213**, 85–91.

Palermo, G., Joris, H., Devroey, P. & Van Steirteghem, A. C. (1992). Pregnancies after intracytoplasmic injection of single spermatozoon into an oocyte. *Lancet*, **340**, 17–18.

Relethford, J. H. & Harpending, H. C. (1994). Craniometric variation, genetic theory, and modern human origins. *American Journal of Physical Anthropology*, **95**, 249–70.

Riccardi, V. M. (1988). American paternal age data for selected years from 1876 to 1981. *Neurofibromatosis,* 1, 93–9.

Robinson, J. S., Seamark, R. P. & Owens, J. A. (1994). Placental function. *Australian and New Zealand Journal of Obstetrics and Gynaecology,* 34, 240–6.

Ruggiu, M., Speed, R., Taggart, M., McKay, S. J., Kilanowski, F., Saunders, P., Dorin, J. & Cooke, H. J. (1997). The mouse DAZLA gene encodes a cytoplasmic protein essential for gametogenesis. *Nature,* 389, 73–7.

Sagan, C. (1996). *The demon haunted world: science as a candle in the dark.* New York: Ballantine Books.

Schill, W. B. (1995). Survey of medical therapy in andrology. *International Journal of Andrology,* 18, 56–62.

Schill, W. B., Parsch, E. M. & Miska, W. (1994). Inhibition of angiotensin converting enzyme – a new concept of medical treatment of male infertility. *Fertility and Sterility,* 61, 1123–8.

Schirren, C. (1996). Andrology – development and future – critical remarks after 45 years of medical practice. *Andrologia,* 28, 137–40.

Schoysman, R. (1981). Epididymal causes of male infertility: pathogenesis and management. In *Pathology and pathophysiology of the epididymis,* vol. 8 ed. C. Bollack & A. Clavert pp. 102–13. Basle: Karger.

Seamark, R. F. & Robinson, J. S. (1995). Potential health problems stemming from assisted reproduction programmes. *Human Reproduction,* 10, 1321–2.

Setchell, B. P. (1997). Sperm counts in semen of farm animals 1932–1995. *International Journal of Andrology,* 20, 209–14.

Seuanez, H. N., Carothers, A. O., Martin, D. E. & Short, R. V. (1977). Morphological abnormalities in the shape of spermatozoa of man and the great apes. *Nature,* 270, 345–7.

Short, R. V. (1997). The testis – the witness of the mating system, the site of mutation and the engine of desire. *Acta Paediatrica,* 86, 3–7.

Silber, S. J., Van Steirteghem, A., Nagy, Z., Liu, J. E., Tournaye, H. & Devroey, P. (1996). Normal pregnancies resulting from testicular sperm extraction and intracytoplasmic sperm injection for azoospermia due to maturation arrest. *Fertility and Sterility,* 66, 110–17.

Steinberger, E. & Rodrigues-Rigau, L. J. (1983). The infertile couple. *Journal of Andrology,* 4, 111–18.

Swann, K. & Lai, F. A. (1997). A novel signalling mechanism for generating Ca^{2+} oscillations at fertilization in mammals. *Bioessays,* 19, 371–8.

Tournaye, H. & Van Steirteghem, A. (1997). Controversies in science: intracytoplasmic sperm injection. ICSI concerns do not outweigh its benefits. *Journal of NIH Research,* 9, 35–40.

Tournaye, H., Staessen, C., Liebaers, I., Van Assche, E., Devroey, P., Bonduelle, M. & Van Steirteghem, A. (1996). Testicular sperm recovery in nine 47,XXY Klinefelter patients. *Human Reproduction,* 11, 1644–9.

Uehara, T. & Yanagimachi, R. (1976). Microsurgical injection of spermatozoa into hamster eggs with subsequent transformation of sperm nuclei into male pronuclei. *Biology of Reproduction,* 15, 467–70.

Vogt, P. H., Edelmann, A., Kirsch, S., Henegariu, O., Hirschmann, P., Kiesewetter, F., Kohn, F. M., Schill, W. B., Farah, S., Ramos, C., Hartmann, M.,

Hartschuh, W., Meschede, D., Behre, H. M., Castel, A., Nieschlag, E., Weidner, W., Grone, H. J., Jung, A., Engel, W. & Haidl, G. (1996). Human Y chromosome azoospermia factors (AZF) mapped to different subregions in Yq11. *Human Molecular Genetics*, **5**, 933–43.

Wilding, M. & Dale, B. (1997). Sperm factor – what is it and what does it do? *Molecular Human Reproduction*, **3**, 269–73.

Yanagimachi, R. (1995). Is an animal model needed for intracytoplasmic sperm injection (ICSI) and other assisted reproduction technologies? *Human Reproduction*, **10**, 2525–6.

Index